Blood Transfusion

Blood Transfusion

Edited by **Martha Roper**

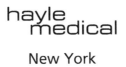

hayle
medical

New York

Published by Hayle Medical,
30 West, 37th Street, Suite 612,
New York, NY 10018, USA
www.haylemedical.com

Blood Transfusion
Edited by Martha Roper

International Standard Book Number: 978-1-63241-059-7 (Hardback)

Printed in the United States of America.

Contents

Preface   IX

Part 1   **ABO in the Context of Blood Transfusion**   1

Chapter 1   **ABO in the Context of Blood Transfusion and Beyond**   3
Emili Cid, Sandra de la Fuente,
Miyako Yamamoto and Fumiichiro Yamamoto

Part 2   **Blood Transfusion in Medicine and Surgery**   23

Chapter 2   **Blood Transfusion Practices in Major Orthopaedic Surgery**   25
Saqeb B. Mirza, Sukhmeet S. Panesar and
Douglas G. Dunlop

Chapter 3   **Transfusion Reduction in Orthopedic Surgery**   51
Ruud H.G.P. van Erve and Alexander C. Wiekenkamp

Chapter 4   **Blood Transfusion Therapy in High Risk Surgical Patients**   73
João Manoel Silva Junior and Alberto Mendonça P. Ferreira

Chapter 5   **Scope of Blood Transfusion in Obstetrics**   83
Subhayu Bandyopadhyay

Chapter 6   **Uterine Atony: Management Strategies**   97
Pei Shan Lim, Mohamad Nasir Shafiee,
Nirmala Chandralega Kampan, Aqmar Suraya Sulaiman,
Nur Azurah Abdul Ghani, NorAzlin Mohamed Ismail,
Choon Yee Lee, Mohd Hashim Omar and
Muhammad Abdul Jamil Mohammad Yassin

Chapter 7   **Effects of Blood Transfusion on
Retinopathy of Prematurity**   **129**
Ebrahim Mikaniki, Mohammad Mikaniki and
Amir Hosein Shirzadian

Part 3   **Preventing Transfusion Transmitted Infections**   **141**

Chapter 8   **Implicating the Need for
Serological Testing of Borna Disease Virus and
Dengue Virus During Blood Transfusion**   **143**
S. Gowri Sankar and A. Alwin Prem Anand

Chapter 9   **Transfusion-Transmitted
Bacterial, Viral and Protozoal Infections**   **163**
Pankaj Abrol and Harbans Lal

Chapter 10   **Human T-Lymphotropic Viruses (HTLV)**   **175**
Marina Lobato Martins,
Rafaela Gomes Andrade, Bernardo Hinkelmann Nédir
and Edel Figueiredo Barbosa-Stancioli

Part 4   **Alternative Strategies to Allogenic Blood Transfusion**   **189**

Chapter 11   **Autotransfusion: Therapeutic
Principles, Efficacy and Risks**   **191**
A.W.M.M. Koopman-van Gemert

Chapter 12   **Bloodless Medicine and Surgery**   **209**
Nathaniel I. Usoro

Chapter 13   **Impact of Acute Normovolemic
Hemodilution in Organ and Cell Structure**   **223**
D.A. Otsuki, D.T. Fantoni and J.O.C. Auler Junior

Chapter 14   **Cryopreservation of Blood**   **233**
Miloš Bohoněk

Part 5   **Immunomodulatory Effects of Blood Transfusion**   **243**

Chapter 15   **Effect of Blood Transfusion
on Subsequent Organ Transplantation**   **245**
Puneet K. Kochhar, Pranay Ghosh and Rupinder Singh Kochhar

Chapter 16   **Posthepatic Manipulative Blood Extraction
with Blood Transfusion Alleviates Liver
Transplant Ischemia/Reperfusion Injury and
Its Induced Lung Injury**   **255**
Changku Jia

Permissions

List of Contributors

Preface

Blood transfusion is a process principally used to treat various medical conditions. This book deals with the applications of blood transfusion in diverse clinical surroundings. It discusses significant issues like the fundamental theories regarding ABO blood group system in blood transfusion, the use of transfusion in a variety of clinical surroundings, among others. It also deals with transfusion transmitted diseases, different techniques for allotransplantation and immunomodulatory effects of blood transfusion. The book covers various aspects of blood transfusion and will provide valuable information to its readers.

All of the data presented henceforth, was collaborated in the wake of recent advancements in the field. The aim of this book is to present the diversified developments from across the globe in a comprehensible manner. The opinions expressed in each chapter belong solely to the contributing authors. Their interpretations of the topics are the integral part of this book, which I have carefully compiled for a better understanding of the readers.

At the end, I would like to thank all those who dedicated their time and efforts for the successful completion of this book. I also wish to convey my gratitude towards my friends and family who supported me at every step.

Editor

Part 1

ABO in the Context of Blood Transfusion

ABO in the Context of Blood Transfusion and Beyond

Emili Cid, Sandra de la Fuente,
Miyako Yamamoto and Fumiichiro Yamamoto
*Institut de Medicina Predictiva i
Personalitzada del Càncer (IMPPC), Badalona, Barcelona,
Spain*

1. Introduction

ABO histo-blood group system is widely acknowledged as one of the antigenic systems most relevant to blood transfusion, but also cells, tissues and organs transplantation. This chapter will illustrate a series of subjects related to blood transfusion but will also give an overview of ABO related topics such as its genetics, biochemistry and its association to human disease as well as a historical section. We decided not to include much detail about the related Lewis oligosaccharide antigens which have been reviewed extensively elsewhere (Soejima & Koda 2005) in order to focus on ABO and allow the inclusion of novel and exciting developments.

ABO group	A/B antigens on red blood cells	Anti-A/-B in serum	Genotype
O	None	Anti-A and Anti-B	O/O
A	A	Anti-B	A/A or A/O
B	B	Anti-A	B/B or B/O
AB	A and B	None	A/B

Table 1. Simple classification of ABO phenotypes and their corresponding genotypes.

As its simplest, the ABO system is dictated by a polymorphic gene (ABO) whose different alleles encode for a glycosyltransferase (A or B) that adds a monosaccharide (N-acetyl-D-galactosamine or D-galactose, respectively) to a specific glycan chain, except for the protein O which is not active. The 3 main alleles: A, B and O are inherited in a classical codominant Mendelian fashion (with O being recessive) and produce, when a pair of them are combined in a diploid cell, the very well known four phenotypic groups (see Table 1). Being one of the first known and easily detectable polymorphic traits in humans, it has been extensively studied as a historical background illustrates.

2. History

Various advancements in both blood storage and serology have contributed to the development of safe blood transfusion. One of the key events that brought transfusion medicine forward was the discovery of the ABO blood group system. The first successful attempts of human to human blood transfusion already started in the 18th century, but it was an unsafe process in which some patients died. It was not until 1900 when the Austrian pathologist, Karl Landsteiner discovered the ABO blood group system, which opened the door for performing safe blood transfusions (Landsteiner, 1900).

Landsteiner separated the cell components and the sera of blood samples from different individuals, including his own blood, and mixed them in various combinations. He observed that in some combinations red blood cells (RBCs) agglutinated. According to these agglutination patterns, Landsteiner classified the individuals in three different groups. These blood groups were called A, B and C (later called the blood group O). One year later, Decastello and Sturli described one new group, the AB blood group (von Decastello & Sturli, 1902).

Landsteiner theorized that the RBCs possessed two different markers (antigens A and B) able to react with the corresponding sera antibodies (anti-A and anti-B), and as opposite to many other blood group systems such as the Rh system, the presence of the antibodies against A or B occurs naturally in individuals that do not express the antigens. The serum from an individual with A type RBCs present antibodies against the B antigen, so it is able to agglutinate B and AB type RBCs, but not his own type. The serum from B type individuals agglutinates A and AB type RBCs. Finally, the serum from O group can agglutinate A, B and AB RBCs because it contains both anti-A and anti-B antibodies while the serum of AB group do not have reactivity towards none of these antigens. This phenomenon was later known as Landsteiner's Law.

From that first discovery of the ABO system, new developments took place relatively fast during the following years. On 1908, Epstein and Ottenberg suggested that the blood groups could be an inherited character (Epstein & Ottenberg, 1908). That was confirmed in 1910 by von Dungern and Hirszfeld who showed that inheritance of the A and B antigens obeyed Mendel's laws (von Dungern & Hirszfeld, 1910). In fact, ABO was one of the first genetic markers to be used in paternity testing and forensic medicine.

To explain the mode of inheritance, Berstein proposed, in 1924, the one gene locus-three alleles model. He assumed that the A, B and O genes were alleles at the same ABO genetic locus and that the A and B alleles were co-dominant against the recessive O allele (Crow, 1993).

Already by 1926, it was shown that A and B antigens were not restricted to the surface of erythrocytes. They were also found in semen and saliva, and four years later, Putkonen and Lehrs discovered that the ability to secrete these antigens was genetically independent from the ABO gene and inheritable in a classical dominant Mendelian manner (Putkonen, 1930).

In 1950s, two research groups, one led by Kabat and another group led by Watkins and Morgan elucidated the chemical nature of ABH substances (H antigens were found abundantly in individuals with blood group type O) (Kabat, 1956; Morgan, 1960; Watkins, 1981). They determined that they were oligosaccharide antigens and also pointed out the biochemical difference between A (with a terminal N-acetylgalactosamine) and B (with galactose instead) substances. Moreover, they demonstrated that the ABO blood group system antigens were not the primary gene products (i. e. protein antigens), but were the result of enzymatic reactions producing carbohydrate chains. In the following years various works established the tissue distribution of these antigens and their changes during embryonic development (Ravn & Dabelsteen, 2000).

Between 1970 and 1980, the metabolic pathways leading to the biosynthesis of ABH antigens were established (Watkins, 1981) and in 1976, the ABO locus was localized and assigned to chromosome 9q34 (Ferguson-Smith et al., 1976).

In 1990, after the purification of the soluble form of human A transferase by Clausen and collaborators (Clausen et al., 1990), Yamamoto and his group were able to clone the cDNAs for A glycosyltransferase first (Yamamoto et al., 1990b) and afterwards those for the B glycosyltransferase and the O protein and elucidated the molecular basis for the synthesis of A and B antigens (Yamamoto et al., 1990a). Since the original description of the main alleles (A1, B, O) many others have been described by them and other groups and they have been annotated and included in public databases.

Together with the amino acid substitutions between A and B transferases, as well as the mutations causing a decrease or ablation of the enzymatic activity in A/B weak subgroup alleles and O alleles, the determination of their 3-D structure has facilitated a better understanding of the structure-functional relationship of these transferases (Patenaude et al., 2002).

3. Biochemistry and structure

A and B antigens share the same structure except for a terminal sugar bound by an α1-3 glycosidic linkage to galactose (see Fig. 1). In the case of A antigen the last sugar is N-acetylgalactosamine (GalNAc) while in the case of B antigen the last sugar is galactose (Gal).

If these two terminal sugars are eliminated from the common structure the corresponding antibodies lose their reactivity. Therefore these sugars are immunodominant within the epitope. The H antigen is the natural precursor of A and B antigen and its fucose residue is required for A and B glycosyltransferases to recognize it as the acceptor and transfer GalNAc or Gal to its terminal Gal. In the case of O individuals it rests without further elongation.

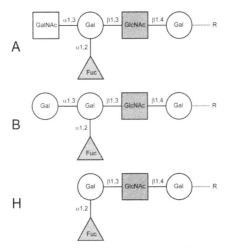

Fig. 1. ABH antigens of Type 2 core structure are schematically drawn showing their chemical composition and the nature of their glycosidic bonds. GalNAc, Gal, GlcNAc and Fuc stand for N-acetylgalactosamine, galactose, N-acetylglucosamine and fucose respectively. R represents the reducing end of the carbohydrate chain.

These antigens reside at the end of carbohydrate structures of variable length. Depending on the disaccharide precursor core chain on which ABH determinants are synthesized, they can be further divided into different types:

Type 1: Galβ1->3GlcNAcβ1-> R

Type 2: Galβ1->4GlcNAcβ1-> R

Type 3: Galβ1->3GalNAcα1-> R

Type 4: Galβ1->3GalNAcβ1-> R

Type 5: Galβ1->3Galβ1-> R

Type 6: Galβ1->4Glcβ1-> R

The internal reducing end of these precursors is bound to carrier molecules (R) of diverse nature: oligosaccharides, glycolipids or glycoproteins (Clausen & Hakomori, 1989). Types 1 through 4 are found on RBCs although Type 2 is the most common on those cells, while Type 6 is present in free oligosaccharides and some tissues (renal vein, intestinal cells) (Björk et al., 1987; Holgersson et al., 1990). Finally Type 5 is synthetic and it was utilized in the characterization of monoclonal antibodies against ABH (Oriol et al., 1990). In turn, these antigens can be present on the cell membrane bound to embedded glycoproteins or glycolipids or also forming part of these glycoconjugates but suspended in fluids as plasma or exocrine secretions and finally as free oligosaccharides without any protein or lipid carrier.

3.1 Carrier molecules

ABH substances are present on glycoproteins as terminal structures of two main types of protein modifying glycans: N-glycans and O-glycans. N-glycans are highly branched oligosaccharides attached to the amide nitrogen of asparagine through an N-acetylglucosamine residue while O-glycans, which could be simple or complex structures, are attached to the hydroxyl oxygen atom of serine or threonine residues through N-acetylgalactosamine sugar.

On RBCs, ABH antigens are present as terminal modifications of N-glycans. The most abundant glycoproteins carrying these ABH determinants are the anion exchange protein band 3, and the glucose transport protein band 4.5, as well as the urea transporter and the water channel AQP1 (aquaporin-1), which are the carrier of blood groups Kidd and Colton, respectively (Fukuda & Fukuda, 1981; Smith et al., 1994; Lucien et al., 2002). The other most abundant red cell glycoprotein, glycophorin A, on which the MNS blood group resides, does not appear to carry any ABH antigen.

Apart from glycoproteins, ABH antigens are also found as terminal modifications of glycolipids. Before 1980, it was generally considered that most of ABH determinants on RBCs were actually carried on glycosphingolipids but after that year several studies demonstrated that glycoproteins were the main carriers (Finne et al., 1980). ABH antigens on lipids are carried predominantly by glycosphingolipids. These molecules consist of a carbohydrate chain attached to ceramide, and according to the nature of the internal carbohydrate chain they are classified into six different series:

Lacto series:	Galβ1->3GlcNAcβ1->3Galβ1->4Glcβ1->Cer
Neolacto series:	Galβ1->4GlcNAcβ1->3Galβ1->4Glcβ1->Cer
Ganglio series:	Galβ1->3GalNAcβ1->4Galβ1->4Glcβ1->Cer
Isoganglio series:	Galβ1->3GalNAcβ1->3Galβ1->4Glcβ1->Cer
Globo series:	GalNAcβ1->3Galα1->4Galβ1->4Glcβ1->Cer
Isoglobo series:	GalNAcβ1->3Galα1->3Galβ1->4Glcβ1->Cer

On each of these structures ABH antigens can be added to the terminal sugar being the most common the Lacto and the Neolacto series.

Additionally, free oligosaccharides containing ABH activity are also found in milk and urine. In this case, these glycans are synthesized mostly from Type 6 precursor chain (Kobata et al., 1978; Lundblad, 1978).

3.2 Antigen distribution

ABH antigens were discovered on RBCs but are also present in many other tissues. For that reason they are also called histo-blood group antigens. In blood, apart from RBCs, platelets also present these antigens although in variable quantities depending on the individuals and their blood group. ABH antigens are detected on endothelial cells and epithelia from the lung and the gastrointestinal tract and also on the lining of the urinary and reproductive tracts. The presence of the antigens is therefore relevant for cell, tissue or organ transplantation (reviewed in (Ravn & Dabelsteen, 2000)).

4. ABO gene and the A and B antigens biosynthesis

We mentioned before that these glycan antigens are not directly encoded by genes. The A and B antigens are synthesized by enzymatic reactions catalyzed by two different enzymes called glycosyltransferases (transferases), the A transferase (α1,3-N-acetyl-D-galactosaminyltransferase) and the B transferase (α1,3-D-galactosyltransferase), respectively. Both, A and B transferases catalyze the last step on the synthesis of A and B antigen adding a GalNAc or a Gal to a precursor chain, the H antigen, by an identical α1-3 glycosidic linkage (for a review in glycosyltransferase biochemistry see (Hakomori, 1981)).

The gene is located in the long arm of chromosome 9 (9q34) and extends over more than 18 kilobases (kb). The gene has the coding sequence distributed in 7 exons, being the last one the largest. The glycosyltransferase catalytic domain is encoded in the last two exons. The 3'UTR region contains repetitive sequences that could be involved in the mRNA stability. Promoter activity resides in the gene sequence just upstream of the transcription initiation site (Yamamoto et al., 1995).

Probing cDNA libraries obtained from human adenocarcinoma cell lines of different ABO phenotypes, we successfully defined the main alleles. It was concluded that the distinct donor nucleotide-sugar specificity between A and B transferases is the result of 7 substitutions out of 1062 coding nucleotides, and only 4 of them resulting in amino acid substitutions (Arginine, Glycine, Leucine and Glycine in A transferase and Glycine, Serine, Methionine and Alanine for B transferase at codons 176, 235, 266, 268) (Yamamoto et al., 1990a).

Together with previous mutagenic studies (Yamamoto & McNeill 1996), the elucidation of the 3-D structure of the glycosyltransferases has allowed to clarify the roles of these amino acids (Patenaude et al., 2002) (see Fig. 2). The amino acid residues at codons 266 and 268 are directly involved in the recognition and binding of the sugar portion of the nucleotide-sugar donor substrates in the glycosyltransferase reaction. The amino acid residue at codon 176 is relatively far from the catalytic center, while the amino acid residue at codon 235 is at a middle distance.

The O allele encodes a non-functional glycosyltransferase enzyme. Most of O alleles contained a single nucleotide deletion at the 261 position, relatively close to the N-terminal of the coding sequence, resulting in a codon frameshift starting from amino acid 88 in the protein sequence, which causes the production of a truncated non-functional protein. This truncated protein has no catalytic domain and its mRNA transcript is less stable (O'Keefe & Dobrovic, 1996).

The antigen biosynthesis realized by the active glycosyltransferases takes place in the Golgi apparatus. These transferases are classified as type II transmembrane proteins as their structures follow the common pattern of a short transmembrane domain followed by a stem region and a catalytic domain within the Golgi lumen. The 3-D structure showed that the catalytic site is composed of two main domains. The N-terminal domain recognizes the nucleotide-sugar donor substrate. In the case of the A allele, which encodes for an α1,3-N-acetylgalactosaminyltransferase, the sugar donor is uridine diphosphate-N-acetyl-D-galactosamine (UDP-GalNAc) while the B gene product, an α1,3-galactosyltransferase transfers galactose from UDP-galactose. The C-terminal domain binds to the acceptor substrate, the fucosylated galactosyl residue of the H antigen.

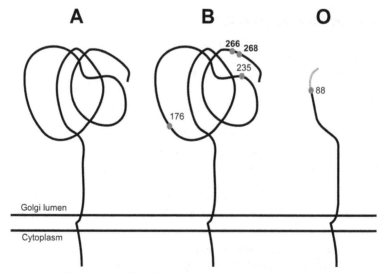

Fig. 2. Schematics with the main alleles' products and their modified residues. The different amino acids are numbered on B, in boldface the ones defining the sugar donor specificity, while in O the first amino acid after the frameshift is indicated and the alternative translation is in grey.

Since the discovery of the major alleles numerous polymorphisms/mutations have been described for the ABO gene (Yamamoto, 2004). The majority of these variations are nucleotide changes resulting in amino acid substitutions or a single nucleotide deletion/insertion and correlate well with the presence of specific subgroup phenotypes. At the moment the total number of alleles deposited in the ABO system section of the Blood Group Antigen Gene Mutation Database (dbRBC at NCBI http://www.ncbi.nlm.nih.gov/gv/mhc/xslcgi.cgi?cmd=bgmut/home) has surpassed 270 and considering the rapid advancement of next-generation sequencing, this number is going to increase in the coming years.

5. Subgroups of A and B

Many weak subgroups have been described for A group and a lower number for B group. These rare phenotypes account for a minority of individuals. Different strategies have been developed to test for these less common occurrences when the results of forward and reverse tests do not match or other inconsistencies are found (genetic for example).

The first subgroups to be recognized were A_1 and A_2. In 1910, Dungern and Hirszfeld noticed differences in the amount of A antigen expression present in A individuals (von Dungern & Hirszfeld, 1910). It was also observed that serum from B group blood presented two different antibodies reacting to A RBCs. One general anti-A that was able to react towards all A erythrocytes, and one specific to A_1. A_1 phenotype is characterized by the presence of a higher number of A antigen when compared to A_2 (Rochant et al., 1976). The A^1 allele is dominant over A^2 and encodes for an A transferase with higher affinity and reactivity for the substrates of the reaction (UDP-GalNAc and H-antigen/2'-fucosyllactose) than the A_2 transferase (Schachter et al., 1973).

Other subgroups of A include weak expressors of the antigen (A_3, A_{end}, A_{finn}, A_{bantu}, A_x, A_m, A_y, A_{el}) and the intermediate phenotype between A_1 and A_2, A_{int}. Cartron developed a method to assess the relative agglutinability of cells by radiolabelled anti-A antibodies. This quantification permitted to classify the phenotypes in respect to RBC A antigen expression and demonstrated substantial individual variation within the subgroups (Cartron et al., 1974). Further characterization includes the determination of anti-A or anti-A_1, the A transferase activity in serum, and the presence of A and/or H antigens in saliva.

The B phenotype does not present so many variants and they are more difficult to cluster in coherent groups so the weak variants have been classified by similarity to A subgroups. They are B_3, B_x, B_m, B_{el} and B_w and present various degrees of B transferase activity in plasma and secretions and weak B antigen expression.

It has to be pointed out that the phenotypic classifications do not completely correlate genetically as different weak alleles may be included in each subgroup and some have not been included in any of the existing categories (polymorphisms reviewed in (Yip, 2002)).

An interesting phenomenon has been reported, which was recognized by not adhering to classic Mendelian type of inheritance. Usually, the expression of A and B antigens is specified by two separate A and B alleles, one derived from the mother and the other one derived from the father. That is known as a common AB phenotype (*trans*-AB). However, in unusual cases of AB phenotype the expression of both A and B antigens is apparently specified by a single gene derived from either one of the parents resulting in what it is referred to as cis-AB (Yamamoto et al., 1993a; Yazer et al., 2006).

A similar phenomenon named B(A) was reported when weak A reactivity was demonstrated using a monoclonal anti-A reagents on the blood of certain B-type individuals. It appears that small quantities of A antigens, in addition to larger quantities of B antigens, were produced by special B transferase. Various different alleles for both cis-AB and B(A) have been found (Yamamoto et al., 1993b).

The assignment to these subgroups and its confirmation requires further tests than forward and reverse typing and may include the detection of the transferase activity in serum, the detection of antigens in saliva and/or genetic confirmation.

6. H and Secretor genes and related phenotypes

A and B antigen are synthesized on the same common fucosylated precursor, the H antigen. This precursor is produced by the transfer of an L-fucose residue from guanosine diphosphate (GDP)-L-fucose to the C-2 position of the terminal galactose of Type 1 or 2 core precursor chains using an α1-2 glycosidic bond. There are two α1,2-L-fucosyltransferases that are able to catalyze this reaction, encoded by two genes, FUT1 (H) and FUT2(Se). Both produce H-active structures but their expression is tissue-dependent. On one hand, the Hh system is a blood group on its own and it is closely related to ABO. On the other hand, the product of the Secretor gene allows the ABH antigens to be present in secretions and therefore it is also of relevance. Both genes and the related phenotypes will be discussed briefly.

6.1 Hh

H-transferase, the product of FUT1 is primarily present in tissues derived from ectoderm and mesoderm and is responsible for the synthesis of RBCs, bone marrow, vascular endothelium, skin and primary sensory neurons H antigens.

FUT1 and FUT2 share about 70% sequence identity and are 35 kb apart on the long arm of chromosome 19 (19q13.3). FUT1 gene consists of 4 exons, and the catalytic region is contained in the last one. Only one transcript has been described and it is translated into a 365 amino acid long protein. In addition, FUT1 has a preferential affinity for Type 2 acceptor substrate than for Type 1.

Some FUT1 alleles producing H-deficient phenotypes have been described due to different types of mutations, mostly missense mutations, but also to deletions causing frameshifts in the coding region. Those without or reduced enzymatic activity (h alleles) are the cause of the Bombay and para-Bombay phenotypes. The Bombay phenotype is characterized by the total absence of H antigen on RBCs and secretions irrespectively of the ABO status. These individuals are typed as O by the routine ABO typing because the A or B transferases, even if present, cannot synthesize their products due to the absence of precursor. These phenotypes are very uncommon but can be locally relevant (Mollicone et al., 1995).

6.2 Secretor (Se/se)

In 1926, it was found that ABH antigens were present, in soluble form, in seminal fluid and saliva. It was observed that the ability to secrete those antigens was genetically independent of ABO.

The locus controlling the secretion of ABH substances is called Secretor. The capacity to secrete (Se) is inherited as a dominant trait over the non-secretor phenotype (se). Se and se are alleles of the endodermal α1,2-fucosyltransferase gene (FUT2). Secretor-transferase, the product of FUT2, is active in tissue of endodermal origin and is responsible for Type 1 and 2 H structures. In secretor individuals of the appropriate ABO group, ABH antigens are detected in secretions of the goblet cells and mucous glands of the gastrointestinal tract (saliva, gastric juice, bile, meconium), genitourinary tract (seminal fluid, vaginal secretions, ovarian cyst fluid, urine), and respiratory tract, as well as milk, sweat, tears and amniotic fluid. The Se allele is present in the majority of the population (Race & Sanger, 1975).

In non-secretors se determines the absence of H substance in secretions. Therefore, A and B transferases, which are not under the control of the secretor gene, are not able to catalyze the production of A and B substances in body fluids of non-secretors who lack the H antigen, their acceptor substrate.

FUT2 gene consists of two exons with the entire coding sequence contained in the second exon and encodes a 332 amino acid long enzyme with a higher affinity to Type 1 acceptor substrates. An additional isoform with 11 more amino acid residues at the N-terminus has also been described. The allele containing the nonsense mutation at codon 143 is the most common non-secretor allele of FUT2. That mutation generates a stop codon and produces an early translation termination resulting in a null enzymatic activity. (Kelly et al., 1995; Spitalnik & Spitalnik, 2000)

7. Evolution genetics and homologous genes

The ABO gene has been conserved throughout evolution. Primates present a 95% of amino acid conservation among the ABO transferases. Comparing the partial nucleotide and deduced amino acid sequences of the ABO gene in samples of several species of primates with the human ABO gene, it was found that A to B divergence could have occurred at least in three different occasions during the ABO gene evolution in primates (Saitou & Yamamoto, 1997).

In addition, the ABO gene repertoire of alleles varies between humans and the other primates. For example, in chimpanzees there are only A or O groups, and in gorillas only the B type is found, in contrast with the A, B, AB or O groups in human. ABO groups exist in other mammals other than primates as well. For instance, pigs only show an AO polymorphism (Yamamoto & Yamamoto, 2001), and the mouse ABO gene encodes for an enzyme with dual specificity that is capable of synthesizing both A and B antigens *in vitro*, although in animal tissues the A antigen is primarily detected (Yamamoto et al., 2001). Currently, and thanks to DNA sequencing efforts, ABO orthologous genes have been found in a total of 45 vertebrate species.

In addition to A and B transferases, additional enzymes exist with similar specificities. The genes encoding these glycosyltransferases have some similarity and are evolutionary related with the ABO gene. They are classified into the α1,3- Gal(NAc) transferase family (or GT6 family). They are α1,3-galactosyltransferase (α1,3GalT), isogloboside b3 synthase (iGb3S), and Forssman glycolipid synthase (FS).

α1,3GalT transferase is encoded by the GGTA1 gene and catalyses the transfer of galactose to another galactose to form the α-galactosyl epitope (Galα1-3Gal-). As opposite to A and B transferases, α1,3GalT utilizes acceptor substrates lacking a fucose linked to the galactose. This enzyme activity is present in many mammalian species including some primates, but excluding Old World monkeys and anthropoid apes, such as humans. These species instead possess the antibody against the α-galactosyl epitope (Macher & Galili, 2008). On humans the GGTA1 gene was shown to contain frameshift and nonsense mutations, abolishing the enzymatic activity (Shaper et al., 1992).

IGb3S synthesizes iGb3 ceramide (Galα1-3Galβ1-4GlcCer) and it is encoded by the A3GALT2 gene. This enzyme transfers a galactose using the UDP-galactose as a donor substrate (Keusch et al., 2000). Conversely, FS is encoded by the GBGT1 gene and is responsible for the synthesis of Forssman antigen (GalNAcα1-3GalNAcβ1-3Galα1-4Galβ1-4GlcCer) using a UDP-GalNAc as a donor substrate (Haslam & Baenziger, 1996).

Apart from vertebrates some bacteria are also capable of synthesizing A or B antigens. In the case of *Escherichia coli* strain O86 high B activity was detected on its *O*-lipopolysaccharide antigen. Non-vertebrate A/B transferases genes have been identified in many other bacteria and also in one cyanophage. Based on the fact that there are no homologous genes found in species between vertebrates and bacteria, the possibility of horizontal transfer was proposed (Brew et al., 2010).

8. Natural antibodies against ABH

ABO is the only blood group system that in a natural and consistent manner has antibodies present in sera of people who lack the corresponding antigen from their red blood cells. With the exception of newborn infants under 5 months, deviations from this rule are extremely rare and related to disease. These antibodies are detected at about 3 months and increase their titer until the 5th to 10th year of life. Neonates may present the IgG type of ABO antibodies that have maternal origin, because IgG antibodies can cross the placenta. However in some occasions the fetus can produce by himself the IgM type of ABO antibodies. In adults they are mostly IgM although some may be IgG or IgA. The ABO antibodies may also be found in various body fluids including saliva, milk, cervical secretions, tears, and cysts.

The widely held hypothesis to explain the presence of these alloantibodies is that they are formed in response to terminal carbohydrates that share structural homology with A and B antigens present in the organism. These could derive from bacteria cell walls from normal intestinal microbial flora or be of animal origin and introduced through the diet. This view is supported by the fact that the levels of anti-A and anti-B antibodies seem to be influenced mostly by environmental factors, and genetics have a minor role.

Sera from A individuals contain anti-B antibody while B individuals' sera contain two types of antibody against A antigens. The first is anti-A and the second one is specific towards A_1 RBCs. Anti-A reacts with both A_1 and A_2 cells whereas the second only does with A_1 RBCs. Anti-A_1 is also present in some A_2 and A_2B individuals (Landsteiner & Levine, 1926). Group O people produce an antibody, anti-A,B able to cross-react with both A and B RBCs. It has been proposed that this antibody binds to a common structure shared by A and B antigens. This has been confirmed using human monoclonal analysis. Anti-A,B isotype is mainly IgG but some IgM or IgA may be present (Klein et al., 2005). Bombay (O_h) and para-Bombay type individuals also present a very potent anti-H antibody. That is the reason they can only be transfused with blood of their own type as RBCs from all the main groups will be destroyed due to the presence of the H antigen (Le Pendu et al., 1986).

9. ABO typing

In the reverse typing, the detection of antibodies against the A or B antigens in sera is performed using RBCs of known type (A_1 and B) that have been available for many years. But, forward ABO typing procedures changed completely with the invention of the hybridoma technology and the production of monoclonal antibodies. Reagents to better type blood donors were created. Nowadays, monoclonal antibodies to detect A and B antigens are routinely used in transfusion and clinical medicine and detailed descriptions are found in specialized reports. Very potent anti-A antibodies are able to agglutinate A_x RBCs helping in the detection of rare subgroups. They have also been very helpful in determining the structure of the precursor chains bound to A determinants. Also anti-B, anti-A,B and anti-H have been produced.

Lectins are proteins of non-immune origin able to bind sugars and therefore agglutinate cells or precipitate glycoconjugates carrying specific saccharides. Their binding to glycans can be inhibited by mono- or oligosaccharides. The nature of these sugar inhibitors is used to identify the specificity of the lectin as it is assumed that they are binding to the same site as the cell surface antigens. For reviews see (Bird, 1989; Nilsson 2007).

DBA, from *Dolichos biflorus* is specific for terminal N-acetylgalactosamine and has been extensively used to differentiate A_1 from A_2 subgroup RBCs. At precise dilutions A_1 and A_1B cells react positively while A_2 and A_2B do not. This property has been attributed to the avidity of the lectin rather than to qualitative differences between A_1 and A_2 antigens (Furukawa et al., 1985). There are fewer examples of B-specific lectins. As the specificity of these lectins depends on the terminal D-galactose determinant, they may cross-react with other antigens containing similar residues, i.e P, P1 and P^k (Voak et al., 1974). The most used reagent to detect secretor status in saliva from O group individuals is *Ulex europaeus* lectins which recognize the H antigen. Two lectins are present in the seeds of this species: UEA I is inhibited by L-fucose while UEA II is not. UEA II seems to recognize not only the terminal L-fucose but also a subterminal N-acetylglucosamine. The fucose requirement for reactivity of both lectins was corroborated by their failure to react against α-L-fucosidase-treated O cells (Matsumoto & Osawa, 1970).

Technical improvements have also allowed the detection and quantification of the antigens and the correspondent antibodies by other techniques than hemagglutination, such as cytofluorometry or ELISA and are being used to detect ABO histo-blood antigens in other organs and tissues.

10. ABO genotyping

Within the immunology related fields, HLA and ABO were two of the first genes to which DNA-based genotyping was applied. Many alleles encoding for variants of the main ABO alleles have been discovered and annotated and also in many cases their frequency in various world populations is also known. In any case, ABO typing based only on DNA techniques faces a very unique drawback. The O alleles are mostly the result of inactivating mutations of A[1]. Only those which are known can be detected by regular genotyping methods that otherwise will miss any novel ones. Complete sequencing of the donor/recipient genome is about to solve the problem of undetected mutations which arise from only sequencing some exons or RFLP strategies. But still, there are cases in which mutations in non-coding regions can produce aberrant messengers, as the formation of a new splicing site, or changes in expression levels if they are located in promoter or enhancer regions. Confusion over non-deleterious SNPs and novel mutations is going to arise with the introduction of these new technologies, and therefore forward and/or reverse typing are not going to disappear from blood bank facilities (Anstee, 2009; Reid & Denomme 2011).

Numerous methods have been established to determine the ABO genotype from genomic DNA (reviewed in (Olsson et al., 2001)). They are mostly designed to detect three to six of the most common alleles but many are not able to predict many subgroup, nondeletional, cis-AB and B(A) alleles, or hybrid alleles. A wrongly assigned blood type can be of serious consequence not only in blood transfusion but also for transplantation. Screening strategies taking into account these rare alleles have been implemented (Hosseini-Maaf et al., 2007). But for the most of the small/medium clinical setting microsequencing has been developed allowing a faster and reliable identification of the six major alleles. High-throughput techniques are able to detect more described mutations/alleles but they are considerably more expensive (Ferri & Pelotti, 2009).

11. Non-infectious adverse effects of ABO incompatibility

Many efforts have been devoted to avoid the transmission of pathogens during transfusion. But incompatibility barriers associated with ABO may cause clinical symptoms derived from mismatched ABO phenotypes.

11.1 ABO hemolytic disease of the newborn

Rh antigens are the most common blood group antigens associated with hemolytic disease of the newborn (HDN) but this disease also occurs as a result of ABO incompatibility between group O mothers carrying a group A, B or AB fetus (recently reviewed by Roberts (Roberts, 2008)). Even though the ABO incompatibility between mother and fetus should affect around a 20% of all pregnancies (in the case of European descent parents) only in very few instances they become symptomatic. Moreover, in many of those manifested cases this incompatibility only results in very mild symptoms and requires no treatment. In a small number of cases, phototherapy or antibody-inhibition by soluble oligosaccharides have been used.

A very minor fraction of these mothers produces a high quantity of IgG antibodies in place of the common IgM antibodies. The IgG isotype can pass through the placenta to the fetal circulation causing hemolysis of fetal RBCs and therefore fetal anemia and HDN. Although very uncommon, cases of ABO HDN have been reported in infants born to mothers with blood groups A and B. In contrast to Rh disease, about half of the cases of ABO HDN occur in a firstborn baby and ABO HDN does not become much severer after further pregnancies.

11.2 Erroneous transfusion

Even now, erroneous ABO incompatible transfusion is still an important cause for morbidity and mortality associated with transfusions, together with other non-ABO hemolytic transfusion reactions (HTR), transfusion-related acute lung injury (TRALI), transfusion associated circulatory overload (TACO), and bacterial contamination. The year 2010 report from the United Kingdom SHOT hemovigilance system showed a 2% of all the cases of incompatible transfusion corresponding to the ABO system (SHOT, 2010). A similar report from the USA FDA published in 2009 indicated that 9% of all fatal cases during transfusion were due to ABO mismatched HTR (FDA, 2009). Fortunately, many reports have shown that about 50 percent of ABO-mismatched recipients do not show any obvious sign of a transfusion reaction. The reason for this lack of symptoms is not known but if resistance mechanisms are involved, their elucidation could lead to the improvement of transplantation strategies.

Studies on ABO-compatible, but not ABO-identical, blood transfusions have shown an increased risk of death in recipients of ABO-mismatched platelet concentrates. As mentioned before, platelets also express ABH antigens in variable amounts. It has been shown though that platelets coming from A_2 individuals do not express H or A antigens and can be used as "universal". The biochemical reason for this phenomenon is not known yet (Cooling et al., 2005).

11.3 ABO mismatched transplantations

ABO-mismatching has also been investigated in transplantation recipients. In the case of hematopoietic stem cell transplantation, ABO incompatibility has not been associated with a shortened overall survival or increased mortality related to transplantation. However, transplantation of solid organs with ABO-incompatibility has a more modest success rate depending on the age of the recipient. Infants tolerate much better this incompatibility as demonstrated in heart transplantation probably due to B-cell immature response. Immunosuppressive drugs are the hallmark treatment after any kind of transplantation as they are able to reduce or eliminate rejection reactions. These molecules together with apheresis and monoclonal antibody therapies are of help in ABO-mismatched transplantation (Nydegger et al., 2005; Nydegger et al., 2007).

12. ABO and diseases

Many associations have been reported between specific ABO alleles and different susceptibility to several diseases such as vascular and cardiovascular diseases, diverse infections, and also cancer. For many years studies compared the incidence of a disease within each of the blood groups and it became apparent that some kind of association existed between some diseases and particular blood types. More recently genome-wide association studies have taken over and in a bias-free manner have linked polymorphisms of the ABO locus to different diseases (reviewed in Yamamoto et al., 2011)(Fig. 3).

Relating cardiovascular and vascular disease it is known that the ABO groups are a major determinant modulating the plasma levels of two coagulation factors: factor VIII (FVIII) and von Willebrand factor (vWF). Non-O blood group individuals have approximately 25%

lower levels of these glycoproteins. It was already known that there was a higher incidence of both arterial and venous thrombotic disease in A, B or AB individuals compared with O group individuals. This has been confirmed by GWAS results showing decreased risk for venous thromboembolism among individuals of O and A₂ groups (Tregouet et al., 2009).

There have also been studies aimed to understand different associations of ABO with pathogenic infections like Noroviruses because of the fact that many bacteria or viruses utilize glycosylated proteins as cell surface receptors for attachment. The interactions between host receptors and pathogen predict that these associations are very dependent on the receptor selectivity. Actually, many classical etiological studies identified links between ABO and peptic ulcer, cholera, or malaria (Mourant et al., 1978). These associations are currently being reassessed by the newer genomic approaches. In the case of malaria, a recent GWAS has not found strong association with ABO although the same samples exhibited the association by targeted analysis (Jallow et al., 2009).

But one of the most striking associations found is the increased susceptibility of non-O blood type individuals to pancreatic cancer. For both stomach and pancreatic cancer this difference in incidence was already known from targeted studies. Recently though, in the case of pancreatic cancer a GWAS has confirmed this association and ranked first a single nucleotide polymorphism in the ABO gene discriminating O- and non-O alleles with the highest score (Amundadottir et al., 2009). It is obvious that the presence of non-O alleles does not cause cancer, but nonetheless they might be favoring the carcinogenic process in a subtle but steady manner.

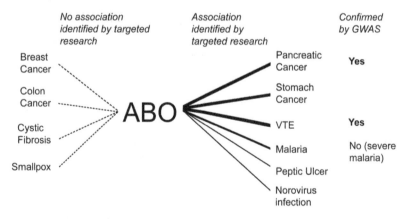

Fig. 3. Diseases associated with ABO polymorphisms were first detected by targeted research and some of these associations have been confirmed by GWAS. Other studies also found no association with other diseases.

As we mentioned before, the expression of ABH antigens is not constant. It undergoes alterations during cellular differentiation, development and aging as well as pathologic phenomena, as occurs in carcinogenesis. In the case of ABO it has been known for many years that tumors may reduce the expression of A or B antigens and that process is part of the global changes that cancer cause in glycosylation (Hakomori, 1999). Some of these changes are already being used as diagnostic markers but as more studies are brought forward more are going to be added.

13. Enzyme-converted O RBCs

O RBCs can be transfused to individuals of any ABO group type as they are not going to react with any of the alloantibodies. Therefore, in case of a surplus of A or B blood it would be advantageous to be able to convert it to O. One of the most promising strategies to achieve this has been the use of glycosidases able to enzymatically remove the terminal sugar (N-acetylgalactosamine in the case of A or galactose for B). There have been advancements with the use of bacterial glycosidases and this line of research is still being pursued actively (Olsson & Clausen, 2008).

14. Conclusion

The ABO histo-blood group system is a major player in transfusion/transplantation and regeneration medicine. For years, investigations in this field have been pushing forward developments in different scientific areas. New typing procedures and strategies to cross the ABO incompatibility barriers are improving blood banking and transfusion. Moreover, basic research focused on this system contributes to a better understanding of a range of topics, from genomics to pathological processes. We anticipate that newer technologies will bring individual genome sequencing to a daily routine in the coming years and that will affect not only ABO genotyping but also many other medical issues. GWAS will increase the links of ABO to other diseases, giving the opportunity to researchers to start to tackle one of the most fundamental, and unanswered questions about ABO, the function of the antigens in physiological and pathological conditions by studying the molecular mechanisms underlying those associations.

15. Acknowledgment

We thankfully acknowledge the financial support of the Institut of Medicina Predictiva i Personalitzada del Càncer.

16. References

Amundadottir, L., Kraft, P., Stolzenberg-Solomon, R. Z., Fuchs, C. S., Petersen, G. M., Arslan, A. A., et al. (2009). Genome-wide association study identifies variants in the ABO locus associated with susceptibility to pancreatic cancer. *Nature Genetics*, Vol. 41, No. 9, pp. 986-990. ISSN 1546-1718

Anstee, D. J. (2009). Red cell genotyping and the future of pretransfusion testing. *Blood*, Vol. 114, No. 2, pp. 248-256. ISSN 1528-0020

Bird, G. W. (1989). Lectins in immunohematology. *Transfusion Medicine Reviews*, Vol. 3, No. 1, pp. 55-62. ISSN 0887-7963

Björk, S., Breimer, M. E., Hansson, G. C., Karlsson, K. A., & Leffler, H. (1987). Structures of blood group glycosphingolipids of human small intestine. A relation between the expression of fucolipids of epithelial cells and the ABO, Le and Se phenotype of the donor. *Journal of Biological Chemistry*, Vol. 262, No. 14, pp. 6758-6765. ISSN: 0021-9258

Brew, K., Tumbale, P., & Acharya, K. R. (2010). Family 6 glycosyltransferases in vertebrates and bacteria: inactivation and horizontal gene transfer may enhance mutualism between vertebrates and bacteria. *Journal of Biological Chemistry*, Vol. 285, No. 48, pp. 37121-37127. ISSN 1083-351X

Cartron, J. P., Gerbal, A., Hughes-Jones, N. C., & Salmon, C. (1974). 'Weak A' phenotypes. Relationship between red cell agglutinability and antigen site density. *Immunology*, Vol. 27, No. 4, pp. 723-727. ISSN 0019-2805

Clausen, H., & Hakomori, S. (1989). ABH and related histo-blood group antigens; immunochemical differences in carrier isotypes and their distribution. *Vox Sanguinis*, Vol. 56, No. 1, pp. 1-20. ISSN 0042-9007

Clausen, H., White, T., Takio, K., Titani, K., Stroud, M., Holmes, E., et al. (1990). Isolation to homogeneity and partial characterization of a histo-blood group A defined Fuc alpha 1-2Gal alpha 1-3-N-acetylgalactosaminyltransferase from human lung tissue. *Journal of Biological Chemistry*, Vol. 265, No. 2, pp. 1139-1145. ISSN 0021-9258

Cooling, L. L., Kelly, K., Barton, J., Hwang, D., Koerner, T. A., & Olson, J. D. (2005). Determinants of ABH expression on human blood platelets. *Blood*, Vol. 105, No. 8, pp. 3356-3364. ISSN 0006-4971

Crow, J. F. (1993). Felix Bernstein and the first human marker locus. *Genetics,*Vol. 133, No. 1, pp. 4-7. ISSN 0016-6731

Epstein, A. A., & Ottenberg, R. (1908). Simple method of performing serum reactions. *Proceedings of the New York Pathological Society*, Vol. 8, pp. 117-123.

Ferguson-Smith, M. A., Aitken, D. A., Turleau, C., & de Grouchy, J. (1976). Localisation of the human ABO: Np-1: AK-1 linkage group by regional assignment of AK-1 to 9q34. *Human Genetics*, Vol. 34, No. 1, pp. 35-43. ISSN 0340-6717

Ferri, G., & Pelotti, S. (2009). Multiplex ABO genotyping by minisequencing. *Methods in Molecular Biology*, Vol. 496, pp. 51-58. ISSN 1064-3745

Finne, J., Krusius, T., Rauvala, H., & Jarnefelt, J. (1980). Molecular nature of the blood-group ABH antigens of the human erythrocyte membrane. *Revue Francaise de Transfusion et Immuno-Hematologie*, Vol. 23, No. 5, pp. 545-552. ISSN 0338-4535

Food and Drug Administration. (2009). Fatalities Reported to FDA Following Blood Collection and Transfusion: Annual Summary for Fiscal Year 2009. Silver Spring, USA.

Fukuda, M., & Fukuda, M. N. (1981). Changes in cell surface glycoproteins and carbohydrate structures during the development and differentiation of human erythroid cells. *Journal of Supramolecular Structure and Cellular Biochemistry*, Vol. 17, No. 4, pp. 313-324. ISSN 0275-3723

Furukawa, K., Mattes, M. J., & Lloyd, K. O. (1985). A1 and A2 erythrocytes can be distinguished by reagents that do not detect structural differences between the two cell types. *Journal of Immunology*, Vol. 135, No. 6, pp. 4090-4094. ISSN 0022-1767

Hakomori, S. (1981). Blood group ABH and Ii antigens of human erythrocytes: chemistry, polymorphism, and their developmental change. *Seminars in Hematology*, Vol. 18, No. 1, pp. 39-62. ISSN 0037-1963

Hakomori, S. (1999). Antigen structure and genetic basis of histo-blood groups A, B and O: their changes associated with human cancer. *Biochimica et Biophysica Acta*, Vol. 1473, No. 1, pp. 247-266. ISSN 0006-3002

Haslam, D. B., & Baenziger, J. U. (1996). Expression cloning of Forssman glycolipid synthetase: a novel member of the histo-blood group ABO gene family. *Proceedings of the National Academy of Sciences U S A*, Vol. 93, No. 20, pp. 10697-10702. ISSN 0027-8424

Holgersson, J., Clausen, H., Hakomori, S., Samuelsson, B. E., & Breimer, M. E. (1990). Blood group A glycolipid antigen expression in kidney, ureter, kidney artery, and kidney vein from a blood group A¹Le(a-b+) human individual. Evidence for a novel blood group A heptaglycosylceramide based on a type 3 carbohydrate chain. *Journal of Biological Chemistry*, Vol. 265, No. 34, pp. 20790-20798. ISSN 0021-9258

Hosseini-Maaf, B., Hellberg, A., Chester, M. A., & Olsson, M. L. (2007). An extensive polymerase chain reaction-allele-specific polymorphism strategy for clinical ABO blood group genotyping that avoids potential errors caused by null, subgroup, and hybrid alleles. *Transfusion*, Vol. 47, No. 11, pp. 2110-2125. ISSN 0041-1132

Jallow, M., Teo, Y. Y., Small, K. S., Rockett, K. A., Deloukas, P., Clark, T. G., et al. (2009). Genome-wide and fine-resolution association analysis of malaria in West Africa. *Nature Genetics*, Vol. 41, No. 6, pp. 657-665. ISSN 1546-1718

Kabat, E. A. (1956). *Blood group substances; their chemistry and immunochemistry*, Academic Press. New York, USA

Kelly, R. J., Rouquier, S., Giorgi, D., Lennon, G. G., & Lowe, J. B. (1995). Sequence and expression of a candidate for the human Secretor blood group alpha(1,2)fucosyltransferase gene (FUT2). Homozygosity for an enzyme-inactivating nonsense mutation commonly correlates with the non-secretor phenotype. *Journal of Biological Chemistry*, Vol. 270, No. 9, pp. 4640-4649. ISSN 0021-9258

Keusch, J. J., Manzella, S. M., Nyame, K. A., Cummings, R. D., & Baenziger, J. U. (2000). Expression cloning of a new member of the ABO blood group glycosyltransferases, iGb3 synthase, that directs the synthesis of isoglobo-glycosphingolipids. *Journal of Biological Chemistry*, Vol. 275, No. 33, pp. 25308-25314. ISSN 0021-9258

Klein, H. G., Mollison, P. L., & Anstee, D. J. (2005). *Mollison's blood transfusion in clinical medicine* (11th ed.). Blackwell, ISBN 0632064544, Malden, USA.

Kobata, A., Yamashita, K., & Tachibana, Y. (1978). Oligosaccharides from human milk. *Methods in Enzymology*, Vol. 50, pp. 216-220. ISSN 0076-6879

Landsteiner, K. (1900). Zur Kenntnis der antifermentativen, lytischen und agglutinierenden Wirkungen des Blutserums und der Lymphe. *Zentralblatt Bakteriologie*, Vol. 27, pp.357-362.

Landsteiner, K., & Levine, P. (1926). On the Cold Agglutinins in Human Serum. *The Journal of Immunology*, Vol. 12, No. 6, pp. 441-460.

Le Pendu, J., Lambert, F., Gerard, G., Vitrac, D., Mollicone, R., & Oriol, R. (1986). On the specificity of human anti-H antibodies. *Vox Sanguinis*, Vol. 50, No. 4, pp. 223-226. ISSN 0042-9007

Lucien, N., Sidoux-Walter, F., Roudier, N., Ripoche, P., Huet, M., Trinh-Trang-Tan, M. M., et al. (2002). Antigenic and functional properties of the human red blood cell urea transporter hUT-B1. *Journal of Biological Chemistry*, Vol. 277, No. 37, pp. 34101-34108. ISSN 0021-9258

Lundblad, A. (1978). Oligosaccharides from human urine. *Methods in Enzymology*, Vol. 50, pp. 226-235. ISSN 0076-6879

Macher, B. A., & Galili, U. (2008). The Galalpha1,3Galbeta1,4GlcNAc-R (alpha-Gal) epitope: a carbohydrate of unique evolution and clinical relevance. *Biochimica et Biophysica Acta*, Vol. 1780, No. 2, pp. 75-88. ISSN 0006-3002

Matsumoto, I., & Osawa, T. (1970). Purification and characterization of a Cytisus-type Anti-H(O) phytohemagglutinin from Ulex europeus seeds. *Archives of Biochemistry and Biophysics*, Vol. 140, No. 2, pp. 484-491. ISSN 0003-9861

Mollicone, R., Cailleau, A., & Oriol, R. (1995). Molecular genetics of H, Se, Lewis and other fucosyltransferase genes. *Transfusion clinique et biologique*, Vol. 2, No. 4, pp. 235-242. ISSN 1246-7820

Morgan, W. T. (1960). A contribution to human biochemical genetics; the chemical basis of blood-group specificity. *Proceedings of the Royal Society B: Biological Sciences*, Vol. 151, pp 308-347. ISSN 0080-4649

Mourant, A. E., Kopeć, A. C., & Domaniewska-Sobczak, K. (1978). *Blood groups and diseases: a study of associations of diseases with blood groups and other polymorphisms.* Oxford University Press. ISBN 0192641700, Oxford, New York, USA.

Nilsson, C. L. (2007). *Lectins : analytical technologies* (1st ed.). Elsevier. ISBN 9780444530776 Boston, Massachusetts, USA

Nydegger, U., Mohacsi, P., Koestner, S., Kappeler, A., Schaffner, T., Carrel, T., et al. (2005). ABO histo-blood group system-incompatible allografting. *International Immunopharmacology*, Vol. 5, No. 1, pp. 147-153. ISSN 1567-5769

Nydegger, U. E., Riedler, G. F., & Flegel, W. A. (2007). Histoblood groups other than HLA in organ transplantation. *Transplantation Proceedings*, Vol. 39, No. 1, pp. 64-68. ISSN 0041-1345

O'Keefe, D. S., & Dobrovic, A. (1996). Decreased stability of the O allele mRNA transcript of the ABO gene. *Blood*, Vol. 87, No. 7, pp. 3061-3062. ISSN 0006-4971

Olsson, M. L., & Clausen, H. (2008). Modifying the red cell surface: towards an ABO-universal blood supply. *British Journal of Haematology*, Vol. 140, No. 1, pp. 3-12. ISSN 1365-2141

Olsson, M. L., Irshaid, N. M., Hosseini-Maaf, B., Hellberg, A., Moulds, M. K., Sareneva, H., et al. (2001). Genomic analysis of clinical samples with serologic ABO blood grouping discrepancies: identification of 15 novel A and B subgroup alleles. *Blood*, Vol. 98, No. 5, pp. 1585-1593. ISSN 0006-4971

Oriol, R., Samuelsson, B. E., & Messeter, L. (1990). ABO antibodies - serological behaviour and immuno-chemical characterization. *Journal of Immunogenetics*, Vol. 17, No. 4-5, pp. 279-299. ISSN 0305-1811

Patenaude, S. I., Seto, N. O., Borisova, S. N., Szpacenko, A., Marcus, S. L., Palcic, M. M., et al. (2002). The structural basis for specificity in human ABO(H) blood group biosynthesis. *Nature Structural Biology*, Vol. 9, No. 9, pp. 685-690. ISSN 1072-8368

Putkonen, T. (1930). Über die gruppenspezifischen Eigenschaften Verschiedener Korperflussigkeiten. *Acta Soc Med Fenn Duodecim Ser A*, Vol. 14, pp. 113-153.

Race, R. R., & Sanger, R. (1975). *Blood groups in man* (6th ed.). Blackwell Scientific Publications. ISBN: 0632004312, Oxford, Philadelphia, USA.

Ravn, V., & Dabelsteen, E. (2000). Tissue distribution of histo-blood group antigens. *Acta Pathologica, Microbiologica et Immunologica Scandinavica*, Vol. 108, No. 1, pp. 1-28. ISSN 0903-4641

Reid, M. E., & Denomme, G. A. (2011). DNA-based methods in the immunohematology reference laboratory. *Transfusion and Apheresis Science*, Vol. 44, No. 1, pp. 65-72. ISSN 1473-0502

Roberts, I. A. (2008). The changing face of haemolytic disease of the newborn. *Early Human Development,* Vol. 84, No. 8, pp. 515-523. ISSN 0378-3782

Rochant, H., Tonthat, H., Henri, A., Titeux, M., & Dreyfus, B. (1976). Abnormal distribution of erythrocytes A1 antigens in preleukemia as demonstrated by an immunofluorescence technique. *Nouvelle revue francaise d'hematologie; blood cells,* Vol. 17, No. 1-2, pp. 237-255.

Saitou, N., & Yamamoto, F. (1997). Evolution of primate ABO blood group genes and their homologous genes. *Molecular Biology and Evolution,* Vol. 14, No. 4, 399-411. ISSN 0737-4038

Schachter, H., Michaels, M. A., Tilley, C. A., Crookston, M. C., & Crookston, J. H. (1973). Qualitative differences in the N-acetyl-D-galactosaminyltransferases produced by human A1 and A2 genes. *Proceedings of the National Academy of Sciences U S A,* Vol. 70, No. 1, pp. 220-224. ISSN 0027-8424

Shaper, N. L., Lin, S. P., Joziasse, D. H., Kim, D. Y., & Yang-Feng, T. L. (1992). Assignment of two human alpha-1,3-galactosyltransferase gene sequences (GGTA1 and GGTA1P) to chromosomes 9q33-q34 and 12q14-q15. *Genomics,* Vol. 12, No. 3, pp. 613-615. ISSN 0888-7543

Smith, B. L., Preston, G. M., Spring, F. A., Anstee, D. J., & Agre, P. (1994). Human red cell aquaporin CHIP. I. Molecular characterization of ABH and Colton blood group antigens. *Journal of Clinical Investigation,* Vol. 94, No. 3, pp. 1043-1049. ISSN 0021-9738

Soejima, M., & Koda, Y. (2005). Molecular mechanisms of Lewis antigen expression. *Legal Medicine (Tokyo),* Vol. 7, No. 4, pp. 266-269. ISSN 1344-6223

Spitalnik, P. F., & Spitalnik, S. L. (2000). Human blood groups antigens and antibodies. Part 1: Carbohydrate determinants. In: *Hematology: Basic Principles and Practice,* R. Hoffman, E. J. Benz, B. Furie & S. J. Shattil (Eds.), pp. 2188-2196. Churchill Livingstone. Philadelphia, USA.

SHOT (2010). SHOT 2010 Report, Manchester, UK.

Tregouet, D. A., Heath, S., Saut, N., Biron-Andreani, C., Schved, J. F., Pernod, G., et al. (2009). Common susceptibility alleles are unlikely to contribute as strongly as the FV and ABO loci to VTE risk: results from a GWAS approach. *Blood,* Vol. 113, No. 21, pp. 5298-5303. ISSN 1528-0020

Voak, D., Todd, G. M., & Pardoe, G. I. (1974). A study of the serological behaviour and nature of the anti-B-P-Pk activity of Salmonidae roe protectins. *Vox Sanguinis,* Vol. 26, No. 2, pp. 176-188. ISSN 0042-9007

von Decastello, A., & Sturli, A. (1902). Über die Isoagglutinie im Serum gesunder und kranker Menschen. *Münchener Medizinische Wochenschrift,* Vol. 26, pp. 1090-1095.

von Dungern, E., & Hirszfeld, L. (1910). Über Vererbung gruppenspezifischer Strukturen des Blutes. *Z Immun Forsch Exper Ther,* Vol. 6, pp. 284-292.

Watkins, W. M. (1981). Biochemistry and genetics of the ABO, Lewis, and P blood group systems., In: *Advances in Human Genetics* (Vol. 10). H. Harris & K. Hirschhorn (Eds.), pp 1-136. Plenum Press, New York, USA.

Yamamoto, F. (2004). Review: ABO blood group system -ABH oligosaccharide antigens, anti-A and anti-B, A and B glycosyltransferases, and ABO genes. *Immunohematology,* Vol. 20, No. 1, pp 3-22. ISSN 0894-203X

Yamamoto, F., Cid, E., Yamamoto, M., & Blancher, A. (2011). ABO Research in the Modern Era of Genomics. *Transfusion Medicine Reviews,* Epub: September 22nd. ISSN 1532-9496

Yamamoto, F., Clausen, H., White, T., Marken, J., & Hakomori, S. (1990a). Molecular genetic basis of the histo-blood group ABO system. *Nature*, Vol. 345, No. 6272, pp. 229-233. ISSN 0028-0836

Yamamoto, F., Marken, J., Tsuji, T., White, T., Clausen, H., & Hakomori, S. (1990b). Cloning and characterization of DNA complementary to human UDP-GalNAc: Fuc alpha 1-2Gal alpha 1-3GalNAc transferase (histo-blood group A transferase) mRNA. *Journal of Biological Chemistry*, Vol. 265, No. 2, pp. 1146-1151. ISSN 0021-9258

Yamamoto, F., & McNeill, P. D. (1996). Amino acid residue at codon 268 determines both activity and nucleotide-sugar donor substrate specificity of human histo-blood group A and B transferases: In vitro mutagenesis study. *Journal of Biological Chemistry*, Vol. 271, No. 18, pp. 10515-10520. ISSN 0021-9258

Yamamoto, F., McNeill, P. D., & Hakomori, S. (1995). Genomic organization of human histo-blood group ABO genes. *Glycobiology*, Vol. 5, No. 1, pp. 51-58. ISSN 0959-6658

Yamamoto, F., McNeill, P.D., Kominato, Y., Yamamoto, M., Hakomori, S. Ishimoto, S., Nishida, S., Shima, M. & Fujimura, Y. (1993a). Molecular genetic analysis of the ABO blood group system: 2. *cis*-AB alleles. *Vox Sanguinis*, Vol. 64, No. 2, pp. 120-123. ISSN 0042-9007

Yamamoto, F., McNeill, P. D., Yamamoto, M., Hakomori, S., & Harris, T. (1993b). Molecular genetic analysis of the ABO blood group system: 3. Ax and B(A) alleles. *Vox Sanguinis*, Vol. 64, No. 3, pp. 171-174. ISSN 0042-9007

Yamamoto, F., & Yamamoto, M. (2001). Molecular genetic basis of porcine histo-blood group AO system. *Blood*, Vol. 97, No. 10, pp. 3308-3310. ISSN 0006-4971

Yamamoto, M., Lin, X. H., Kominato, Y., Hata, Y., Noda, R., Saitou, N., et al. (2001). Murine equivalent of the human histo-blood group ABO gene is a *cis*-AB gene and encodes a glycosyltransferase with both A and B transferase activity. *Journal of Biological Chemistry*, Vol. 276, No. 17, pp. 13701-13708. ISSN 0021-9258

Yazer, M. H., Olsson, M. L., & Palcic, M. M. (2006). The cis-AB blood group phenotype: fundamental lessons in glycobiology. *Transfusion Medicine Reviews*, Vol. 20, No. 3, pp. 207-217. ISSN 0887-7963

Yip, S. P. (2002). Sequence variation at the human ABO locus. *Annals of Human Genetics*, Vol. 66 (Pt 1), pp. 1-27. ISSN 0003-4800

Part 2

Blood Transfusion in Medicine and Surgery

Blood Transfusion Practices in Major Orthopaedic Surgery

Saqeb B. Mirza[1], Sukhmeet S. Panesar[2] and Douglas G. Dunlop[3]

[1]Specialist Registrar, University Hospital Southampton,
[2]Special Advisor, National Patient Safety Agency,
[3]Consultant Orthopaedic Surgeon, University Hospital Southampton,
UK

1. Introduction

Blood forms a major component in the management of surgical patients in whom major blood loss is expected. In the past years, transfusion of allogeneic blood has been the mainstay of management of patients who have or are considered to be at risk of major bleeding, particularly in cardiac and orthopaedic surgery where blood loss can often be substantial. Studies have shown that in many countries across the world, over fifty per cent of red cells transfused were in surgical specialties (Cook 1991;Lenfant 1992;Regan 2002). For example, in Canada, 31% of all red cell transfusions were given in cardiac and orthopaedic surgery (Chiavetta 1996).

2. Blood loss in orthopaedic surgery

In primary hip surgery, the blood loss is estimated at 3.2 +/- 1.3 units(Toy 1992) and 4.07 +/- 1.74 grams of haemoglobin(Toy 1992). In revision hip surgery, the blood loss is about 4.0 +/- 2.1 units. In primary knee replacement, the blood loss ranges from 1000-1500mls and can average 3.85 +/- 1.4 grams of haemoglobin(Keating 1998;Mylod, Jr 1990) and may be higher in cementless knee replacements(Hays 1988). Transfusion rates of 2.0 +/- 1.8 units for primary THR and 2.9 +/- 2.3 units for revision THRs have been documented(Bae 2001). The rates for knee replacements are not well studied but are estimated at 1 – 2 units for primary surgery and can be up to 3-4 units for revision surgery(Callaghan 2000).

Other settings which present major blood loss scenarios in orthopaedic surgery include:

- Pelvic surgery
- Tumour surgery
- Bilateral primary joint replacement

3. Predictors of allogeneic blood transfusion

A series of studies covering a heterogeneous population of over 10,000 patients has attempted to define certain risk factors that may predict the need for allogeneic blood transfusion. All studies made an attempt to reduce confounding factors and risk factors were shown to be consistent with high levels of statistical significance in their association with the risk of exposure to allogeneic blood.

Preoperative haemoglobin level is one of the main factors associated with risk of transfusion following total joint replacement(de, Jr 1996;Faris 1999) . In a study of 9,482 patients who underwent THR or TKR, Bierbaum *et al* demonstrated that the lower the baseline haemoglobin level, the more probable the transfusion of allogeneic blood(Bierbaum 1999) . Patients with a preoperative haemoglobin of less than 100g/L had a 90% chance of needing a transfusion, those with a level of 100-135g/L had a 15-25% chance of requiring allogeneic blood(Callaghan 2000).

Age over 65 years(Hatzidakis 1998;Hatzidakis 2000) has been shown to increase the risk of being transfused with patients less than 65 years with a haemoglobin of 135g/L or more having only a 3% chance of being transfused.

Other risk factors that have been closely associated with a likelihood of allogeneic transfusion include low weight, small height, female sex, estimated surgical blood loss, whether primary or revision surgery, type of surgery, anticoagulant use, thrombocytopaenia, other comorbidities and bilateral joint surgery(Bierbaum 1999; Borghi 1993; Churchill 1998; Hatzidakis 2000).

4. Risks of allogeneic blood transfusion

The association of allogeneic blood with numerous risks including transfusion transmitted infections (TTIs) has limited its utility in recent years(Klein 2000). Thus, there is now considerable interest in finding ways to avoid allogeneic blood.

1.   Tranfusion transmitted infections (TTIs)

The risks of transfusion transmitted infections have been considerably reduced in the developed world by measures to improve the detection and elimination of infected blood (Goodnough 1999a). The total TTI risk has been estimated at 1:100,000 to 1:1,000,000 in an American population (Kleinman 2000). However in developing countries, there is still a high prevalence of such infections and transfusion services are still inadequately equipped to conduct universal antibody screening (Lackritz 1998; McFarland 1997).

a.   Viral infections
The risks of viral TTIs can be regarded as being very low in the developed world when compared to other life time risks (Glynn 2000;Regan 2000).
The following are estimated risks (Klein 1995;Klein 2000):
Human Immunodeficiency Virus (HIV)   1:1,000,000
Hepatitis B Virus (HBV)   1:100,000
Hepatitis C Virus (HCV)   1:500 to 1:5,000
Human T-Lymphocytic Virus 1 and 2 (HTLV)   1:200,000
Cytomegalovirus (CMV)   1:2,500
A previous retrospective analysis of data from the United States, Australia and Europe found that in repeat donors, seroconversions were detected as follows (Muller-Breitkreutz 2000):

Anti-HIV screening   1:2,323,778
Anti-hepatitis C screening   1:620,754
Hepatitis B screening   1:398,499

Other viral infections such as Guillian-Barre virus C, human herpes virus and TT virus have not to date been shown to be relevant to transfusion practice (Allain 2000).

b. Bacterial infections
    This risk is estimated at 1:400,000 transfusions (The SHOT Committee 2000).

c. Creutzfeld-Jacob disease
    Universal leucodepletion of all blood prepared for transfusion, excluding previously transfused UK donors and excluding donor plasma from fractionation are precautionary measures instituted to prevent the transmission of CJD (Scottish Intercollegiate Guidelines Network 2001).

2. Direct immune injury
    Mild haemolytic reactions range from 1:5,000 to severe haemolytic reactions and anaphylaxis in 1:600,000 (Callaghan 2000).

3. Immunomodulation
    In vitro, allogeneic blood has been shown to have the capacity to depress immune function (Gafter 1992; Kaplan 1984), an effect mediated mainly by transfused white blood cells (Blajchman 1994; Bordin 1994). However, the clinical importance of this effect is poorly understood (Goodnough 1999a). The practice of leucodepletion of blood is now commonplace in developed countries. However, studies have not demonstrated a clear cut clinical benefit of this practice. Randomized control trials using both leucodepleted blood and autologous blood have not demonstrated an increase in either the risk of cancer or infection (Goodnough 2000; Jensen 1998). A meta-analysis of three randomized control trials and two cohort studies where control groups received either leucodepleted blood or autologous transfusion found no significant differences in cancer recurrence (McAlister 1998).

4. Procedural/clerical error
    The blood transfusion process can be complex and crosses many disciplines and professions, with one study identifying over forty steps between the patient and their transfusion, all of which involve the potential for human error(Will 1996). Clerical error has been estimated at 1:25,000 (AuBuchon 1996). Serious complications including coagulopathy, renal failure, intravascular haemolysis, admission to ITU, persistent viral infection and death have been estimated at 1:67,000 (Scottish Intercollegiate Guidelines Network 2001; The SHOT Committee 2000). These risks can be controlled by using safe protocols for transfusion, for example those recommended by the British Committee for Standards in Haematology.

5. Risks of perioperative anaemia

Some studies have shown that surgical morbidity and mortality are inversely correlated with preoperative haemoglobin levels (Carson 1988;Spence 1998). The rate of fatal complications due to anaemia in sixteen reports of the surgical management of Jehovah's witnesses has been reported at 0.5-1.5% (Kearon 1997). A retrospective survey of a similar patient population indicated that when confounding factors were taken into account, mortality does not increase as haemoglobin falls to 80g/L (Carson 1996; Carson 1998a).

However, below this level, ninety per cent received transfusions and thus it is hard to comment on the effect of anaemia on mortality at haemoglobin below this level.

Substantial perioperative blood loss is common in major orthopaedic surgery and patients are often elderly with a high prevalence of ischaemic heart disease. Consequently, many who are undergoing major orthopaedic surgery will be at high risk of cardiovascular complications (Neill 2000). The incidence of anaemia increases with age (Ania 1997) and is four to six times greater than can be predicted by clinical symptoms in the over 65 year age group (Ania 1997).

Perioperative anaemia in the elderly is not without morbidity and includes fatigue, tachycardia, hypotension, dyspnoea and impaired level of consciousness (Spence 1998) and can be associated with decreased vigour, potentially prolonging the duration of hospital stay (Bierbaum 1999;Keating 1999) and affecting quality of life. Indeed a correlation between muscle strength and haematocrit levels suggests that haematocrit may be a valuable objective measure of vigour in patients undergoing major orthopaedic surgery (Keating 1999).

In patients with known cardiovascular comorbidity, severe preoperative anaemia can be associated with a massive increase in mortality. Carson *et al* (Carson 1996) reported that the 30-day mortality rate in patients with preoperative Hb levels of less than 60g/L was 33.3% compared with 1.3% for those with levels in excess of 120g/L.

Observational studies and consensus statements suggest that the elderly and those with a poor cardiovascular reserve or major cardiovascular comorbidity or peripheral vascular disease are less tolerant to perioperative anaemia and should therefore be transfused at a higher haemoglobin level(Carson 1998a).

6. Transfusion thresholds

In an attempt to provide optimal patient management balanced with patient safety, it is now common practice for clinicians to define transfusion thresholds of haemoglobin below which level the patient's haemoglobin should not fall during the perioperative period.

6.1 Preoperative thresholds

It is known that preoperative anaemia increases the likelihood of allogeneic transfusion (Spence 1990) and hence an attempt should be made to correct the haemoglobin level prior to a major orthopaedic operation where inevitably, a substantial amount of blood loss is expected or anticipated. When patients refuse a blood transfusion, for example due to religious convictions, the preoperative haemoglobin level becomes all so important as a determinant of operative outcome, particularly in the elderly and those with major cardiovascular comorbidity (Carson 1996;Spence 1990). Usually, a preoperative lower limit of 100g/L is taken prior to major orthopaedic surgery, in spite of there being little evidence for this arbitrary level (Scottish Intercollegiate Guidelines Network 2001).

6.2 Intraoperative thresholds

Accurate measurement of intraoperative blood loss is difficult. Rapid intraoperative measurement of haemoglobin levels using near-patient testing may improve safety margins and avoid unnecessary transfusions (Loo 1997;Smetannikov 1996). However, intraoperative measurements must be interpreted in the context of a multifaceted clinical assessment of the patient in real time intraoperatively. This should include a clinical evaluation of blood volume status, on-going and anticipated postoperative bleeding (de Andrade Jr 1996, Welch 1992).

6.3 Postoperative thresholds

Experimental data from animal studies (Spahn 1992; Spahn 1994) indicate electrocardiographic changes occur between the haemoglobin levels of 50-70g/L and in one study in healthy humans during normovolaemic haemodilution, adequate oxygen delivery to tissues was sustained down to a haemoglobin level level of 50g/L (Weiskopf 1998).

A large randomized control trial performed over 800 patients admitted to intensive care (Hebert 1999) where patients were randomized to a haemoglobin level of 70-90g/L or 100-120g/L transfusion thresholds showed no significant differences in 30-60 day mortality or severe ventricular dysfunction between the two groups. However, caution is recommended in extrapolating these figures from the critical care setting to patients having routine elective orthopaedic surgery. Another large retrospective study of surgical patients found that, allowing for confounding factors, there was no definite difference in mortality using a lower threshold of either 80g/L or 100g/L as a transfusion threshold (Carson 1998a).

Guidelines and consensus statements have consistently expressed the transfusion threshold as a range between 70g/L and 100g/L, with clinical indicators further defining the need to transfuse in between these levels (Anon 1996; Simon 1998; Spence 1995).

A small randomized control trial involving elderly patients with fractured necks of femur found no difference in mortality in patients transfused when symptomatic or with a haemoglobin of less than 80g/L compared with the haemoglobin maintained at 10g/L(Carson 1998b). This study was limited by its inadequate analytical power to show significant differences in mortality and myocardial events(Scottish Intercollegiate Guidelines Network 2001). Most guidelines and consensus statements propose a higher transfusion threshold of 80-90g/L for those who are elderly, with cardiovascular comorbidity or peripheral vascular disease, rather than the lower level of 70-80g/L (Hebert 1999; Hill 2002).

7. Blood sparing strategies

Blood sparing strategies should be considered in every patient undergoing major blood loosing surgery in orthopaedics. In addition, special situations where these can be considered and may indeed be the only alternative include Jehovah's witnesses, those with multiple antibodies and those with serious anxieties about allogeneic blood transfusion.

Strategies include the following:

- Preoperative autologous blood donation (PABD)
- Acute normovolaemic haemodilution (ANH)
- Surgical technique
- Anaesthetic techniques
- Pharmacological therapies

- Increase RBC production – erythropoietin
- Reduce bleeding – antifibrinolytics, topical haemostatic agents, recombinant factor VII
- Cell salvage
  - Intraoperative
  - Postoperative

7.1 Surgical technique

Adherence to prescribed guidelines for maintaining haemostasis such as electrocautery and argon beam coagulation may reduce perioperative blood loss(Spence 1995).

7.2 Anaesthetic techniques

Specialist anaesthetic techniques such as hypotensive anaesthesia (Sharrock et al. 1993), regional anaesthesia (Carson 1998a; Dauphin 1997) and euthermia (Schmied 1996; Schmied 1998) may reduce surgical bleeding in arthroplasty surgery. For example, in one study, a difference in mean arterial pressure of 10mmHg significantly reduced mean intraoperative blood loss from 263mls to 179mls on average in patients undergoing primary THR (Sharrock 1993).

7.3 Preoperative autologous blood donation (PABD)

This entails the patient donating a unit of blood every week for 3-5 weeks preoperatively. This has been demonstrated to be safe and effective in the elective surgical setting and is widely practiced in a number of countries. 20 years ago, less than 5% participated in PABD before elective surgery in the United States and Canada. Today it ranges from 50-75% depending on the centre (Goodnough 1999b).

In orthopaedic surgery patients it has been used safely in elderly populations with diverse comorbidities (Kleinman 2000). However, it is recommended that patients should be stratified according to the risk of requiring a transfusion and should be considered if the likelihood of transfusion exceeds 50%.

The effectiveness of PABD in reducing patient exposure to allogeneic blood has been studied in a meta-analysis of six randomized control trials and nine well conducted cohort studies (Forgie 1998). Patients who pre-donated blood were less likely to receive allogeneic blood but autologous donors were statistically more likely to undergo any kind of transfusion, allogeneic or autologous. This is to say that PABD reduced allogeneic blood exposure albeit increasing the total number of transfusion episodes.

In another study, when the presenting haemoglobin was 110-145g/L in men and 130-145g/L in women, PABD was shown to reduce the expected number of patients exposed to allogeneic blood to less than 20% of the total (Hatzidakis 2000;Nuttall 2000).

Over collection of blood is a problem with PABD and often results in routine collection of more blood than is needed for the average patient(Keating 2002). When the presenting haemoglobin is between 110-145g/L (Voak 1994) PABD is unnecessary and limiting PABD to two units for joint replacement is usually sufficient to avoid most allogeneic blood exposure(Bierbaum 1999;Churchill 1998). The magnitude and rate of patient response to compensatory erythropoiesis to replace lost red cells has also generally been overestimated(Goodnough 1999b) and can result in preoperative anaemia. A study of 225 patients estimated that compensatory erythropoiesis resulted in preoperative red cell production of 351mls compared with a mean loss of 522mls from weekly donated autologous blood (Kasper 1997). The degree of compensatory erythropoiesis is also dependant on initial iron stores (Goodnough 1995) and it may be necessary to supplement patients with iron.

Although its use has increased substantially over the past decade, it can be associated with risks such as ischaemic events and complications severe enough to require hospitalization (Popovsky 1995). Although rare, bacterial contamination of stored autologous units can rarely cause sepsis and death (Dodd 1992; Roth 2000) and is also subject to all the potential clerical/procedural errors as allogeneic blood albeit avoiding the hazards of TTIs and immunological hazards associated with allogeneic transfusion. It also requires a weekly commitment from the patient and involves a weekly appointment at the donation site, in addition to staffing, other practical issues and related costs of the PABD programme. There have been reports of potential reduction in the risk of postoperative deep vein thrombosis in TKR (Anders 1996) and THR (Bae 2001) but the current evidence is too weak to confirm this.

7.4 Acute normovolaemic haemodilution (ANH)

This is the removal of whole blood and the restoration of blood volume with acellular fluid shortly before anticipated significant surgical blood loss. Mathematical models indicate that ANH is only suitable for a minority of patients (Kick 1997). These include healthy adults in whom a relatively low target haemoglobin, both intraoperatively and postoperatively is acceptable, with an anticipated blood loss of greater than 50% and a relatively high starting haemoglobin (Goodnough 1998). The maximum volume of blood that can be withdrawn depends on the preoperative haemoglobin, the lowest acceptable intraoperative haemoglobin level and the estimated blood loss(Brecher 1997;Cohen 1995;Kick 1997).

The real evidence for the benefit of ANH is equivocal. A meta-analysis of ANH trials (Bryson 1998) found that allogeneic transfusion was reduced when more than 1000mls was withdrawn. There was a significant reduction in the average number of allogeneic units transfused, though not in the number of patients exposed to allogeneic blood. However, when trials without a transfusion protocol were excluded from the analysis, no significant benefit was identified in terms of reducing allogeneic transfusion.

7.4.1 ANH versus PABD

A randomized study comparing the above two blood sparing strategies found no differences in either calculated red cell savings or exposure to allogeneic transfusion, prompting the authors to suggest that ANH should be preferred to PABD on the basis of lower cost and less potential for transfusion errors (Monk 1998). However, issues of patient selection, theatre time, staff training and technical expertise and organisational issues that surround an effective ANH programme need to be factored into the equation.

ANH does have its advantages. In contrast to PABD, it does not require testing to screen for TTIs and is therefore less costly. There is virtually no risk of bacterial contamination or administrative error that could lead to blood group incompatibility and does not require additional time investment from patients to donate blood (Monk 1995).

7.5 Erythropoietin (EPO)

The effect of EPO in minimizing exposure to allogeneic blood compared to placebo has been studied in patients undergoing orthopaedic (Faris 1998;Laupacis 1998), cardiac (Laupacis 1998) and colonic cancer surgery (Kettelhack 1998; Qvist 1999). In excess of 1000 patients were randomized and an overall significant reduction in allogeneic transfusion occurred in orthopaedic patients. Post-operative transfusion fell from between 40-60% in controls to 10-20% in EPO treated patients.

De Andrade *et al* (deAndrade, Jr. 1996) stratified 316 patients into those presenting with haemoglobins above and below 130g/L. In the EPO group a significant reduction (45-16%) in allogeneic transfusion rate was observed in those with a presenting haemoglobin of less than 130g/L as opposed to a non-significant reduction in patients with a haemoglobin of more than 130g/L. This finding has been confirmed by subgroup analysis in other studies (Anon 1993;Faris 1996).

In those with objections to allogeneic transfusion, for example Jehovah's witnesses, EPO may have a significant role in preparing these patients for surgery involving substantial blood loss (Gaudiani 1991).

Little evidence of side effects of EPO have been found(Faught 1998) and no trial or meta-analysis has been of sufficient power to detect important adverse effects at low incidence. In some studies concerns about increased risk of thrombosis were present in patients with a baseline haemoglobin of 130g/L but were similar to controls when the haemoglobin was 100-130g/L (de Andrade, Jr. 1996). Due to perceived thrombotic risk and the risk of uncontrolled hypertension, trials involving EPO have had very strict entry criteria. Despite this, studies have suggested no major increased thrombotic or hypertensive risk (Faught 1998). With a 50% rise in haematocrit during EPO treatment, some units recommend venesection.

7.5.1 PABD and erythropoietin

When PABD was used with EPO, a meta-analysis of 11 orthopaedic and cardiac randomized studies enrolling 825 patients found a statistically significant decrease in the proportion of patients transfused with allogeneic blood (Laupacis 1997). EPO-supported PABD individuals are also able to donate significantly more units than standard PABD (Mercuriali 1998;Price 1996;Rau 1998) and also had a higher day-of-surgery haemoglobin level (Cazenave 1997;de Andrade 1997). However, adequate iron status must be maintained through supplementation in patients receiving EPO (Adamson 1994).

7.6 Aprotinin

Aprotinin has been investigated for hip and knee replacements (D'Ambrosio 1999;Hayes 1996;Murkin 1995) and revisions (Murkin 1995), knee replacements (Thorpe 1994), spinal surgery (Lentschener 1999) and tumour surgery (Capdevila 1998). A reduction in blood loss of between 25-60% was demonstrated. However, a Canadian study reported an increased risk of death in cardiac surgery patients treated with aprotinin compared with tranexamic acid and aminocaproic acid and this led to the market suspension of this drug(Fergusson 2008).

7.7 Antifibrinolytic drugs (Tranexamic acid and aminocaproic acid)

These inhibit fibrinolysis by binding to the lysine-binding sites of plasminogen to fibrin. They have been used in TKR patients who have had their operations under tourniquet control. In this situation, local fibrinolytic activity may be enhanced and may cause post-operative bleeding on release of the tourniquet (Murphy 1993; Petaja 1987). A reduction in blood loss of between 43-54% as well as a significant reduction in the total number of units transfused and the number of patients exposed to allogeneic blood has been demonstrated in a series of randomized control studies where the antifibrinolytic drug was given prior to tourniquet release (Benoni 1995; Benoni 1996; Hiippala 1995; Hiippala 1997; Jansen 1999; Zohar 1999). Concerns about the potential risks of thrombosis (Hiippala 1997; Howes 1996) have not been borne out by these studies, but studies have been small. In clinical practice, their use is usually reserved for those patients where other blood sparing techniques cannot be used and where major blood loss is anticipated.

7.8 Desmopressin (DDAVP)

This has been used to prevent bleeding in other types of surgery but has had no effect on reducing blood loss or allogeneic transfusion requirements in THR or TKR (Karnezis 1994; Schott 1995).

7.9 Topical haemostatic agents

Topically active agents that have been used include thrombin, collagen and fibrin glue. A gelatin matrix containing thrombin was shown to stop bleeding in cardiac surgery patients within 10 minutes in 94% of patients(Oz 2000). Fibrin glue made with highly concentrated human fibrinogen and clotting factors does not depend on platelet or clotting factor levels to be effective. The use of fibrin tissue adhesive has been shown to significantly reduce mean postoperative blood loss from 878-360mls in TKR (Levy 1999).

7.10 Recombinant factor VIIa

Recombinant factor VII is produced from a line of baby hamster kidney cells with an amino acid sequence identical to that of endogenous factor VII (Thim 1988) and becomes active after forming a complex with tissue factor. Following this factors IX and X are activated and a thrombin burst is induced, leading to a quicker formation of a fibrin clot at the site of vascular injury (Rizoli 2006), and also binds to the surface of thrombin-activated platelets, activating factor X directly independent of tissue factor (Monroe 1997).

In Europe, recombinant factor VII (rVIIa) has been licensed for the treatment of and for the prevention of further bleeding episodes in patients with congenital haemophilia with inhibitors to coagulation factors VIII or IX, patients with congenital haemophilia who are expected to have a high anamnestic response to factor VIII or IX administration, patients with acquired haemophilia, patients with congenital factor VII deficiency and some patients with Glanzman's thromboaesthenia with past/present resistance to platelet transfusions (Rodriguez-Merchan 2004). Although life expectancy in haemophiliac patients is now getting closer to that of the normal population (Darby 2007), the significant burden of joint disease does have an impact on their quality of life (Scalone 2006), with problems such as joint instability, muscle atrophy and flexion contractures (Gringeri 2003). One study showed that 24% of males with haemophilia aged 14-35years were reliant on a wheelchair (Morfini 2007).

Data from an international series of 108 patients of elective orthopaedic surgery performed in seven countries revealed that 19% were involved in hip and knee arthroplasty. 80% had good results with a further 5% having fair results reported (Rodriguez-Merchan 2004). Another study of patients given an initial bolus dose followed by a continuous infusion revealed an overall good final outcome in all cases (Ludlam 2003). The optimal dose and whether bolus or infusions are better still remains to be established (Obergfell 2008). The outcome of 10 major orthopaedic operations in five comprehensive care centres in the United Kingdom and Ireland in haemophilia patients has shown good results with bolus doses (Giangrande 2009). Intraoperative haemostasis was found to be satisfactory in all 10 operations. Two cases had postoperative bleeding episodes one of which was managed with an increased bolus dose of rVIIa and the other with an addition of tranexamic acid and the final results were reported as excellent or extremely satisfactory in all cases (Giangrande 2009).

Elective major orthopaedic surgery in patients with haemophilia should be undertaken in comprehensive care centres that have the multidisciplinary expertise and facilities according to the consensus protocols (Giangrande 2009). Management in these centres have demonstrated a survival benefit compared to non-specialist centres (Soucie 2000). Topical application of fibrin sealant during the intraoperative period to minimize capillary ooze and the use of vasoconstrictors and antifibrinolytics can be used to enhance the effect of rVIIa and improve haemostasis (Schulman 1998). Activated prothrombin complex concentrate (aPCC) has also been used to cover surgical procedures in haemophilia patients with inhibitors (Dimichele 2006;Goudemand 2004;Hvid 2002;Negrier 1997;Tjonnfjord 2004) and data suggests similar efficacy to rVIIa, albeit having the risk of an anamnestic rise in antibody titre (Schulman 1998), a risk not present with rVIIa. Current guidelines give equal merit to rVIIa and aPCC in managing bleeding in haemophilia (Hay 2006). Costs to cover this type of surgery can be prohibitive although they may be recovered in the long term through abolition of bleeding episodes. One pharmacokinetic study calculating the break-even time (time after surgery when cost is completely offset by savings resulting from avoiding bleeding episodes) ranging from 5-9 years (Lyseng-Williamson 2007).

Recombinant factor VII has also been used to treat coagulopathic trauma patients. rVIIa functions by triggering an enhanced coagulation response dependant on multiple agents in the clotting cascade. Thus, to increase its efficacy, the mechanisms that lead to coagulopathy in trauma patients need to be corrected before its administration, including administering FFP and maintaining fibrinogen levels at >0.1mg/dL using cryoprecipitate and platelet transfusions to maintain platelet count > 50,000/mm^3, correcting hypothermia and acidosis (Gunter, Jr 2008; Holcomb 2008; Meng 2003; Sperry 2008). In two parallel randomized placebo- controlled blinded studies of 301 patients experiencing blunt or penetrating trauma, patients with blunt trauma who were managed with rVIIa required fewer PRBC transfusions than patients randomized to placebo. The need for massive transfusion was also significantly reduced in these patients (Boffard 2005). Two other trials have also demonstrated a decreased mortality in trauma patients who received rVIIa. In the combat setting, 30 day mortality in patients requiring massive transfusion was reduced from 51% to 31% (Spinella 2008). A mortality benefit has also been demonstrated in the civilian major trauma setting in patients requiring massive transfusion secondary to trauma (Rizoli 2006). In the military setting, some of the proposed criteria for the use of factor rVIIa are haemorrhage induced hypotension, base deficit of >6mEq/L, difficult to control bleeding associated with hypothermia, clinically coagulopathic bleeding or INR > 1.5, the need for damage control measures, the need for fresh whole blood, anticipated or actual PRBC transfusion of > 4 units or significant surgical haemorrhage (Nessen 2008) and some of these may well be indications for rVIIa in the civilian setting as well (Holcomb 2007).

Complications of rVIIa in the trauma setting have also been studied with 9.4% experiencing thrombotic complications (Boffard 2005). This contraindicates it in patients with symptomatic vaso-occlusive disease (angina, claudication, deep venous thrombosis, pulmonary embolism, cerebral or myocardial infarction) within 30 days prior to traumatic injury.

8. Cell salvage

Cell salvage has been shown to have some benefit in reducing the exposure to allogeneic blood. Seven orthopaedic trials with a total of 427 patients between them reported on data for volume of allogeneic blood transfused. For the patients that were randomized to cell salvage, there was an average saving of 0.82 units of red blood cells per patient (Carless 2010).

The Cochrane Collaboration review which included 67 cell salvage trials in both cardiac and orthopaedic surgery with a total of 6025 patients, indicated that overall, the use of cell salvage reduced the rate of allogeneic blood transfusion by a relative 38%, although heterogeneity between studies was significant (Carless 2010). Of the trials included in the Cochrane review, 32 involved orthopaedic surgery, demonstrating a larger reduction in orthopaedic trials than any other trials with regards to the number of patients exposed to red blood cell transfusion (Carless 2010). When cell salvage was used in orthopaedic surgery, the risk of exposure to allogeneic transfusion was reduced by 54% compared to only 22% in cardiac surgery.

8.1 Intra-operative cell salvage

This is intra-operative collection of cells that are washed prior to retransfusion. Larger volumes can be transfused in comparison to post-operative blood salvage (Goodnough 1999b;Paravicini 1983) with cell washing devices being able to provide the equivalent of 10 units of blood per hour. This can be used in patients with substantial blood loss in major orthopaedic surgery, providing less costly, immediately available blood (Goodnough 1999b).

However, there is a considerable capital cost of the basic equipment and it is estimated that at least two units need to be recovered per patient for it to be cost effective to run(Goodnough 1999b). The recommendation is to use it in patients where intra-operative blood loss of 1000-1500mls is anticipated (Gargaro 1991;Schmied 1998;Slagis 1991;Wilson 1989). It can be used in pelvic surgery and revision arthroplasty where infection has been ruled out and should not be used in bacterial contamination or tumour surgery (Napier 1997).

8.2 Post-operative cell salvage

This involves collecting blood from surgical drains followed by retransfusion. The blood is filtered to eliminate larger aggregates but not bacteria (Gannon 1991; Kristensen 1992; Martin 1992). Complications of unwashed blood have included hypertension, hypothermia, upper airway oedema and coagulopathy (Southern 1995). Because the recovered blood is diluted, defibrinated and partially haemolysed and contains cytokines, there is generally a threshold of blood that can be transfused by this method. This is usually not more than 1500mls. The risk of bacterial contamination/infective colonization increases with time and it is generally recommended that recovered blood should not be transfused later than six hours after collection. The safety and efficacy of post-operative cell salvage also remains somewhat controversial (Faris 1991;Ritter 1994) and due to high cost and questionable benefit, some have recommended its use to be limited to cases in which a large post-operative blood loss is anticipated.

However, studies have shown that it can reduce exposure to allogeneic blood if no autologous pre-donated blood is available (Ayers 1995;Knight 1998;Newman 1997) and may further reduce allogeneic exposure when autologous blood is available (Xenakis 1997). Forty six trials in the Cochrane review reported the use of post-operative cell salvage and included 4361 patients. 2209 were randomized to post-operative cell salvage. The risk of allogeneic blood exposure was reduced on average by 37% in those patients treated with post-operative cell salvage compared to controls. However, significant heterogeneity was present amongst the studies included.

8.3 Washed versus unwashed blood

27 trials in the Cochrane review studied washed cell salvage while 40 investigated unwashed cell salvage. Overall when cell salvage was conducted with devices that washed the blood, the relative risk of exposure to red cell transfusion was only marginally lower than that with unwashed blood salvage and for orthopaedic trials, this difference was insignificant (Carless 2010). Again these results must be interpreted with caution due to significant heterogeneity between studies.

8.4 Volume of blood transfused

32 trials reported on the volume of allogeneic blood transfused and included 2321 orthopaedic and cardiac patients. 1172 patients were randomized to cell salvage. Although overall, the use of cell salvage reduced the volume of red cells transfused by 0.68 units, greater reductions than this were observed in trials involving orthopaedic surgery compared to cardiac surgery (Carless 2010).

8.5 Other complications

It has been thought that post-operative cell salvage may increase the rate of infection and wound complications in orthopaedic surgery. This has not been borne out in the 16 trials involving 1462 patients of whom 1011 were randomized to cell salvage (Carless 2010). Likewise, the relative risk of developing any thrombus including deep vein thrombosis, stroke and non-fatal myocardial infarction in patients treated with cell salvage was not significantly different compared to controls (Carless 2010).

Principle findings from the systematic review appear to suggest that the efficacy of cell salvage in reducing the need for allogeneic transfusion appear to be greatest in the setting of orthopaedic surgery where the risk of exposure to allogeneic transfusion was reduced by 54% compared to 23% in cardiac surgery. However, these results should be interpreted with caution as most of the trials were un-blinded leading to a potential source of bias in favour of cell salvage, in addition to heterogeneity between the studies considered (Carless 2010).

8.6 Cost considerations

A recent cost effectiveness analysis indicated that cell salvage was cost effective compared to all other transfusion strategies except ANH (Davies 2006). The study indicated that the net benefit of cell salvage was between £112 and £359 per person, compared with the allogeneic blood transfusion strategy, PABD, PABD and EPO, Fibrin sealants, antifibrinolytics and EPO. It also estimated a blood saving of between 6,500 and 320,000 units of allogeneic blood per year (Davies 2006). The economic viability of cell salvage has been suggested by other studies as well (Mirza 2007). However, cost analysis should also be interpreted with caution as in many instances, neither the cost of the technology/manpower needed to execute this activity have been taken into account, nor have the capital cost of the cell saver devices.

9. Conclusions

Orthopaedic surgery often involves a substantial volume of blood loss. Blood is a scarce resource and developing a rational approach to transfusion in orthopaedic surgery involves the following:

- Individual assessment of patient risk for transfusion
- Estimating anticipated blood loss
- Pre-operative haemoglobin assessment
- Determining patient-specific transfusion triggers according to age, risk factors and comorbidities
- Optimizing operative and anaesthetic techniques
- Developing transfusion practice standards and institutional guidelines
- Determining the most appropriate blood conservation technique or option according to individual patient characteristics, operation and circumstances and local protocols and resources

The true value of avoiding allogeneic blood transfusion remains debateable. However, concerns over the safety of allogeneic transfusion have led to the development of new techniques of blood conservation. Preoperative assessment of estimated blood loss and transfusion risk and consideration of alternatives to allogeneic blood are now key to optimizing blood management. The growing evidence on the efficacy of transfusion triggers means that a more conservative approach to transfusion is recommended in patients with cardiovascular risk factors (Carson 1998b;Carson 2002). However, surgeons must be discriminating in the method of blood sparing strategy used by carefully considering individual patient condition, specific surgical practices and potential for adverse events. The choice of intervention that best minimizes patient exposure to allogeneic blood transfusion is not clear cut with the current evidence. The evidence and safety of ANH and PABD is generally regarded as being of indifferent quality due to lack of blinding outcomes and heterogeneity between studies. However, they have been shown to have blood sparing effects. Cell salvage appears to be justified in orthopaedic surgery although again there is significant heterogeneity between existing studies. Surgeon preference, availability and cost primarily determine what alternative to allogeneic blood transfusion is used. Large multicentre randomized studies are needed to answer questions about the safety and efficacy of the various alternatives to allogeneic blood transfusion.

10. References

1993. Effectiveness of perioperative recombinant human erythropoietin in elective hip replacement. Canadian Orthopedic Perioperative Erythropoietin Study Group. *Lancet*, 341, (8855) 1227-1232 available from: PM:8098389

Practice guidelines for blood component therapy: A report by the American Society of Anesthesiologists tsk force on blood component therapy. Anesthesiology 84, 732-747. 1996. Ref Type: Generic

Adamson, J.W. 1994. The relationship of erythropoietin and iron metabolism to red blood cell production in humans. *Semin.Oncol.*, 21, (2 Suppl 3) 9-15 available from: PM:8202725

Allain, J.P. 2000. Emerging viral infections relevant to transfusion medicine. *Blood Rev.*, 14, (4) 173-181 available from: PM:11124105

Anders, M.J., Lifeso, R.M., Landis, M., Mikulsky, J., Meinking, C., & McCracken, K.S. 1996. Effect of preoperative donation of autologous blood on deep-vein thrombosis following total joint arthroplasty of the hip or knee. *J.Bone Joint Surg.Am.*, 78, (4) 574-580 available from: PM:8609136

Ania, B.J., Suman, V.J., Fairbanks, V.F., Rademacher, D.M., & Melton, L.J., III 1997. Incidence of anemia in older people: an epidemiologic study in a well defined population. *J.Am.Geriatr.Soc.*, 45, (7) 825-831 available from: PM:9215333

AuBuchon, J.P. & Littenberg, B. 1996. A cost-effectiveness analysis of the use of a mechanical barrier system to reduce the risk of mistransfusion. *Transfusion*, 36, (3) 222-226 available from: PM:8604506

Ayers, D.C., Murray, D.G., & Duerr, D.M. 1995. Blood salvage after total hip arthroplasty. *J.Bone Joint Surg.Am.*, 77, (9) 1347-1351 available from: PM:7673284

Bae, H., Westrich, G.H., Sculco, T.P., Salvati, E.A., & Reich, L.M. 2001. The effect of preoperative donation of autologous blood on deep-vein thrombosis after total hip arthroplasty. *J.Bone Joint Surg.Br.*, 83, (5) 676-679 available from: PM:11476304

Benoni, G., Carlsson, A., Petersson, C., & Fredin, H. 1995. Does tranexamic acid reduce blood loss in knee arthroplasty? *Am.J.Knee.Surg.*, 8, (3) 88-92 available from: PM:7552611

Benoni, G. & Fredin, H. 1996. Fibrinolytic inhibition with tranexamic acid reduces blood loss and blood transfusion after knee arthroplasty: a prospective, randomised, double-blind study of 86 patients. *J.Bone Joint Surg.Br.*, 78, (3) 434-440 available from: PM:8636182

Bierbaum, B.E., Callaghan, J.J., Galante, J.O., Rubash, H.E., Tooms, R.E., & Welch, R.B. 1999. An analysis of blood management in patients having a total hip or knee arthroplasty. *J.Bone Joint Surg.Am.*, 81, (1) 2-10 available from: PM:9973048

Blajchman, M.A. 1994. An overview of the mechanism of action of antithrombin and its inherited deficiency states. *Blood Coagul.Fibrinolysis*, 5 Suppl 1, S5-11 available from: PM:8186357

Boffard, K.D., Riou, B., Warren, B., Choong, P.I., Rizoli, S., Rossaint, R., Axelsen, M., & Kluger, Y. 2005. Recombinant factor VIIa as adjunctive therapy for bleeding control in severely injured trauma patients: two parallel randomized, placebo-controlled, double-blind clinical trials. *J.Trauma*, 59, (1) 8-15 available from: PM:16096533

Bordin, J.O., Heddle, N.M., & Blajchman, M.A. 1994. Biologic effects of leukocytes present in transfused cellular blood products. *Blood*, 84, (6) 1703-1721 available from: PM:8080981

Borghi, B., Bassi, A., de, S.N., Laguardia, A.M., & Formaro, G. 1993. Autotransfusion: 15 years experience at Rizzoli Orthopaedic Institute. *Int.J.Artif.Organs*, 16 Suppl 5, 241-246 available from: PM:8013998

Brecher, M.E., Monk, T., & Goodnough, L.T. 1997. A standardized method for calculating blood loss. *Transfusion*, 37, (10) 1070-1074 available from: PM:9354828

Bryson, G.L., Laupacis, A., & Wells, G.A. 1998. Does acute normovolemic hemodilution reduce perioperative allogeneic transfusion? A meta-analysis. The International Study of Perioperative Transfusion. *Anesth.Analg.*, 86, (1) 9-15 available from: PM:9428843

Callaghan, J.J. & Spitzer, A.I. 2000. Blood management and patient specific transfusion options in total joint replacement surgery. *Iowa Orthop.J.*, 20, 36-45 available from: PM:10934623

Capdevila, X., Calvet, Y., Biboulet, P., Biron, C., Rubenovitch, J., & d'Athis, F. 1998. Aprotinin decreases blood loss and homologous transfusions in patients undergoing major orthopedic surgery. *Anesthesiology*, 88, (1) 50-57 available from: PM:9447855

Carless, P.A., Henry, D.A., Moxey, A.J., O'Connell, D., Brown, T., & Fergusson, D.A. 2010. Cell salvage for minimising perioperative allogeneic blood transfusion. *Cochrane.Database.Syst.Rev.* (4) CD001888 available from: PM:20393932

Carson, J.L., Duff, A., Berlin, J.A., Lawrence, V.A., Poses, R.M., Huber, E.C., O'Hara, D.A., Noveck, H., & Strom, B.L. 1998a. Perioperative blood transfusion and postoperative mortality. *JAMA*, 279, (3) 199-205 available from: PM:9438739

Carson, J.L., Duff, A., Poses, R.M., Berlin, J.A., Spence, R.K., Trout, R., Noveck, H., & Strom, B.L. 1996. Effect of anaemia and cardiovascular disease on surgical mortality and morbidity. *Lancet*, 348, (9034) 1055-1060 available from: PM:8874456

Carson, J.L., Hill, S., Carless, P., Hebert, P., & Henry, D. 2002. Transfusion triggers: a systematic review of the literature. *Transfus.Med.Rev.*, 16, (3) 187-199 available from: PM:12075558

Carson, J.L., Poses, R.M., Spence, R.K., & Bonavita, G. 1988. Severity of anaemia and operative mortality and morbidity. *Lancet*, 1, (8588) 727-729 available from: PM:2895260

Carson, J.L., Terrin, M.L., Barton, F.B., Aaron, R., Greenburg, A.G., Heck, D.A., Magaziner, J., Merlino, F.E., Bunce, G., McClelland, B., Duff, A., & Noveck, H. 1998b. A pilot randomized trial comparing symptomatic vs. hemoglobin-level-driven red blood cell transfusions following hip fracture. *Transfusion*, 38, (6) 522-529 available from: PM:9661685

Cazenave, J.P., Irrmann, C., Waller, C., Sondag, D., Baudoux, E., Genetet, B., Laxenaire, M.C., Dupont, E., Sundal, E., Obrist, R., & Stocker, H. 1997. Epoetin alfa facilitates presurgical autologous blood donation in non-anaemic patients scheduled for orthopaedic or cardiovascular surgery. *Eur.J.Anaesthesiol.*, 14, (4) 432-442 available from: PM:9253573

Chiavetta, J.A., Herst, R., Freedman, J., Axcell, T.J., Wall, A.J., & van Rooy, S.C. 1996. A survey of red cell use in 45 hospitals in central Ontario, Canada. *Transfusion*, 36, (8) 699-706 available from: PM:8780664

Churchill, W.H., McGurk, S., Chapman, R.H., Wallace, E.L., Bertholf, M.F., Goodnough, L.T., Kao, K.J., Olson, J.D., Woodson, R.D., & Surgenor, D.M. 1998. The Collaborative Hospital Transfusion Study: variations in use of autologous blood account for hospital differences in red cell use during primary hip and knee surgery. *Transfusion*, 38, (6) 530-539 available from: PM:9661686

Cohen, J.A. & Brecher, M.E. 1995. Preoperative autologous blood donation: benefit or detriment? A mathematical analysis. *Transfusion*, 35, (8) 640-644 available from: PM:7631403

Cook, S.S. & Epps, J. 1991. Transfusion practice in central Virginia. *Transfusion*, 31, (4) 355-360 available from: PM:1902337

D'Ambrosio, A., Borghi, B., Damato, A., D'Amato, G., Antonacci, D., & Valeri, F. 1999. Reducing perioperative blood loss in patients undergoing total hip arthroplasty. *Int.J.Artif.Organs*, 22, (1) 47-51 available from: PM:10098585

Darby, S.C., Kan, S.W., Spooner, R.J., Giangrande, P.L., Hill, F.G., Hay, C.R., Lee, C.A., Ludlam, C.A., & Williams, M. 2007. Mortality rates, life expectancy, and causes of death in people with hemophilia A or B in the United Kingdom who were not infected with HIV. *Blood*, 110, (3) 815-825 available from: PM:17446349

Dauphin, A., Raymer, K.E., Stanton, E.B., & Fuller, H.D. 1997. Comparison of general anesthesia with and without lumbar epidural for total hip arthroplasty: effects of epidural block on hip arthroplasty. *J.Clin.Anesth.*, 9, (3) 200-203 available from: PM:9172026

Davies, L., Brown, T.J., Haynes, S., Payne, K., Elliott, R.A., & McCollum, C. 2006. Cost-effectiveness of cell salvage and alternative methods of minimising perioperative allogeneic blood transfusion: a systematic review and economic model. *Health Technol.Assess.*, 10, (44) iii-x, 1 available from: PM:17049141

de, A., Jr., Jove, M., Landon, G., Frei, D., Guilfoyle, M., & Young, D.C. 1996. Baseline hemoglobin as a predictor of risk of transfusion and response to Epoetin alfa in orthopedic surgery patients. *Am.J.Orthop.(Belle.Mead NJ)*, 25, (8) 533-542 available from: PM:8871751

de, P.C., Mermillod, B., Hoffmeyer, P., & Beris, P. 1997. Recombinant human erythropoietin as adjuvant treatment for autologous blood donation in elective surgery with large blood needs (> or = 5 units): a randomized study. *Transfusion*, 37, (7) 708-714 available from: PM:9225934

Dimichele, D. & Negrier, C. 2006. A retrospective postlicensure survey of FEIBA efficacy and safety. *Haemophilia.*, 12, (4) 352-362 available from: PM:16834734

Dodd, R.Y. 1992. The risk of transfusion-transmitted infection. *N.Engl.J.Med.*, 327, (6) 419-421 available from: PM:1625717

Faris, P.M. & Ritter, M.A. 1998. Epoetin alfa. A bloodless approach for the treatment of perioperative anemia. *Clin.Orthop.Relat Res.* (357) 60-67 available from: PM:9917701

Faris, P.M., Ritter, M.A., & Abels, R.I. 1996. The effects of recombinant human erythropoietin on perioperative transfusion requirements in patients having a major orthopaedic operation. The American Erythropoietin Study Group. *J.Bone Joint Surg.Am.*, 78, (1) 62-72 available from: PM:8550681

Faris, P.M., Ritter, M.A., Keating, E.M., & Valeri, C.R. 1991. Unwashed filtered shed blood collected after knee and hip arthroplasties. A source of autologous red blood cells. *J.Bone Joint Surg.Am.*, 73, (8) 1169-1178 available from: PM:1890117

Faris, P.M., Spence, R.K., Larholt, K.M., Sampson, A.R., & Frei, D. 1999. The predictive power of baseline hemoglobin for transfusion risk in surgery patients. *Orthopedics*, 22, (1 Suppl) s135-s140 available from: PM:9927114

Faught, C., Wells, P., Fergusson, D., & Laupacis, A. 1998. Adverse effects of methods for minimizing perioperative allogeneic transfusion: a critical review of the literature. *Transfus.Med.Rev.*, 12, (3) 206-225 available from: PM:9673005

Fergusson, D.A., Hebert, P.C., Mazer, C.D., Fremes, S., MacAdams, C., Murkin, J.M., Teoh, K., Duke, P.C., Arellano, R., Blajchman, M.A., Bussieres, J.S., Cote, D., Karski, J., Martineau, R., Robblee, J.A., Rodger, M., Wells, G., Clinch, J., & Pretorius, R. 2008. A comparison of aprotinin and lysine analogues in high-risk cardiac surgery. *N.Engl.J.Med.*, 358, (22) 2319-2331 available from: PM:18480196

Forgie, M.A., Wells, P.S., Laupacis, A., & Fergusson, D. 1998. Preoperative autologous donation decreases allogeneic transfusion but increases exposure to all red blood cell transfusion: results of a meta-analysis. International Study of Perioperative Transfusion (ISPOT) Investigators. *Arch.Intern.Med.*, 158, (6) 610-616 available from: PM:9521225

Gafter, U., Kalechman, Y., & Sredni, B. 1992. Induction of a subpopulation of suppressor cells by a single blood transfusion. *Kidney Int.*, 41, (1) 143-148 available from: PM:1534385

Gannon, D.M., Lombardi, A.V., Jr., Mallory, T.H., Vaughn, B.K., Finney, C.R., & Niemcryk, S. 1991. An evaluation of the efficacy of postoperative blood salvage after total joint arthroplasty. A prospective randomized trial. *J.Arthroplasty*, 6, (2) 109-114 available from: PM:1875200

Gargaro, J.M. & Walls, C.E. 1991. Efficacy of intraoperative autotransfusion in primary total hip arthroplasty. *J.Arthroplasty*, 6, (2) 157-161 available from: PM:1875207

Gaudiani, V.A. & Mason, H.D. 1991. Preoperative erythropoietin in Jehovah's Witnesses who require cardiac procedures. *Ann.Thorac.Surg.*, 51, (5) 823-824 available from: PM:2025093

Giangrande, P.L., Wilde, J.T., Madan, B., Ludlam, C.A., Tuddenham, E.G., Goddard, N.J., Dolan, G., & Ingerslev, J. 2009. Consensus protocol for the use of recombinant activated factor VII [eptacog alfa (activated); NovoSeven] in elective orthopaedic surgery in haemophilic patients with inhibitors. *Haemophilia.*, 15, (2) 501-508 available from: PM:19187194

Glynn, S.A., Kleinman, S.H., Schreiber, G.B., Busch, M.P., Wright, D.J., Smith, J.W., Nass, C.C., & Williams, A.E. 2000. Trends in incidence and prevalence of major transfusion-transmissible viral infections in US blood donors, 1991 to 1996. Retrovirus Epidemiology Donor Study (REDS). *JAMA*, 284, (2) 229-235 available from: PM:10889598

Goodnough, L.T. 2000. The case against universal WBC reduction (and for the practice of evidence-based medicine). *Transfusion*, 40, (12) 1522-1527 available from: PM:11134574

Goodnough, L.T., Brecher, M.E., Kanter, M.H., & AuBuchon, J.P. 1999a. Transfusion medicine. First of two parts--blood transfusion. *N.Engl.J.Med.*, 340, (6) 438-447 available from: PM:9971869

Goodnough, L.T., Brecher, M.E., Kanter, M.H., & AuBuchon, J.P. 1999b. Transfusion medicine. Second of two parts--blood conservation. *N.Engl.J.Med.*, 340, (7) 525-533 available from: PM:10021474

Goodnough, L.T., Monk, T.G., & Brecher, M.E. 1998. Acute normovolemic hemodilution should replace the preoperative donation of autologous blood as a method of autologous-blood procurement. *Transfusion*, 38, (5) 473-476 available from: PM:9633561

Goodnough, L.T., Price, T.H., & Parvin, C.A. 1995. The endogenous erythropoietin response and the erythropoietic response to blood loss anemia: the effects of age and gender. *J.Lab Clin.Med.*, 126, (1) 57-64 available from: PM:7602235

Goudemand, J., Tagariello, G., & Lopaciuk, F. 2004. Cases of surgery in high-responder haemophilia patients. *Haemophilia.*, 10 Suppl 2, 46-49 available from: PM:15385046

Gringeri, A., Mantovani, L.G., Scalone, L., & Mannucci, P.M. 2003. Cost of care and quality of life for patients with hemophilia complicated by inhibitors: the COCIS Study Group. *Blood*, 102, (7) 2358-2363 available from: PM:12816859

Gunter, O.L., Jr., Au, B.K., Isbell, J.M., Mowery, N.T., Young, P.P., & Cotton, B.A. 2008. Optimizing outcomes in damage control resuscitation: identifying blood product ratios associated with improved survival. *J.Trauma*, 65, (3) 527-534 available from: PM:18784564

Hatzidakis, A. M., Mendlick, R. M., & McKillip, T. The effect of preoperative autologous donation and other factors on the frequency of transfusion after total joint arthroplasty. 65th Annual Meeting of the AAOS, New Orleans . 1998. Ref Type: Generic

Hatzidakis, A.M., Mendlick, R.M., McKillip, T., Reddy, R.L., & Garvin, K.L. 2000. Preoperative autologous donation for total joint arthroplasty. An analysis of risk factors for allogenic transfusion. *J.Bone Joint Surg.Am.*, 82, (1) 89-100 available from: PM:10653088

Hay, C.R., Brown, S., Collins, P.W., Keeling, D.M., & Liesner, R. 2006. The diagnosis and management of factor VIII and IX inhibitors: a guideline from the United Kingdom Haemophilia Centre Doctors Organisation. *Br.J.Haematol.*, 133, (6) 591-605 available from: PM:16704433

Hayes, A., Murphy, D.B., & McCarroll, M. 1996. The efficacy of single-dose aprotinin 2 million KIU in reducing blood loss and its impact on the incidence of deep venous thrombosis in patients undergoing total hip replacement surgery. *J.Clin.Anesth.*, 8, (5) 357-360 available from: PM:8832445

Hays, M.B. & Mayfield, J.F. 1988. Total blood loss in major joint arthroplasty. A comparison of cemented and noncemented hip and knee operations. *J.Arthroplasty*, 3 Suppl, S47-S49 available from: PM:3199139

Hebert, P.C., Wells, G., Blajchman, M.A., Marshall, J., Martin, C., Pagliarello, G., Tweeddale, M., Schweitzer, I., & Yetisir, E. 1999. A multicenter, randomized, controlled clinical trial of transfusion requirements in critical care. Transfusion Requirements in Critical Care Investigators, Canadian Critical Care Trials Group. *N.Engl.J.Med.*, 340, (6) 409-417 available from: PM:9971864

Hiippala, S., Strid, L., Wennerstrand, M., Arvela, V., Mantyla, S., Ylinen, J., & Niemela, H. 1995. Tranexamic acid (Cyklokapron) reduces perioperative blood loss associated with total knee arthroplasty. *Br.J.Anaesth.*, 74, (5) 534-537 available from: PM:7772427

Hiippala, S.T., Strid, L.J., Wennerstrand, M.I., Arvela, J.V., Niemela, H.M., Mantyla, S.K., Kuisma, R.P., & Ylinen, J.E. 1997. Tranexamic acid radically decreases blood loss and transfusions associated with total knee arthroplasty. *Anesth.Analg.*, 84, (4) 839-844 available from: PM:9085968

Hill, S.R., Carless, P.A., Henry, D.A., Carson, J.L., Hebert, P.C., McClelland, D.B., & Henderson, K.M. 2002. Transfusion thresholds and other strategies for guiding allogeneic red blood cell transfusion. *Cochrane.Database.Syst.Rev.* (2) CD002042 available from: PM:12076437

Holcomb, J.B., Jenkins, D., Rhee, P., Johannigman, J., Mahoney, P., Mehta, S., Cox, E.D., Gehrke, M.J., Beilman, G.J., Schreiber, M., Flaherty, S.F., Grathwohl, K.W., Spinella, P.C., Perkins, J.G., Beekley, A.C., McMullin, N.R., Park, M.S., Gonzalez, E.A., Wade, C.E., Dubick, M.A., Schwab, C.W., Moore, F.A., Champion, H.R., Hoyt, D.B., & Hess, J.R. 2007. Damage control resuscitation: directly addressing the early coagulopathy of trauma. *J.Trauma*, 62, (2) 307-310 available from: PM:17297317

Holcomb, J.B., Wade, C.E., Michalek, J.E., Chisholm, G.B., Zarzabal, L.A., Schreiber, M.A., Gonzalez, E.A., Pomper, G.J., Perkins, J.G., Spinella, P.C., Williams, K.L., & Park, M.S. 2008. Increased plasma and platelet to red blood cell ratios improves outcome in 466 massively transfused civilian trauma patients. *Ann.Surg.*, 248, (3) 447-458 available from: PM:18791365

Howes, J.P., Sharma, V., & Cohen, A.T. 1996. Tranexamic acid reduces blood loss after knee arthroplasty. *J.Bone Joint Surg.Br.*, 78, (6) 995-996 available from: PM:8951024

Hvid, I. & Rodriguez-Merchan, E.C. 2002. Orthopaedic surgery in haemophilic patients with inhibitors: an overview. *Haemophilia.*, 8, (3) 288-291 available from: PM:12010425

Jansen, A.J., Andreica, S., Claeys, M., D'Haese, J., Camu, F., & Jochmans, K. 1999. Use of tranexamic acid for an effective blood conservation strategy after total knee arthroplasty. *Br.J.Anaesth.*, 83, (4) 596-601 available from: PM:10673876

Jensen, L.S. 1998. Benefits of leukocyte-reduced blood transfusions in surgical patients. *Curr.Opin.Hematol.*, 5, (6) 376-380 available from: PM:9814642

Kaplan, J., Sarnaik, S., Gitlin, J., & Lusher, J. 1984. Diminished helper/suppressor lymphocyte ratios and natural killer activity in recipients of repeated blood transfusions. *Blood*, 64, (1) 308-310 available from: PM:6234037

Karnezis, T.A., Stulberg, S.D., Wixson, R.L., & Reilly, P. 1994. The hemostatic effects of desmopressin on patients who had total joint arthroplasty. A double-blind randomized trial. *J.Bone Joint Surg.Am.*, 76, (10) 1545-1550 available from: PM:7929503

Kasper, S.M., Gerlich, W., & Buzello, W. 1997. Preoperative red cell production in patients undergoing weekly autologous blood donation. *Transfusion*, 37, (10) 1058-1062 available from: PM:9354825

Kearon, C. & Hirsh, J. 1997. Management of anticoagulation before and after elective surgery. *N.Engl.J.Med.*, 336, (21) 1506-1511 available from: PM:9154771

Keating, E.M. & Meding, J.B. 2002. Perioperative blood management practices in elective orthopaedic surgery. *J.Am.Acad.Orthop.Surg.*, 10, (6) 393-400 available from: PM:12470041

Keating, E.M., Meding, J.B., Faris, P.M., & Ritter, M.A. 1998. Predictors of transfusion risk in elective knee surgery. *Clin.Orthop.Relat Res.* (357) 50-59 available from: PM:9917700

Keating, E.M., Ranawat, C.S., & Cats-Baril, W. 1999. Assessment of postoperative vigor in patients undergoing elective total joint arthroplasty: a concise patient- and caregiver-based instrument. *Orthopedics*, 22, (1 Suppl) s119-s128 available from: PM:9927112

Kettelhack, C., Hones, C., Messinger, D., & Schlag, P.M. 1998. Randomized multicentre trial of the influence of recombinant human erythropoietin on intraoperative and postoperative transfusion need in anaemic patients undergoing right hemicolectomy for carcinoma. *Br.J.Surg.*, 85, (1) 63-67 available from: PM:9462386

Kick, O. & Daniel, E. 1997. Mathematical considerations in the practice of acute normovolemic hemodilution. *Transfusion*, 37, (2) 141-143 available from: PM:9051087

Klein, H.G. 1995. Allogeneic transfusion risks in the surgical patient. *Am.J.Surg.*, 170, (6A Suppl) 21S-26S available from: PM:8546242

Klein, H.G. 2000. Transfusion safety: avoiding unnecessary bloodshed. *Mayo Clin.Proc.*, 75, (1) 5-7 available from: PM:10630750

Kleinman, S.H. & Busch, M.P. 2000. The risks of transfusion-transmitted infection: direct estimation and mathematical modelling. *Baillieres Best.Pract.Res.Clin.Haematol.*, 13, (4) 631-649 available from: PM:11102281

Knight, J.L., Sherer, D., & Guo, J. 1998. Blood transfusion strategies for total knee arthroplasty: minimizing autologous blood wastage, risk of homologous blood transfusion, and transfusion cost. *J.Arthroplasty*, 13, (1) 70-76 available from: PM:9493540

Kristensen, P.W., Sorensen, L.S., & Thyregod, H.C. 1992. Autotransfusion of drainage blood in arthroplasty. A prospective, controlled study of 31 operations. *Acta Orthop.Scand.*, 63, (4) 377-380 available from: PM:1529683

Lackritz, E.M. 1998. Prevention of HIV transmission by blood transfusion in the developing world: achievements and continuing challenges. *AIDS*, 12 Suppl A, S81-S86 available from: PM:9632988

Laupacis, A. & Fergusson, D. 1997. Drugs to minimize perioperative blood loss in cardiac surgery: meta-analyses using perioperative blood transfusion as the outcome. The International Study of Peri-operative Transfusion (ISPOT) Investigators. *Anesth.Analg.*, 85, (6) 1258-1267 available from: PM:9390590

Laupacis, A. & Fergusson, D. 1998. Erythropoietin to minimize perioperative blood transfusion: a systematic review of randomized trials. The International Study of

Peri-operative Transfusion (ISPOT) Investigators. *Transfus.Med.*, 8, (4) 309-317 available from: PM:9881425

Lenfant, C. 1992. Transfusion practice should be audited for both undertransfusion and overtransfusion. *Transfusion*, 32, (9) 873-874 available from: PM:1471253

Lentschener, C., Cottin, P., Bouaziz, H., Mercier, F.J., Wolf, M., Aljabi, Y., Boyer-Neumann, C., & Benhamou, D. 1999. Reduction of blood loss and transfusion requirement by aprotinin in posterior lumbar spine fusion. *Anesth.Analg.*, 89, (3) 590-597 available from: PM:10475286

Levy, O., Martinowitz, U., Oran, A., Tauber, C., & Horoszowski, H. 1999. The use of fibrin tissue adhesive to reduce blood loss and the need for blood transfusion after total knee arthroplasty. A prospective, randomized, multicenter study. *J.Bone Joint Surg.Am.*, 81, (11) 1580-1588 available from: PM:10565650

Loo, S. & Low, T.C. 1997. Perioperative transfusion strategies: a national survey among anaesthetists. *Ann.Acad.Med.Singapore*, 26, (2) 193-199 available from: PM:9208073

Ludlam, C.A., Smith, M.P., Morfini, M., Gringeri, A., Santagostino, E., & Savidge, G.F. 2003. A prospective study of recombinant activated factor VII administered by continuous infusion to inhibitor patients undergoing elective major orthopaedic surgery: a pharmacokinetic and efficacy evaluation. *Br.J.Haematol.*, 120, (5) 808-813 available from: PM:12614214

Lyseng-Williamson, K.A. & Plosker, G.L. 2007. Recombinant factor VIIa (eptacog alfa): a pharmacoeconomic review of its use in haemophilia in patients with inhibitors to clotting factors VIII or IX. *Pharmacoeconomics.*, 25, (12) 1007-1029 available from: PM:18047387

Martin, J.W., Whiteside, L.A., Milliano, M.T., & Reedy, M.E. 1992. Postoperative blood retrieval and transfusion in cementless total knee arthroplasty. *J.Arthroplasty*, 7, (2) 205-210 available from: PM:1613532

McAlister, F.A., Clark, H.D., Wells, P.S., & Laupacis, A. 1998. Perioperative allogeneic blood transfusion does not cause adverse sequelae in patients with cancer: a meta-analysis of unconfounded studies. *Br.J.Surg.*, 85, (2) 171-178 available from: PM:9501809

McFarland, W., Mvere, D., Shandera, W., & Reingold, A. 1997. Epidemiology and prevention of transfusion-associated human immunodeficiency virus transmission in sub-Saharan Africa. *Vox Sang.*, 72, (2) 85-92 available from: PM:9088075

Meng, Z.H., Wolberg, A.S., Monroe, D.M., III, & Hoffman, M. 2003. The effect of temperature and pH on the activity of factor VIIa: implications for the efficacy of high-dose factor VIIa in hypothermic and acidotic patients. *J.Trauma*, 55, (5) 886-891 available from: PM:14608161

Mercuriali, F., Inghilleri, G., Biffi, E., Colotti, M.T., Vinci, A., & Oriani, G. 1998. Epoetin alfa in low hematocrit patients to facilitate autologous blood donation in total hip replacement: a randomized, double-blind, placebo-controlled, dose-ranging study. *Acta Haematol.*, 100, (2) 69-76 available from: PM:9792935

Mirza, S.B., Campion, J., Dixon, J.H., & Panesar, S.S. 2007. Efficacy and economics of postoperative blood salvage in patients undergoing elective total hip replacement. *Ann.R.Coll.Surg.Engl.*, 89, (8) 777-784 available from: PM:17999819

Monk, T.G. & Goodnough, L.T. 1998. Acute normovolemic hemodilution. *Clin.Orthop.Relat Res.* (357) 74-81 available from: PM:9917703

Monk, T.G., Goodnough, L.T., Birkmeyer, J.D., Brecher, M.E., & Catalona, W.J. 1995. Acute normovolemic hemodilution is a cost-effective alternative to preoperative autologous blood donation by patients undergoing radical retropubic prostatectomy. *Transfusion*, 35, (7) 559-565 available from: PM:7631387

Monroe, D.M., Hoffman, M., Oliver, J.A., & Roberts, H.R. 1997. Platelet activity of high-dose factor VIIa is independent of tissue factor. *Br.J.Haematol.*, 99, (3) 542-547 available from: PM:9401063

Morfini, M., Haya, S., Tagariello, G., Pollmann, H., Quintana, M., Siegmund, B., Stieltjes, N., Dolan, G., & Tusell, J. 2007. European study on orthopaedic status of haemophilia patients with inhibitors. *Haemophilia.*, 13, (5) 606-612 available from: PM:17880451

Muller-Breitkreutz, K. 2000. Results of viral marker screening of unpaid blood donations and probability of window period donations in 1997. EPFA Working Group on Quality Assurance. *Vox Sang.*, 78, (3) 149-157 available from: PM:10838515

Murkin, J.M., Shannon, N.A., Bourne, R.B., Rorabeck, C.H., Cruickshank, M., & Wyile, G. 1995. Aprotinin decreases blood loss in patients undergoing revision or bilateral total hip arthroplasty. *Anesth.Analg.*, 80, (2) 343-348 available from: PM:7529467

Murphy, W.G., Davies, M.J., & Eduardo, A. 1993. The haemostatic response to surgery and trauma. *Br.J.Anaesth.*, 70, (2) 205-213 available from: PM:7679584

Mylod, A.G., Jr., France, M.P., Muser, D.E., & Parsons, J.R. 1990. Perioperative blood loss associated with total knee arthroplasty. A comparison of procedures performed with and without cementing. *J.Bone Joint Surg.Am.*, 72, (7) 1010-1012 available from: PM:2384499

Napier, J.A., Bruce, M., Chapman, J., Duguid, J.K., Kelsey, P.R., Knowles, S.M., Murphy, M.F., Williamson, L.M., Wood, J.K., Lee, D., Contreras, M., Cross, N., Desmond, M.J., Gillon, J., Lardy, A., & Williams, F.G. 1997. Guidelines for autologous transfusion. II. Perioperative haemodilution and cell salvage. British Committee for Standards in Haematology Blood Transfusion Task Force. Autologous Transfusion Working Party. *Br.J.Anaesth.*, 78, (6) 768-771 available from: PM:9215035

Negrier, C., Goudemand, J., Sultan, Y., Bertrand, M., Rothschild, C., & Lauroua, P. 1997. Multicenter retrospective study on the utilization of FEIBA in France in patients with factor VIII and factor IX inhibitors. French FEIBA Study Group. Factor Eight Bypassing Activity. *Thromb.Haemost.*, 77, (6) 1113-1119 available from: PM:9241742

Neill, F., Sear, J.W., French, G., Lam, H., Kemp, M., Hooper, R.J., & Foex, P. 2000. Increases in serum concentrations of cardiac proteins and the prediction of early postoperative cardiovascular complications in noncardiac surgery patients. *Anaesthesia*, 55, (7) 641-647 available from: PM:10919418

Nessen, S., Lounsbury, D., & Hetz, S. 2008, "Vascular Trauma," *In War Surgery in Afghanistan and Iraq: A Series of Cases, 2003-2007.*, S. Nessen, Lounsbury DE, & Hetz SP, eds., Washigton DC: Falls Church, VA, United States Army, Office of the Surgeon General and Washington DC, Walter Reed Army Medical Center, Borden Institute, pp. 317-359.

Newman, J.H., Bowers, M., & Murphy, J. 1997. The clinical advantages of autologous transfusion. A randomized, controlled study after knee replacement. *J.Bone Joint Surg.Br.*, 79, (4) 630-632 available from: PM:9250753

Nuttall, G.A., Santrach, P.J., Oliver, W.C., Jr., Ereth, M.H., Horlocker, T.T., Cabanela, M.E., Trousdale, R.T., & Schroeder, D.R. 2000. Possible guidelines for autologous red blood cell donations before total hip arthroplasty based on the surgical blood order equation. *Mayo Clin.Proc.*, 75, (1) 10-17 available from: PM:10630751

Obergfell, A., Auvinen, M.K., & Mathew, P. 2008. Recombinant activated factor VII for haemophilia patients with inhibitors undergoing orthopaedic surgery: a review of the literature. *Haemophilia.*, 14, (2) 233-241 available from: PM:18081827

Oz, M.C., Cosgrove, D.M., III, Badduke, B.R., Hill, J.D., Flannery, M.R., Palumbo, R., & Topic, N. 2000. Controlled clinical trial of a novel hemostatic agent in cardiac surgery. The Fusion Matrix Study Group. *Ann.Thorac.Surg.*, 69, (5) 1376-1382 available from: PM:10881808

Paravicini, D., Frisch, R., Stinnesbeck, B., & Lawin, P. 1983. [Intraoperative autotransfusion in extensive orthopedic interventions]. *Z.Orthop.Ihre Grenzgeb.*, 121, (3) 278-282 available from: PM:6613270

Petaja, J., Myllynen, P., Myllyla, G., & Vahtera, E. 1987. Fibrinolysis after application of a pneumatic tourniquet. *Acta Chir Scand.*, 153, (11-12) 647-651 available from: PM:3124428

Popovsky, M.A., Whitaker, B., & Arnold, N.L. 1995. Severe outcomes of allogeneic and autologous blood donation: frequency and characterization. *Transfusion*, 35, (9) 734-737 available from: PM:7570932

Price, T.H., Goodnough, L.T., Vogler, W.R., Sacher, R.A., Hellman, R.M., Johnston, M.F., Bolgiano, D.C., & Abels, R.I. 1996. Improving the efficacy of preoperative autologous blood donation in patients with low hematocrit: a randomized, double-blind, controlled trial of recombinant human erythropoietin. *Am.J.Med.*, 101, (2A) 22S-27S available from: PM:8928704

Qvist, N., Boesby, S., Wolff, B., & Hansen, C.P. 1999. Recombinant human erythropoietin and hemoglobin concentration at operation and during the postoperative period: reduced need for blood transfusions in patients undergoing colorectal surgery-- prospective double-blind placebo-controlled study. *World J.Surg.*, 23, (1) 30-35 available from: PM:9841760

Rau, B., Schlag, P.M., Willeke, F., Herfarth, C., Stephan, P., & Franke, W. 1998. Increased autologous blood donation in rectal cancer by recombinant human erythropoietin (rhEPO). *Eur.J.Cancer*, 34, (7) 992-998 available from: PM:9849445

Regan, F. & Taylor, C. 2002. Blood transfusion medicine. *BMJ*, 325, (7356) 143-147 available from: PM:12130612

Regan, F.A., Hewitt, P., Barbara, J.A., & Contreras, M. 2000. Prospective investigation of transfusion transmitted infection in recipients of over 20 000 units of blood. TTI Study Group. *BMJ*, 320, (7232) 403-406 available from: PM:10669443

Ritter, M.A., Keating, E.M., & Faris, P.M. 1994. Closed wound drainage in total hip or total knee replacement. A prospective, randomized study. *J.Bone Joint Surg.Am.*, 76, (1) 35-38 available from: PM:8288663

Rizoli, S.B. & Chughtai, T. 2006. The emerging role of recombinant activated Factor VII (rFVIIa) in the treatment of blunt traumatic haemorrhage. *Expert.Opin.Biol.Ther.*, 6, (1) 73-81 available from: PM:16370916

Rizoli, S.B., Nascimento, B., Jr., Osman, F., Netto, F.S., Kiss, A., Callum, J., Brenneman, F.D., Tremblay, L., & Tien, H.C. 2006. Recombinant activated coagulation factor VII and bleeding trauma patients. *J.Trauma*, 61, (6) 1419-1425 available from: PM:17159685

Rodriguez-Merchan, E.C., Wiedel, J.J., Wallny, T., Caviglia, H., Hvid, I., Berntorp, E., Rivard, G.E., Goddard, N.N., & Querol, F. 2004. Elective orthopedic surgery for hemophilia patients with inhibitors: New opportunities. *Semin.Hematol.*, 41, (1 Suppl 1) 109-116 available from: PM:14872431

Roth, V.R., Arduino, M.J., Nobiletti, J., Holt, S.C., Carson, L.A., Wolf, C.F., Lenes, B.A., Allison, P.M., & Jarvis, W.R. 2000. Transfusion-related sepsis due to Serratia liquefaciens in the United States. *Transfusion*, 40, (8) 931-935 available from: PM:10960519

Scalone, L., Mantovani, L.G., Mannucci, P.M., & Gringeri, A. 2006. Quality of life is associated to the orthopaedic status in haemophilic patients with inhibitors. *Haemophilia.*, 12, (2) 154-162 available from: PM:16476090

Schmied, H., Kurz, A., Sessler, D.I., Kozek, S., & Reiter, A. 1996. Mild hypothermia increases blood loss and transfusion requirements during total hip arthroplasty. *Lancet*, 347, (8997) 289-292 available from: PM:8569362

Schmied, H., Schiferer, A., Sessler, D.I., & Meznik, C. 1998. The effects of red-cell scavenging, hemodilution, and active warming on allogenic blood requirements in patients undergoing hip or knee arthroplasty. *Anesth.Analg.*, 86, (2) 387-391 available from: PM:9459254

Schott, U., Sollen, C., Axelsson, K., Rugarn, P., & Allvin, I. 1995. Desmopressin acetate does not reduce blood loss during total hip replacement in patients receiving dextran. *Acta Anaesthesiol.Scand.*, 39, (5) 592-598 available from: PM:7572006

Schulman, S., d'Oiron, R., Martinowitz, U., Pasi, J., Briquel, M.E., Mauser-Bunschoten, E., Morfini, M., Ritchie, B., Goudemand, J., Lloyd, J., McPherson, J., Negrier, C., Peerlinck, K., Petrini, P., & Tusell, J. 1998. Experiences with continuous infusion of recombinant activated factor VII. *Blood Coagul.Fibrinolysis*, 9 Suppl 1, S97-101 available from: PM:9819037

Scottish Intercollegiate Guidelines Network. Perioperative blood transfusion for elective surgery. 2001. Ref Type: Generic

Sharrock, N.E., Mineo, R., Urquhart, B., & Salvati, E.A. 1993. The effect of two levels of hypotension on intraoperative blood loss during total hip arthroplasty performed under lumbar epidural anesthesia. *Anesth.Analg.*, 76, (3) 580-584 available from: PM:8452271

Simon, T.L., Alverson, D.C., AuBuchon, J., Cooper, E.S., DeChristopher, P.J., Glenn, G.C., Gould, S.A., Harrison, C.R., Milam, J.D., Moise, K.J., Jr., Rodwig, F.R., Jr., Sherman, L.A., Shulman, I.A., & Stehling, L. 1998. Practice parameter for the use of red blood cell transfusions: developed by the Red Blood Cell Administration Practice Guideline Development Task Force of the College of American Pathologists. *Arch.Pathol.Lab Med.*, 122, (2) 130-138 available from: PM:9499355

Slagis, S.V., Benjamin, J.B., Volz, R.G., & Giordano, G.F. 1991. Postoperative blood salvage in total hip and knee arthroplasty. A randomised controlled trial. *J.Bone Joint Surg.Br.*, 73, (4) 591-594 available from: PM:1906472

Smetannikov, Y. & Hopkins, D. 1996. Intraoperative bleeding: a mathematical model for minimizing hemoglobin loss. *Transfusion*, 36, (9) 832-835 available from: PM:8823461

Soucie, J.M., Nuss, R., Evatt, B., Abdelhak, A., Cowan, L., Hill, H., Kolakoski, M., & Wilber, N. 2000. Mortality among males with hemophilia: relations with source of medical care. The Hemophilia Surveillance System Project Investigators. *Blood*, 96, (2) 437-442 available from: PM:10887103

Southern, E.P., Huo, M.H., Mehta, J.R., & Keggi, K.J. 1995. Unwashed wound drainage blood. What are we giving our patients? *Clin.Orthop.Relat Res.* (320) 235-246 available from: PM:7586832

Spahn, D.R., Smith, L.R., McRae, R.L., & Leone, B.J. 1992. Effects of acute isovolemic hemodilution and anesthesia on regional function in left ventricular myocardium with compromised coronary blood flow. *Acta Anaesthesiol.Scand.*, 36, (7) 628-636 available from: PM:1279924

Spahn, D.R., Smith, L.R., Schell, R.M., Hoffman, R.D., Gillespie, R., & Leone, B.J. 1994. Importance of severity of coronary artery disease for the tolerance to normovolemic hemodilution. Comparison of single-vessel versus multivessel stenoses in a canine model. *J.Thorac.Cardiovasc.Surg.*, 108, (2) 231-239 available from: PM:8041171

Spence, R.K. 1995. Surgical red blood cell transfusion practice policies. Blood Management Practice Guidelines Conference. *Am.J.Surg.*, 170, (6A Suppl) 3S-15S available from: PM:8546244

Spence, R.K. 1998. Anemia in the patient undergoing surgery and the transfusion decision. A review. *Clin.Orthop.Relat Res.* (357) 19-29 available from: PM:9917696

Spence, R.K., Carson, J.A., Poses, R., McCoy, S., Pello, M., Alexander, J., Popovich, J., Norcross, E., & Camishion, R.C. 1990. Elective surgery without transfusion: influence of preoperative hemoglobin level and blood loss on mortality. *Am.J.Surg.*, 159, (3) 320-324 available from: PM:2305940

Sperry, J.L., Ochoa, J.B., Gunn, S.R., Alarcon, L.H., Minei, J.P., Cuschieri, J., Rosengart, M.R., Maier, R.V., Billiar, T.R., Peitzman, A.B., & Moore, E.E. 2008. An FFP:PRBC transfusion ratio >/=1:1.5 is associated with a lower risk of mortality after massive transfusion. *J.Trauma*, 65, (5) 986-993 available from: PM:19001962

Spinella, P.C., Perkins, J.G., McLaughlin, D.F., Niles, S.E., Grathwohl, K.W., Beekley, A.C., Salinas, J., Mehta, S., Wade, C.E., & Holcomb, J.B. 2008. The effect of recombinant activated factor VII on mortality in combat-related casualties with severe trauma and massive transfusion. *J.Trauma*, 64, (2) 286-293 available from: PM:18301188

The SHOT Committee. Serious hazards of transfusion: annual report. 2000. Manchester. Ref Type: Generic

Thim, L., Bjoern, S., Christensen, M., Nicolaisen, E.M., Lund-Hansen, T., Pedersen, A.H., & Hedner, U. 1988. Amino acid sequence and posttranslational modifications of human factor VIIa from plasma and transfected baby hamster kidney cells. *Biochemistry*, 27, (20) 7785-7793 available from: PM:3264725

Thorpe, C.M., Murphy, W.G., & Logan, M. 1994. Use of aprotinin in knee replacement surgery. *Br.J.Anaesth.*, 73, (3) 408-410 available from: PM:7524592

Tjonnfjord, G.E., Brinch, L., Gedde-Dahl, T., & Brosstad, F.R. 2004. Activated prothrombin complex concentrate (FEIBA) treatment during surgery in patients with inhibitors to FVIII/IX. *Haemophilia.*, 10, (2) 174-178 available from: PM:14962207

Toy, P.T., Kaplan, E.B., McVay, P.A., Lee, S.J., Strauss, R.G., & Stehling, L.C. 1992. Blood loss and replacement in total hip arthroplasty: a multicenter study. The Preoperative Autologous Blood Donation Study Group. *Transfusion*, 32, (1) 63-67 available from: PM:1731438

Voak, D., Cann, R., Finney, R.D., Fraser, I.D., Mitchell, R., Murphy, M.F., Napier, J.A., Phillips, P., Rejman, A.J., Waters, A.H., & . 1994. Guidelines for administration of blood products: transfusion of infants and neonates. British Committee for Standards in Haematology Blood Transfusion Task Force. *Transfus.Med.*, 4, (1) 63-69 available from: PM:8012495

Weiskopf, R.B., Viele, M.K., Feiner, J., Kelley, S., Lieberman, J., Noorani, M., Leung, J.M., Fisher, D.M., Murray, W.R., Toy, P., & Moore, M.A. 1998. Human cardiovascular and metabolic response to acute, severe isovolemic anemia. *JAMA*, 279, (3) 217-221 available from: PM:9438742

Welch, H.G., Meehan, K.R., & Goodnough, L.T. 1992. Prudent strategies for elective red blood cell transfusion. *Ann.Intern.Med.*, 116, (5) 393-402 available from: PM:1736773

Will, R.G., Ironside, J.W., Zeidler, M., Cousens, S.N., Estibeiro, K., Alperovitch, A., Poser, S., Pocchiari, M., Hofman, A., & Smith, P.G. 1996. A new variant of Creutzfeldt-Jakob disease in the UK. *Lancet*, 347, (9006) 921-925 available from: PM:8598754

Wilson, W.J. 1989. Intraoperative autologous transfusion in revision total hip arthroplasty. *J.Bone Joint Surg.Am.*, 71, (1) 8-14 available from: PM:2913006

Xenakis, T.A., Malizos, K.N., Dailiana, Z., Koukoubis, T., Zervou, E., Golegou, C., & Soucacos, P.N. 1997. Blood salvage after total hip and total knee arthroplasty. *Acta Orthop.Scand.Suppl*, 275, 135-138 available from: PM:9385289

Zohar, E., Fredman, B., Ellis, M., Luban, I., Stern, A., & Jedeikin, R. 1999. A comparative study of the postoperative allogeneic blood-sparing effect of tranexamic acid versus acute normovolemic hemodilution after total knee replacement. *Anesth.Analg.*, 89, (6) 1382-1387 available from: PM:10589612

3

Transfusion Reduction in Orthopedic Surgery

Ruud H.G.P. van Erve and Alexander C. Wiekenkamp

Beter Lopen, Deventer
The Netherlands

1. Introduction

Clinical research has identified blood transfusion as an independent risk factor for immediate and long-term adverse outcomes, including an increased risk of death, myocardial infarction, stroke, renal failure, infection and malignancy (Rawn, 2008).

Blood transfusion is however widely used in orthopedic surgery although the performed surgery is mostly elective. Since the surgeries can, in the majority of cases, be planned ahead it is possible to reduce the use of blood and blood products by planning their use as well.

In the past few years substantial steps have been taken to reduce the need for blood transfusion. The reduction of blood transfusion can be accomplished by several methods, the most successful of which seems to be a combination of different methods available. (van Erve, 2008). It is best to speak of blood management, which is the philosophy to improve patient outcomes by integrating all available techniques to reduce or eliminate allogeneic blood transfusions (Seeber & Shander, 2007). It should be a patient-centered, multidisciplinary, multimodal, planned approach to patient care (Seeber & Shander, 2007).

In order to reduce the use of blood in orthopedic surgery the following separate steps can be identified. First the patients can be optimized before surgery. Second, the use of blood conserving techniques during surgery is to be applied. These steps are considered as Anaemia and Hemostasis Management. Third, the transfusion triggers can be set as low as possible (Appropriate transfusion practices). Finally, the use of re-transfusion of drainage fluids from the surgical wound can be used (Blood conservation). All these measures should improve patient outcomes. Figure 1 illustrates the interconnection of the different parts of blood management.

In orthopedic surgery the above steps are relatively easy to carry out for there is sufficient time to organize them around the individual patient.

We will discuss all possible measures to be taken to reduce the use of allogeneic blood in orthopedic surgery.

2. Autologous transfusion

Patients can be encouraged to donate their own blood prior to surgery (pre-donation). The use of this technique is limited to surgery that can be planned ahead as it needs adequate planning and time to restore the hemoglobin level while the blood should not be taken too

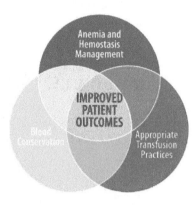

Fig. 1. Organogram as proposed by the Society for the Advancement of Blood Management (SABM)

early in order to have adequate red cell quality. The storage time of the patient's own red cells is the same as for allogeneic transfusions. Pre-donation should be done no more than 40 days before surgery because the storage time of red cells is limited and known to be of utmost importance to the quality of the cells. As most of the surgery done in orthopedics is elective, especially in adult reconstruction, this technique is highly suitable. In trauma surgery this technique is less feasible because of the lack of time to schedule it and the acute need for blood in most major trauma. In trauma surgery other techniques should be used to avoid the use of allogeneic blood. We will discuss these techniques later in this chapter.

Although pre-donated blood is safer than allogeneic blood it is not risk free and besides it is expensive (Domen, 1996). According to Domen the costs per saved quality adjusted life year may be as high as 1 million dollars. Vamvakas and Pineda found the cost effectiveness of pre-donation to be between 2,470 and 3,400,000 dollars per quality adjusted life year saved. The costs of predonation are high because the needs for collection, storage and avoidance of transfusion errors are expensive as well (Vamvakas & Pineda, 2000).

A specialized organization for the use of autologous blood is imperative for the blood has to be specially assigned to every patient individually. For each patient to be assigned his/her own blood an extensive security system is required to reduce the risk of interchanging blood between patients. This makes such a practice expensive. In order to avoid transfusion errors the safety measures for this type of autologous donation have to be the same as for allogeneic transfusion. Its use is therefore limited to hospitals with their own blood banks guaranteeing the safety of the blood harvested from the patients and used for their own re-transfusion when needed.

As the donated blood is not extensively tested for transferable diseases, nor typed and screened, the blood harvested from one patient cannot be used for other patients. Domen found in 1996 that only half of the autologous units collected are actually used. The amount actually needed might even be smaller because physicians in attendance may judge it a waste of good blood not to return the donated blood to the patient, thus giving more transfusions than strictly necessary using restrictive transfusion triggers (Domen, 1996).

Pre-donation includes the risks associated with blood donation in general. In fact all the signs of anemia can occur, dependent on the amount of blood donated and thus on the extent of the surgery planned. The pre-donation procedure introduces an acute iron deficiency anemia with all possible sign and symptoms. Especially in the elderly population, which in orthopedic surgery is the main target group, symptoms may occur. The expected symptoms are fatigue, headaches, faintness, breathlessness, angina, intermittent claudication and palpitations. The claudication will occur in a relative high percentage of the population for many of the orthopedic patients have vascular problems too. Because the pre-donation introduces an iron deficiency anemia it is to be accompanied by iron infusions or erythropoetin to enhance the production of erythrocytes in order to have the hemoglobin and the hematocrit at an appropriate level before surgery.

3. Pre-operative medication

The percentage of patients for major elective orthopedic surgery presenting with marked anemia is 10.5%, using the World Health Organisation (WHO) criteria (Bisbe et al., 2008), while Bierbaum et al found up to 35% hemoglobin levels of 13g/dl or less in patients in the USA (Bierbaum et al., 1999). According to several studies (Goodnough et al., 2011), the postoperative mortality and morbidity increase while the postoperative functional recovery and the quality of life is impaired in the presence of a preoperative anemia (Beattie et al., 2009; Conlon et al., 2008; Gruson et al., 2002).

Preoperative medication can be prescribed to enhance the amount of erythrocytes in the circulation. This can be combined with the previously described pre-donation but can be used separately as well. The trigger for the use of preoperative medication is set to 13.2 g/dl or lower (Goldberg MA et al., 1996). This threshold has to be taken into account to avoid introducing the risk of polycythaemia. If polycytaemia is introduced the risk for thrombosis, haemorrhage and cardiac failure increases. Although the increase of thrombotic or other complications has never been proven (De Andrade et al., 1996; Faris et al., 1996), the risk for thrombosis in orthopedic surgery is high enough without it being increased by medication, especially in hip and knee reconstructive surgery.

Mainly two types of drugs are used; iron and erythropoietin. We will describe these medications below.

3.1 Iron

Intravenous iron can be used to boost the production of erythrocytes and is a component of autotransfusion practice. Especially in pre-donation it is extensively used. It is relatively safe and cheap medication though patients have to be admitted to hospital for the intravenous application. The adverse drug events have been studied by Johnson-Wimbley & Graham and Chertow et al. Some of the additional reported adverse events associated with iron preparations in their studies were hypotension, arthralgias, myalgias, malaise, abdominal pain, nausea, and vomiting. These non life-threatening adverse reactions were more commonly associated with iron dextran and less so with iron sucrose or sodium ferric gluconate (50%, 36%, 35%, respectively) (Johnson-Wimbley & Graham, 2011). The absolute rates of life-threatening adverse drug events were 0.6, 0.9, 3.3 and 11.3 per million for iron sucrose, sodium ferric gluconate complex, lower molecular weight iron dextran and higher molecular weight iron dextran, respectively (Chertow et al., 2006).

In an elaborate review Chritchley & Yenal found adverse events to be rare with slightly higher numbers in high molecular weight iron dextran than in low molecular weight iron dextran (Critchley & Yenal, 2007).

The use of oral iron and of intravenous iron is being intensely studied at the moment. The Society for the Advancement of Blood Management publishes weekly articles of interest in his field at its website (www.SABM.org)

The efficacy of preoperative iron supplementation is mounting. A study of 569 patients undergoing colorectal cancer surgery found that among the 116 patients who were anemic, intraoperative transfusion was needed in a significantly lower proportion of those who received 2 weeks of preoperative oral iron supplementation (200 mg) compared with those who received no iron therapy (9.4% vs 27.4%; $P < .05$) (Okuyama et al, 2005).

According to Serrano-Trenas et al. intra-operatively iron infusion can be administered as successfully as preoperative iron infusions. They compared iron sucrose in hip fracture patients with no iron suppletion and found reduced transfusion requirements in patients with intra-capsular fractures and in those with hemoglobin levels of 12g/dl or more if given 600 mg intravenous iron during the operation (Serrano-Trenas et al., 2011),. They found no difference in mortality, morbidity or length of hospital stay, however (Serrano-Trenas et al., 2011).

3.2 Erythropoietin

Erythopoietin (EPO) is a glycoprotein hormone normally produced in the kidney. The renocortical interstitial cells secrete it in response to reduced oxygen tension in the blood. Erythropoietin functions in the recruitment and differentiation of erythroid progenitor cells, aids in their maintenance and survival, and stimulates the synthesis of Hb (Ersley, 1991). The synthetic Epoetin alfa, the most used administered form of EPO available, is identical to endogenous erythropoietin in its amino acid sequence and biologic activity (Figure 2).

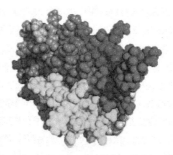

Fig. 2. Eprex molecule, a synthetic erythropoietin alpha (pharmaeurope.com)

Like endogenous erythropoietin, epoetin alfa effectively and safely stimulates synthesis of Hb. The medication can best be administered subcutaneously with 4 injections during the 3 weeks prior to surgery with the last injection given in the operating theater. The subcutaneous method is better than the intravenous administration because the slow release from the depot provides a more sustained plasma level (Ersley, 1991). The amount of erythropoietin given should be 300 IU/kg/day for 15 days peri-operatively or 600 IU/kg in 4 weekly doses beginning 3 weeks prior to surgery (Figure 3).

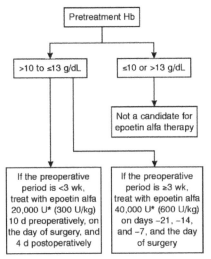

Fig. 3. Treatment algorithm for the use of Epoitin alpha in anemic patients scheduled for elective non-cardiac, non-vascular surgery at high risk for transfusion because of anticipated blood loss (Keating & Meding, 2002).

Erythropoietin should be used in combination with oral or intravenous iron administration to boost the erythrocyte production (García et al., 2009). If erythropoietin is used allogeneic transfusions are markedly reduced. In a prospective observational study of low Hb patients to whom 600 IU/kg EPO in 4 doses was administered, a transfusion percentage of 3.6% was found, while in the low Hb group who did not receive EPO the percentage was 45.2%, and in the normal Hb group 11.9% (Lafosse et al., 2010). The reduction of allogeneic transfusions reached with the administration of EPO was therefore 92% (Lafosse et al., 2010).

Epoietin alfa is expensive but very effective in increasing the Hemoglobin level of the patients by 4g/dl in 4 weeks (if administered 600 IU in 4 subcutaneous injections) which is equivalent to 5 units Red Blood Cells. The Canadian Coordinating Office for Health Technology Assessment performed an economic evaluation of erythropoietin use in surgery in 1998. In their report they state the costs of EPO to be less than 100,000 dollars per gained life year. Assuming 10% of all hip arthroplasty and cardiac bypass surgery patients need EPO they calculated the total costs for the Canadian health care to be 5.9 million dollars annually. These costs were to be made in order to have a potential benefit of 0.12 life years gained for the total population (Otten, 1998). If, however, the use of EPO and autologous transfusion are compared to pre-donation, EPO has better results in the increase of Hb and decrease of allogeneic transfusions (Deutsch, 2006).

4. Peroperative measures

In orthopaedic surgery multiple options are available to help reduce the intra-operative need for allogeneic blood transfusion. Although some methods are very commonly used worldwide, other methods are used less frequently. In this section we will discuss a selection of the major methods in the current orthopedic practice, divided into surgical and anaesthesiological techniques, autologous blood transfusion and anti-fibronolytic drugs.

4.1 Surgical and anaesthesiological techniques

During operation surgical haemostasis should be performed as thoroughly as possible. In orthopedic surgery electrocautery is the most widely used technique. Operations can be performed using a tourniquet and exsanguination to reduce the amount of shed blood. If, and wherever possible, the use of endoscopic techniques can help to reduce the amount of shed blood. The use of anesthesiological techniques such as controlled hypotension, maintenance of normothermia and acute normovolemic dilution can reduce the loss of blood as well.

The usage of tourniquets in total knee arthroplasties is often used to help reduce the intra-operative blood loss (Matziolis et al., 2011; Smith & Hing, 2010; Zhang et al., 2010). Matziolis et. al. found this to be an effective method to reduce intra-operative blood loss (Matziolis et al., 2011). A study by Zhang et. al. found a decrease in intra-operative blood loss, but also a significant increase in post-operative blood loss (Zhang et al., 2010). A systematic review and meta-analysis by Smith and Hing found a significantly reduced level of intra-operative blood loss in patient groups where tourniquets were used, compared to non-tourniquet control groups. They state however, that there was no difference found in total blood loss and complications were more frequent in the tourniquet groups (Smith & Hing, 2010). The usage of tourniquets seems to reduce the amount of blood loss intra-operatively, but it increases the amount of post-operative blood loss. It is therefore useful to take proper post-operative measures, e.g. the use of post-operative autologous reinfusion systems or tranexamic acid. These methods will be discussed later in this chapter.

When using acute normovolemic dilution, patient's blood is withdrawn intra-operatively or shortly before the operation. The withdrawn blood is replaced by an equal volume of crystalloid or colloid solution. In normal circumstances 0,5-1,5 liters of blood are withdrawn from the patients circulation. This makes the blood lost contain less erythrocytes, making the loss of blood less important. The withdrawn blood is always re-transfused as autologous transfusion. Davies et. al. compared different studies and concluded that acute normovolemic dilution may be a cost effective method to decrease the need for allogeneic blood transfusion (Davies et al., 2006). Goodnough et. al. compared the methods of pre-operative autologous blood donation and acute normovolemic hemodilution in patients undergoing total hip arthroplasties. They found acute normovolemic hemodilution to be safe. No differences were found regarding the need for allogeneic blood transfusion in both groups. However, acute normovolemic hemodilution turned out to be significantly more cost effective than pre-operative autologous blood donation (Goodnough et al., 2000).

4.2 Autologous transfusion

The option of intra-operative autologous transfusion is interesting because of the theoretical possibility for re-infusion of infinite amounts of blood. The use of autologous transfusion in orthopedic surgery is useful in large surgeries, i.e. spine and revision surgery, though not in infections and tumor surgeries. Autologous transfusion in smaller surgeries is not practical and expensive.

4.2.1 Washed autologous transfusion

For over 30 years the method of washed autologous transfusion has been used successfully in multiple medical disciplines, especially in surgeries with expected major blood loss. The use of cell saving techniques is warranted to accomplish this. Herein the shed red cells are collected, washed, concentrated and re-infused into the patient. As stated before, the potency of re-infusing large amounts of blood is a great advantage of the cell savers. In orthopedic surgery however, the loss of blood intra- and post-operatively rarely approaches the huge amounts of blood loss in, for instance, cardiac or trauma surgery. In other words, the role of cell saving in orthopedic surgery is limited.

Carless et. al. conclude in their systemic review that cell salvage is an effective tool to reduce the need for allogeneic blood transfusion in both cardiac and orthopaedic surgery. They state however that many studies may have been biased and are therefore difficult to interpret (Carless et al., 2010). It is stated that intra-operative cell salvage is beneficial in surgery when blood loss exceeds 1,000 ml (Lemaire, 2008; Sculco, 1995). Davies et. al. find that cell salvage may be cost effective (Davies et al., 2006). However, it should again be noted that many studies may not be reliable due to biasing.

In their study, Benli IT et al. found higher hematocrit level in patient´s blood when cell salvage was used intra-operatively compared to a control group (Benli et al., 1999). Usage of intra-operative cell salvage also provides advantages regarding post-operative wound infections and the healing process of the wound (Duffy & Neal, 1996; Steinitz et al., 2001; Weber et al., 2005).

The use of allogeneic blood transfusion comes with an increased risk of post-operative wound infections as is shown in two studies (Duffy & Neal, 1996; Steinitz et al., 2001). Duffy finds a decrease in post-operative wound infections when autologous blood is used for transfusion instead of allogeneic blood (Duffy & Neal, 1996). Also, the post-operative wound healing may be positively influenced by using cell salvage, as Weber et. al. find a longer healing process after usage of allogeneic blood transfusion, compared to a control group in which patients did not receive allogeneic blood transfusion (Weber et al., 2005).

The normal way to collect shed blood is using a vacuum suction device. Many studies have been done to identify the best ways of collecting, especially regarding vacuum suction pressure and blood-air contact. Gregoretti found in his study that a vacuum pressure of up to 300 mmHg could be used safely, considering that the levels of potassium, hematocrit and red blood cells did not change significantly when higher pressures than normal (above 150 mmHg) were used (Gregoretti, 1996). He did find however substantial influence of the air-blood contact on the level of hemolysis. A study by Waters et. al. showed that hemolysis increased when a higher vacuum pressure was used in the suction device. Furthermore, they found that suction from flat surfaces also increased the level of hemolysis, when compared to suctioning from a cavity (Waters et al., 2007). They advise diluting the blood with normal saline while it is collected, using minimal vacuum pressure and minimizing the contact between the collected blood and air, both in the suction tube as well as in the collecting device, for this too will increase the amount of hemolysis, thus reducing the quality of the blood. In another study Yazer et al. also conclude that a higher level of air-blood contact increases the level of hemolysis. They also found that hemolysis was decreased by using a vacuum suction device with variable pressure (Yazer et al., 2008).

Another interesting point of debate in cell salvage is the use of it in revision of metal on metal (MoM) hip prosthesis revisions which is increasingly problematic at present in orthopedic surgery. The MoM prostheses, which gained in popularity the past years, have lately proven to shed a lot of metal ions which induce increased levels of mainly Cobalt and Chromium ions in the plasma and full blood of patients and local pseudotumors consisting of large amounts of metal ions in granulomatous tissue surrounding the prostheses causing loosening. If those prostheses are to be revised the metal ions are likely to be sucked into the cell saver with the blood and the plasma components. The metal ions are mostly solved in plasma and incorporated in the leucocytes and thus reintroduced into the patient with the red cells and the leucocytes at retransfusion. Since these ions are known to be carcinogenic and tend to accumulate in the liver, the spleen, the kidneys and the lymphatic system the extra amount of these metal ions introduced in the patients circulation at re-transfusion of the salvaged blood during operation might increase the risk for serious long term complications. The effects of these metals have not been investigated properly since they have not been used in large quantities for long enough to induce carcinomas but the extra load of the ions which is potentially introduced during revision surgery has, potentially, such hazardous consequences that we think we should advise against using cell salvage in the presence of MoM prostheses. More research on this subject is desired.

4.2.2 Non-washed autologous transfusion

Using non-washed blood is a relatively new way to achieve reduction of allogeneic blood transfusion. In this method, shed blood is collected intra-operatively and is to be re-infused into the patients circulation after a filtration process. One has to consider that unwashed intra-operative autologous transfusion differs from the post-operative autologous transfusion, the method we will discuss in the next subsection of this chapter. While collecting the shed blood intra-operatively, large amounts of lipids and bone marrow will also be aspirated into the collecting device. This collateral catch may obstruct the filters of the device, ultimately blocking the system.

The lipids, if not properly filtered, can potentially increase the risk of fatty embolism if introduced in the circulation. The risks of these fatty embolisms have been described extensively in the literature concerning cemented hip prostheses as they are widespread during the preparation of the bone for the prosthesis.

Then there is the theoretical possibility to be considered of tiny bone fragments collected from the surgical wound to rupture the filter in the device or even cause vessel ruptures after being re-infused into the patient's circulation. However, the latter has never been described so far and is very difficult to prove.

The use of non-washed blood from the wound is still under investigation and debate. In three different studies, blood samples are tested after being filtered and considered to be safe when reinfused, regarding potassium, sodium, plasma haemoglobin and systemic haemoglobin levels (Bengtsson et al., 2008; Kvarnström et al., 2008; Stachura et al., 2008). Wiekenkamp et. al. however question the safety of this particular device as they found high levels of plasma haemoglobin (>0.64 g/dl) in their blood samples after filtration (Wiekenkamp et al., 2010). These levels are comparable with levels found by Kvarnström et. al. and Bengtsson et. al., 1.15 g/dl and 1.63 g/dl respectively. Wiekenkamp et. al. continue with an example by stating: a normal person is physically capable to bind 0.03-0.2 g/dl of plasma haemoglobine to haptoglobine. Considering one has the capability to bind 0.2 g/dl and a circulating blood volume of six liters, a maximum of 12.0 g of plasma haemoglobin can be bound. Higher plasma haemoglobin levels will result in saturation of haptoglobine and the risk of binding of plasma haemoglobin to nitric oxide, which will result in dangerous reactive oxide radicals. In this case the maximum level of plasma haemoglobin to safely re-infuse 500 ml of filtered blood, is 2.4 g/dl. Considering that many patients have less binding capabilities, the risk of saturating haptoglobine and therefore endangering the patient with reactive oxide radicals is very real (Wiekenkamp et al., 2010).

4.3 Anti-fibronolytic drugs

The use of medical agents, like tranexamic acid, can be a useful tool to reduce blood loss preoperatively (Erstad 2001a; Erstad 2001b; Henry et al., 2011; Keating, 1999; Lemaire, 2008; Sepah et al., 2011). Anti-fibronolytic drugs are to be given pre-, intra- or post-operatively, depending on the kind of drug that is used. Purpose of using these anti-fibrinolytic agents is decreasing the volume of intra- and post-operative blood loss. Because of the relatively low costs and their successful use in many disciplines, e.g. gynaecology and cardiac surgery, the anti-fibrinolytic drugs are an interesting option in orthopedic surgery.

Henry et. al. found a decrease in blood loss and a lower need for allogeneic red cell transfusion when anti-fibrinolytic drugs were used. Aprotinin showed slightly better results than tranexamic acid or epsilon aminocaproic acid in comparative studies, but also a higher risk of death. No serious adverse effects were found while using tranexamic acid or epsilon aminocaproic acid (Henry et al., 2011). In a retrospective study comparing a group of patients who received tranexamic acid pre- or post-operatively to a group of patients who did not receive tranexamic acid, Sepah et. al. found a significant effect of tranexamic acid. Both the value of the mean Hb-loss and the mean volume of post-operative wound drainage had substantially decreased in the group of patients who received tranexamic acid (Sepah et al., 2011). Den Hartog et. al. compared a group of patients who did receive tranexamic acid intra-operatively with a control group in both total knee and in total hip surgery. In the total knee surgery a 55.6% decrease of blood loss was found post-operatively. In total hip surgery they found a decrease of 20.4%(den Hartog & Roorda, 2011).

In three studies no increased incidence of deep vein thrombosis was found when tranexamic acid is given to patients during total knee replacements (Nielsen & Husted, 2002; Orpen et al., 2006; Zhang et al., 2007). According to Nielsen, the optimal effect is reached by starting with a bolus of 10-15 mg/kg. There seems to be less effect in every dose given on top of the initial dose (Nielsen & Husted, 2002). The three afore mentioned studies conclude that the use of tranexamic acid in total knee replacements is an effective way to reduce post-operative blood loss. Camarasa et. al. find the decrease in blood loss reflected in a reduced requirement for allogeneic blood transfusions (Camarasa et al., 2006). In a study by Good et. al. a decrease in total blood loss was also found when using tranexamic acid in total knee replacements. They state however that the concealed blood loss was not that much influenced when tranexamic acid was used (Good et al., 2003).

In a meta-analysis and systemic review by Sukeik et. al., use of tranexamic acid in patients undergoing total hip replacements was studied. According to Sukeik the use of tranexamic acid reduces the requirement for allogeneic blood transfusion. Furthermore, no significant differences were found between control groups and groups in which tranexamic acid was given, concerning adverse events, such as infection rates or deep vein thrombosis (Sukeik et al., 2011).

Ortega-Andreu et. al. compared a group of patients who received tranexamic acid intra-operatively to a control group, consisting of historical patients who had not received tranexamic acid. The tranexamic acid group showed a decrease in allogeneic transfusion rate, lower visible blood loss and proved to be more cost effective than the control group (Ortega-Andreu et al., 2011).

Given the relatively low costs , the effectiveness and the slight chance of adverse events, it can be stated that usage of tranexamic acid is a safe and reliable way of decreasing the need for allogeneic blood transfusion.

5. Postoperative techniques

Postoperatively it still is possible to reduce further allogeneic transfusion.

5.1 Re-transfusion of wound drain fluids

In orthopedic surgery, especially adult reconstruction surgery, such as hip and knee replacements, most patients lose about 1-1.5 liters of blood during surgery if it is not performed using a tourniquet. Especially in knee surgery the tourniquet can, as previously described, reduce the preoperative bloodloss substantially. If a tourniquet has been used, the patient will still lose some 1-1.5 liter blood from the wound but using postoperative collection techniques this blood can be returned to the patient and thus reduce further allogeneic blood transfusion. In hip surgery the use of a tourniquet is, of course, not possible so the amount of blood, shed during surgery, is higher and the use of drainage fluids to return to the patients is more arguable.

At the end of the operation wound drains may be left behind in the wound to reduce swelling and hematoma formation. The fluid from these drains can be collected and, after filtration, be re-infused to the patient (Hendriks et al., 2009). We conducted several studies concerning the use of these drains and their safety. If such a system is to be used the first choice to be made is the type of system one wants to use. Several types of systems are marketed. The main difference between them is the application of continuous vacuum or intermittent vacuum using a bellow system. A second difference between systems is the filter used to reduce the amount of leucocytes and thrombi. Most systems use standard Sangopur® filters which is a gradual screen filter with pore size of 80 and 40 microns. Some systems use a Pall Lipiguard® Filter, which is a depth filter consisting of polyester screen media with variable pore size with the smallest size being 40 microns. A third difference is the vacuum pressure reached. In the bellow systems the maximum vacuum pressure reached is 90 mmHg, whereas in the continuous vacuum systems the vacuum pressure can be as high as 150 mmHg.

The numerous differences between the systems make comparison difficult and give rise to continuous debate.

5.1.1 Vacuum type and pressure

The vacuum type and especially the vacuum pressure has been the subject of debate between producers. It has not been proven one or the other is better. The erythrocytes seem to be able to survive equally well in 90 as in 150 mmHg vacuum. If the vacuum were a problem at higher values the erythrocytes would burst and thus the plasma hemoglobin would be raised in comparison to low vacuum systems. This seems not to be the case if blood is suctioned from containers (Waters et al., 2007). If suctioned from a flat surface the vacuum pressure does make a difference though it is very small (Yazer et al., 2008). 'Although the variable-pressure device produced a significant reduction in hemolysis during one-pass blood collection, the clinical significance of this reduction is not clear. In relative terms, the variable-pressure device would recover an extra 10 ml of RBCs for every liter of salvaged RBCs, which is negligible compared to the blood loss in major surgery.' The drains used in wound drainage, however, do not suck the blood from a flat surface, but from a cavity, more like the cups used in Water's study previously mentioned. Since the vacuum pressure does not seem to matter if the blood is taken from a cavity the activity of the vacuum on the wound healing as such might be taken into account.

The type of vacuum used has proven differences if the effects on wound healing are compared. Berman et al. proved that 80% of the total drainage is collected within 6 hours post-operatively with a constant suction device, whereas with intermittent suction this is spread over days (Berman et al, 1990). Furthermore they state that a clear advantage to using a continuous vacuum suction device over an intermittent spring-loaded device is seen with respect to hematoma evacuation, wound drainage, wound healing, and possible complications.

There are no proper studies addressing the differences between continuous and intermittent suction in re-transfusion drain models.

5.1.2 Filter type

One point that needs addressing if we speak about filter type is whether or not leucocytes from the wound are to be re-transfused into the patient. Especially in cardiac surgery patients who need more than three blood transfusions, leukocyte depletion by filtration of the allogeneic blood, results in a significant reduction of the postoperative mortality. This effect can only partially be explained by the higher incidence of postoperative infections in those receiving packed cells without buffy coat (van de Watering et al., 1998). Some researchers believe the activated leucocytes do no harm, might even improve wound healing by triggering the body to a generalized activated state of inflammation, thus reducing the amount of infections (Innerhofer et al., 2005). The leucocytes activated in the study of Innerhofer, however, were activated by contact with foreign surfaces, not by the wound itself for he used pre-donated autologous blood and compared that to allogeneic blood. Others believe thus activated leucocytes induce a generalized activation of the immune system which reduces lung function and increases the inflammatory response of the body (Gu et al., 1996). Especially in cardiac surgery the effects of extracorporeal circulation have been extensively investigated. Contact of blood with foreign surfaces, as in the containers of the retransfusion systems, activates complement and leucocytes (Kirklin, 1991), as does the suction of the blood from the surgical wound (Bengtsson &

Lisander, 1990; Sieunarine et al., 1991). Washing the blood, which is done in intra-operative cell salvage, does reduce the complement complexes but in the postoperative systems in which the blood is not washed but only filtered, these activated complement complexes pass some of the filters used. Moonen et al described that filters do have an influence on the quality of retransfused blood. The Pall® filter reduced the amount of leucocytes and thrombocytes more adequate then the Sangopur® filter with the latter allowing more erythrocytes to pass (Moonen et al., 2008). The thrombocytes found in the transfused blood using the Sangopur filter® are, since they are not found with use of the Pall® filter and both filters are 40 microns large, likely to be thrombi and not loose thrombocytes. This might mean that the activated complement complexes, being incorporated in the thrombi, pass the Sangopur® filter, thus activating the body's inflammatory response. Some studies investigating the general reactions of the body to retransfused blood found no transfusion reactions nor fevers when transfused with unwashed, filtered autologous blood. Some chills were found, though (up to 3,1%), with use of a non-leucocyte depleting filter (Athanasoulias et al., 2007; Horstmann et al., 2010). Duchow et al found high levels of factor XIIa, thrombin and fibrin generation markers, and markers of fibrinolysis in the shed blood. After re-transfusion increased levels of these markers together with decreased values for factor XIII and plasminogen were found in the circulation indicative of renewed clot formation and fibrinolysis. These changes were highly significant compared to pre-re-transfusion values of the patient's blood. The unwashed drainage blood contained high levels of pro-coagulation material and induced an activation of the plasma coagulation pathway with renewed clot formation and fibrinolysis in the patients (Duchow et al., 2001). De Jong et al found similar results as they found markedly increased activation of leucocytes and platelets and a distinctive decrease in platelet count of the recipient after infusion, thus potentially favoring thrombosis (de Jong, 2007).

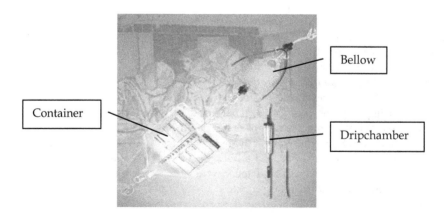

Fig. 4. The Sarstedt retransfusion system

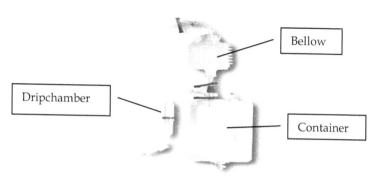

Fig. 5. The Bellovac ABT system

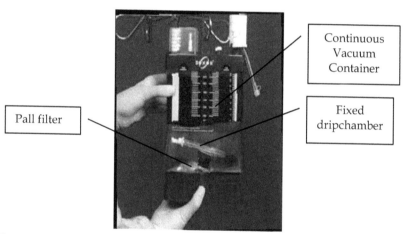

Fig. 6. The Donor system

5.1.3 Total system comparison

No published studies have been done comparing different draining systems for re-transfusion of drain fluids. In a study comparing three systems in a total of 80 patients with 52 hip and 28 knee arthroplaties, a system sold by Sarstedt® (28 patients), which is a bellow system using a stepwise filter of 120 to 10 microns, one from Astra Tech (Bellovac ABT®)(24 patiets), which uses a bellow system and a Sangopur® filter and one from van Straten Medical (Donor®)(28 patients) with a Pall Lipiguard® filter, we tested the Hb, leucocytes, complement C5 and antithrombin 3 (AT3). In the final samples, just before infusing the blood into the patients the measurings were done. Patient characteristics were comparable, and a mean of 484 ml (150-1300 ml) drain fluid was collected. No differences between the systems regarding the amount of drain fluids collected were found. Table 1 shows our findings.

	Sarstedt	Bellovac	Donor
Hb (g/dl)	8.86	11.28	11.44
Leucocytes (x10⁹/l)	3.8	3.4	0.5*
C5 (IE/ml)	78.7	87.7	80.6
AT3 (% of normal)	31.8*	41	37.5

Table 1. Blood component concentrations in the retransfusable blood in the different systems. ($p<0.05$)

As the table shows the levels of AT 3 are substantially lower than normal in blood (0.12 mg/ml), while the levels of C5 are normal and the Hb levels are low. The leucocytes are adequately filtered by the Pall® filter. AT 3 is known to be low after major surgery. Obviously the complement has not been used to activate clotting, not even in the Donor® system which is the only system without heparin coating in the container (van den Boom & van Erve, non published data). The quality of the blood collected in the three systems seems to be comparable although the systems do have different collection mechanisms, (two bellows and one continuous vacuum), different suction pressures (Sarstedt® 70 mmHg, Bellovac ABT® 90 mmHg and Donor® 150 mmHg) and also different filter systems, as previously described.

The choice of system seems to be led by the wish of the physician in attendance to donate the leucocytes and the thrombi back into the patient. Since that is not adequately proven to be good or bad, as mentioned earlier, it remains the choice of the orthopedic surgeon.

5.1.4 Effects of the introduction of re-transfusion of drainage fluid in orthopedic surgery

To determine whether or not the introduction of re-tansfusion of drainage fluid is worthwhile we did a prospective observational study (Hendriks et al., 2009). We compared 195 patients before introduction of the re-transfusion system in our hospital to 175 patients after the introduction of the device. We used the Donor® type drain as described earlier. A restrictive transfusion trigger was used for all patients and patients with a preoperative Hb lower than 13.2 g/dl received EPO (4 doses of 600 IU each). All patients were treated with Acenocoumarol to prevent thrombosis starting the day of surgery (INR targetlevel: 2.5-3.4). Hip and knee arthroplasty patients were evenly distributed between groups as were the other patient characteristics (Table 2). The use of re-transfusion of drainage fluid reduces the use of allogeneic transfusions by 70-98% depending on the type of surgery and the system used.

	Total hip arthoplasty			Total knee arthoplasty		
	No autotra-nsfusion	Autotra-nsfusion	p value	No autotra-nsfusion	autotra-nsfusion	p value
Nr of patients	128	100		67	68	
Male (n/%)	37 (29)	34 (34)	0.41	17 (25)	15 (22)	0.65
Mean age (range)	70.5 (39-95)	69 (46-90)	0.20	71.5 (38-91)	73.7 (53-93)	0.16
Mean nr RBC's (range)	0.4 (0-4)	0.06 (0-2)	<0.01	0.8 (0-6)	0.02 (0-1)	<0.01
Mean volume autotransfusion in ml (range)		409 (0-750)			505(0-1000)	

Table 2. patient characteristics and results of a study into the effects of introductions of an autotransfusion system on the need for allogeneic transfusions in hip and knee arthroplasty patients. (RBC = unit allogeneic blood, p is calculated using χ^2 or t-test)

In a logistic regression analysis in this study the only factor of interest proved to be the use of autologous transfusion.

5.2 Use of a restrictive transfusion trigger

Another important measure to be taken after the operation is the use of a restrictive transfusion trigger. This means that the patient should not be given blood unless the oxygen transport capacity is proven to be lower than the tolerable threshold. The University of Groningen together with the CBO (Centraal Begeleidings Orgaan, Dutch for Central Counseling Bureau) developed a guideline for transfusion which is widely used throughout The Netherlands. It is called 4-5-6 rule (the Hb is expressed in mmol/l in The Netherlands) the international formulation would be: 6.5-8-9.7 rule. The rule is adopted by the national Bloodbank, Sanquin®, and put forward in their transfusion manual (van Rhenen et al., 2011).

This rule uses the ASA class (system developed by the American Society of Anethesiologists) as a guideline to the patient's general health. The ASA class defines the general condition of the patient's health and is used by anesthesiologists worldwide to assess in easy terms the preoperative condition of the patient.

Consider transfusion if the Hb < 6.5 g/dl (Ht: 0,20) and if there is :
   acute blood loss in healthyindividuals (ASA-class I) < 60 years old with
   normovolemia and blood loss in 1 location
   chronic asymptomatic anemia.

Consider transfusion if the Hb < 8 g/dl (Ht: 0,25) and if there is:
   acute blood loss in healthyindividuals (ASA-klasse I) ≥ 60 years old with
   normovolemia and blood loss in1 location
   acute blood loss in healthy individuals < 60 years old with normovolemia and
   blood loss at more than 1 location (polytraumapatients)
   expected blood loss > 500 ml in a patient < 60 years old who will be operated
   upon
   fever
   uncomplicated post-operative period after open heart surgery
   uncomplicated ASA-class II en III

Consider transfusion if the Hb < 9.7 g/dl (Ht: 0,30) and if there is:
   ASA-class IV
   Inability to increase heart minute volume to compensate for
   haemodilution
   sepsis or toxinemia
   serious lungdisease
   symptomatic cerebrovascular disease

Formulated by: University Medical Centre Groningen.
Source: www.cbo.nl/product/richtlijnen/folder20021023121843/bloedkaart.pdf

---

ASA-Classes:
I: healthy individuals;
II: patients with a mild systemic defect, without functional impairment;
III: patients with a seriously impairing systemic defect;
IV: patients with a systemic defect that poses a constant threat for life;
V: patients who are moribund and who will, with or without operation, probably die within 24 hours.

The 4-5-6 rule is an easy to use guide to whether or not transfuse patients based on their capacity to cope with anemia. Several studies showed that postoperative anemia is generally well tolerated as it is in the critically ill. Post-operative anemia after cardiac operations, with hemoglobin levels of 8 to 10 g/dl is well tolerated in patients who have not received a transfusion and induces only a transient impairment of exercise tolerance (Ranucci et al., 2011). Moreover, in critically ill patients a restrictive transfusion trigger is well tolerated (Nichol, 2008) as it is in critically ill children (Lacroix, 2007). The rule of thumb as formulated by the University of Groningen and accepted by the Dutch National Bloodbank and the counseling bureau has proven right in even the critically ill.

For the international community one could consider to change the lower limits from 6.5, 8 and 9.7 to 7, 8 and 10 to make it easier to remember, which is one of the prerequisites for a good rule while still being safe. The limits are thus a little higher than needed, but are comprehensive, easy to remember, easy to use and proven safe. It saves a little less blood than with the limits set more restrictive but the easy application makes the rules more widely acceptable and introducible.

6. Conclusion

In orthopedic surgery, as in other surgeries and in the critically ill, the use of allogeneic blood can be reduced using a wide variety of methods and techniques. All those different methods individually have proven to contribute to the reduction of the use of bank blood. Few if any studies have been done to find out what the combined effect of the introduction of the different methods is. Generally it is assumed the methods and techniques reinforce each other. The additive effect of the used methods is, however, not clear.

The costs of the combination of blood saving methods may, in the end, outweigh the costs of allogeneic blood. It is, however, very difficult to determine the costs of allogeneic blood. In addition to that, the costs are different for every country because of the difference in blood bank systems, salaries and overhead costs.

The effect of hospital admission time has been made clear by Weber et al. who described an increase of hospital admission time of 2.7 days (+/- 0.5 days) per transfused unit of red blood cells in total hip arthroplasty patients(Weber et al., 2005). In a study we performed in 1,422 patients who received a total hip arthroplasty, we found the administration of allogeneic blood to be one of the independent variables in a stepwise regression analysis, for hospital admission time, increasing admission time by 1.78 days per unit Packed cells (p<0.000) (van Erve et al., 2010).

All in all it seems appropriate for all of the above-mentioned measures to be combined to reach the goal set, which is to reduce the administration of allogeneic blood to the minimum.

7. References

Athanasoulias, V. Mavrogenis, AF. Sdrenias, CV. Mitsiokapa, EA. Lourikas, V. Papagelopoulos, PJ & Christodoulou, NA. Post-operative blood salvage and retransfusion in total hip and knee arthroplasty. *J Int Med Res.* 2007;35(2):268-75.

Beattie, WS. Karkouti, K. Wijeysundera, DN & Tait, G. Risk associated with preoperative anemia in noncardiac surgery: a single-center cohort study. *Anesthesiology.* 2009;110(3):574-81.

Bengtsson, A & Lisander, B: Anaphylatoxin and terminal complement complexes in red cell salvage. *Acta Anaethesiol Scand.* 1990;34:339-341.

Bengtsson, A. Bengtson, JP & Kvarnström, A. The safety of Intra-Operative Autologous Transfusion of Filtered Whole Blood in Orthopedic Surgery. *ASA Annual Meeting, Orlando/FL.* 2008 Oct. 18-22.

Benli, IT. Akalin, S. Duman, E. Citak, M & Kis, M. The results of intraoperative autotransfusion in orthopaedic surgery. *Bull Hosp Jt Dis.* 1999;58(4):184-7.

Berman, AT. Fabiano, D. Bosacco, SJ & Weiss, AA. Comparison Between Intermittent (Spring-Loaded) and Continuous Closed Suction Drainage of Orthopedic Wounds. *Orthopedics.* 1990:13(3);309-314.

Bisbe, E. Castillo, J. Sáez, M. Santiveri, X. Ruíz, A & Muños, M. Prevalence of preoperative anemia and hematinic deficiencies in patients scheduled for elective major orthopedic surgery. *Transfusion Alternatives in Transfusion Medicine*, 10:166–173. doi: 10.1111/j.1778-428X.2008.00118.x. 2008.

Bierbaum, BE. Callaghan, JJ. Galante, JO. Rubash, HE. Tooms, RE & Welch, RB. An analysis of blood management in patients having a total hip or knee arthroplasty. *J Bone Joint Surg Am.* 1999;81(1):2-10.

Camarasa, MA. Ollé, G. Serra-Prat, M. Martín, A. Sánchez, M. Ricós, P. Pérez, A. & Opisso, L. Efficacy of aminocaproic, tranexamic acids in the control of bleeding during total knee replacement: a randomized clinical trial. *Br J Anaesth.* 2006;96(5):576-82. Epub 2006 Mar 10.

Carless, PA. Henry, DA. Moxey, AJ. O'Connell, D. Brown, T. & Fergusson, DA. Cell salvage for minimising perioperative allogeneic blood transfusion. *Cochrane Database Syst Rev.* 2010 14;(4):CD001888.

Chertow, GM. Mason, PD. Vaage-Nilsen, O. & Ahlmén, J. Update on adverse drug events associated with parenteral iron. *Nephrol Dial Transplant.* 2006;21(2):378-82. Epub 2005 Nov 11.

Conlon, NP. Bale, EP. Herbison, GP. & McCarroll, M. Postoperative anemia and quality of life after primary hip arthroplasty in patients over 65 years old. *Anesth Analg.* 2008;106(4):1056-61, table of contents.

Critchley, J. & Yenal, D. Adverse events associated with intravenous iron infusion (LMW iron dextran and iron sucrose): a systematic review. *Transfusion Alternative in Transfusion Medicine.* 2007;9(1):8-36.

Davies, L. Brown, TJ. Haynes, S. Payne, K. Elliott, RA. & McCollum, C. Cost-effectiveness of cell salvage and alternative methods of minimising perioperative allogeneic blood transfusion: a systematic review and economic model. *Health Technol Assess.* 2006;10(44):iii-iv, ix-x, 1-210.

De Andrade, JR. Jove, M. Landon, G. Frei, D. Guilfoyle, M. & Young, DC. Baseline hemoglobin as a predictor of risk of transfusion and response to Epoetin alfa in orthopedic surgery patients. *Am J Orthop.* 1996;25:533-542.

De Jong, M. Ray, M. Crawford, S. Whitehouse, SL. & Crawford, RW. Platelet and leukocyte activation in salvaged blood and the effect of its reinfusion on the circulating blood. *Clin Orthop Relat Res.* 2007;456:238-42.

Den Hartog, G. & Roorda, J. Reductie van postoperatief bloedverlies met Cyklokapron bij primaire totale knie en totale heup prothesen. *NTvO.* 2011;18(1):11-14.

Deutsch, A. Spaulding, J. & Marcus, RE. Preoperative epoetin alfa vs autologous blood donation in primary total knee arthroplasty. *J Arthroplasty.* 2006;21(5):628-35.

Domen, RE. Preoperative autologous blood donation: clinical, economic, and ethical issues; *Cleve Clin J Med.* 1996;63(5):295-300.

Duchow, J. Ames, M. Hess, T. & Seyfert, U. Activation of plasma coagulation by retransfusion of unwashed drainage blood after hip joint arthroplasty, a prospective study. *J Arthr.* 2001;16(7):844-849.

Duffy, G. & Neal, KR. Differences in post-operative infection rates between patients receiving autologous and allogeneic blood transfusion: a meta-analysis of published randomized and nonrandomized studies. *Transfusion Medicine.* 1996;6:325-8.

Erslev, AJ. Erythropoietin. *N Engl J Med.* 1991;324:1339-1344

Erstad, BL. Systemic hemostatic medications for reducing surgical blood loss. *Ann Pharmacother.* 2001;35(7):925-934.

Erstad, BL. Antifibrinolytic agents and desmopressin as hemostatic agents in cardiac surgery. *Ann Pharmacother.* 2001;35(9):1075-84.

Faris, PM. Ritter, MA. & Abels, RI. The effects of recombinant human erythropoietin on perioperative transfusion requirements in patients having a major orthopaedic operation: The American Erythropoietin Study Group. *J Bone Joint Surg Am.* 1996;78:62-72.

García-Erce, JA. Cuenca, J. Haman-Alcober, S. Martínez, AA. Herrera, A. & Muñoz, M. Efficacy of preoperative recombinant human erythropoietin administration for reducing transfusion requirements in patients undergoing surgery for hip fracture repair. An observational cohort study. *Vox Sang.* 2009;97(3):260-7. Epub 2009 Jun 3.

Good, L. Peterson, E. & Lisander, B. Tranexamic acid decreases external blood loss but not hidden blood loss in total knee replacement. *Br J Anaesth.* 2003;90(5):596-9.

Goodnough, LT. Despotis, GJ. Merkel, K. & Monk, TG. A randomized trial comparing acute normovolemic hemodilution and preoperative autologous blood donation in total hip arthroplasty. *Transfusion.* 2000;40(9):1054-7.

Goodnough, LT. Maniatis, A. Earnshaw, P. Benoni, G. Beris, P. Bisbe, E. Fergusson, DA. Gombotz, H. Habler, O. Monk, TG. Ozier, Y. Slappendel, R. & Szpalski, M. Detection, evaluation, and management of preoperative anaemia in the elective orthopaedic surgical patient: NATA guidelines. *Br J Anaesth.* 2011;106(1):13–22 doi: 10.1093/bja/aeq361.

Gregoretti, S. Suction-induced hemolysis at various vacuum pressures: implications for intraoperative blood salvage. *Transfusion.* 1996;36 (1):57-60.

Gruson, KI. Aharonoff, GB. Egol, KA. Zuckerman, JD. & Koval, KJ. The relationship between admission hemoglobin level and outcome after hip fracture. *J Orthop Trauma.* 2002;16(1):39-44.

Gu, YJ. De Vries, AJ. Boonstra, PW. & Van Oeveren, W. Leukocyte depletion results in improved lung function and reduced inflammatory response after cardiac surgery. *Jour Thorac Cardiovasc Surg.* 1996;112:494-500.

Hendriks, HGE. Van Erve, RHGP. Salden, H. Van der Zwet, WC. & Barnaart, LFW. Less blood transfusion after the introduction of autotransfusion system in hip and knee replacement [Minder bloedtransfusies na invoering van autotransfusiesysteem bij heup- en knievervanging]. *Ned Tijdschr Geneeskd.* 2009;153:B187. (Dutch).

Henry, DA. Carless, PA. Moxey, AJ. O'Connell, D. Stokes, BJ. Fergusson, DA. & Ker, K. Anti-fibrinolytic use for minimising perioperative allogeneic blood transfusion. *Cochrane Database Syst Rev.* 2011;16;3:CD001886.

Horstmann, WG. Slappendel, R. Van Hellemondt, GG. Castelein, RM. & Verheyen, CCPM. Safety of retransfusion of filtered shed blood in 1819 patients after total hip or knee arthroplasty. *Transfusion Alternatives in Transfusion Medicine.* 2010;11(2):57-64(8).

Innerhofer, P. Klingler, A. Klimmer, C. Fries, D. & Nussbaumer, W. Risk for postoperative infection after transfusion of white blood cell-filtered allogeneic or autologous blood components in orthopedic patients undergoing primary arthroplasty. *Transfusion.* 2005;45(1):103-10.

Johnson-Wimbley, TD. & Graham DY. Diagnosis and management of iron deficiency anemia in the 21st century; *Therap Adv Gastroenterol.* 2011;4(3):177-84.

Keating, EM. Current options and approaches for blood management in orthopaedic surgery. *Instr Course Lect.* 1999;48:655-65.

Keating, EM. Meding, JB. Perioperative Blood Management Practices in Elective Orthopaedic Surgery. *J Am Acad Orthop Surg.* 2002;10(6):393-400.

Kirklin, JK. Prospects for understanding and eliminating the deleterious effects of cardiopulmonary bypass. *Ann Thorac Surg.* 1991;51:529-531.

Kvarnström, A. Schmidt, A. Tylman, M. Jacobsson, M. & Bengtsson, A. Complement split products and proinflammatory cytokines in intraoperatively salvaged unwashed blood during hip replacement: comparison between heparin-coated and non-heparin-coated autotransfusion systems. *Vox Sang.* 2008;95:33-8.

Lacroix, J. Hébert, PC. Hutchison, JS. Hume, HA. Tucci, M. Ducruet, T. Gauvin, F. Collet, JP. Toledano, BJ. Robillard, P. Joffe, A. Biarent, D. Meert, K. & Peters, MJ. TRIPICU Investigators; Canadian Critical Care Trials Group; Pediatric Acute Lung Injury and Sepsis Investigators Network. Transfusion strategies for patients in pediatric intensive care units. *N Engl J Med.* 2007;19;356(16):1609-19.

Lafosse, JM. Minville, V. Chiron, P. Colombani, A. Gris, C. Puorrut, JC. Eychenne, B. & Fourcade, O. Preoperative use of epoietin beta in Total hip replacement: a prospective study. *Arch orth traum surg*. 2010;130(1);41-45, doi:10.1007/s00402-009-0863-3.

Lemaire, R. Strategies for blood management in orthopaedic and trauma surgery. *J Bone Joint Surg Br*. 2008;90(9):1128-36.

Matziolis, D. Perka, C. Hube, R. & Matziolis, G. Influence of tourniquet ischemia on perioperative blood loss after total knee arthroplasty. *Orthopade*. 2011;40(2):178-82.

Moonen, AFCM. Pilot, P. Meijers, WGH. Waelen, RAJ. Leers, MPG. Grimm, B. & Heyligers, IC. Filters in autologous blood retransfusion systems affect the amount of blood cells retransfused in total knee arthroplasty, A pilot study. *Acta Orthop. Belg*. 2008;4:210-215.

Nichol, AD. Restrictive red blood cell transfusion strategies in critical care: does one size really fit all? *Crit Care Resusc*. 2008;10(4):323-7.

Nielsen, RE. & Husted, H. Tranexamic acid reduces blood loss and the need of blood transfusion after knee arthroplasty. *Ugeskr Laeger*. 2002;164(3):326-9.

Orpen, NM. Little, C. Walker, G. & Crawfurd, EJ. Tranexamic acid reduces early post-operative blood loss after total knee arthroplasty: a prospective randomised controlled trial of 29 patients. *Knee*. 2006;13(2):106-10. Epub 2006 Feb 17.

Ortega-Andreu, M. Pérez-Chrzanowska, H. Figueredo, R. & Gómez-Barrena, E. Blood loss control with two doses of tranexamic Acid in a multimodal protocol for total knee arthroplasty. *Open Orthop J*. 2011;5:44-8.

Otten, N. Economic Evaluation of Erythropoietin Use in Surgery. *Ottawa: Canadian Coordinating Office for Health Technology Assessment (CCOHTA)*; 1998.

Ranucci, M. La Rovere, MT. Castelvecchio, S. Maestri, R. Menicanti, L. Frigiola, A. D'Armini, AM. Goggi, C. Tramarin, R. & Febo, O. Postoperative anemia and exercise tolerance after cardiac operations in patients without transfusion: what hemoglobin level is acceptable? *Ann Thorac Surg*. 2011;92(1):25-31. Epub 2011 May 18.

Rawn, J. The Silent Risks of Blood Transfusion. *Current Opinion in Anaesthesiology*. 2008;21(5):664-8.

Sculco, TP. Blood management in orthopedic surgery. *Am J Surg*. 1995;170(6A Suppl):60S-63S.

Seeber, P. & Shander, A. (2007). History and organization of blood management. In: R. Huxley & M. Khan (Eds), *Basics of Blood Management* (Pg. 1). Malden, MA: Blackwell Publishing.

Sepah, YJ. Umer, M. Ahmad, T. Nasim, F. Umer Chaudhry, M. & Umar, M. Use of Tranexamic acid is a cost effective method in preventing blood loss during and after total knee replacement. *J Orthop Surg Res*. 2011;6(1):22.

Serrano-Trenas, JA. Ugalde, PF. Cabello, LM. Chofles, LC. Lázaro, PS. & Benítez, PC. Role of perioperative intravenous iron therapy in elderly hip fracture patients: a single-center randomized controlled trial. *Transfusion*. 2011;51(1):97-104.

Sieunarine, K. Wetherall, J. Lawrence-Brown, MM. Goodman, MA. Prendergast, FJ. & Hellings, M. Levels of complement factor C3 and its activated product, C3a, in operatively salvaged blood. *Aust NZ Jour Surg*. 1991;61:302-395.

Smith, TO. Hing, CB. Is a tourniquet beneficial in total knee replacement surgery? A meta-analysis and systematic review. *Knee.* 2010;17(2):141-7. Epub 2009 Jul 19.

Stachura, A. Król, R. Michalik, D. Pomianowski, S. & Bengtsson, A. Intraoperative collection and transfusion of autologous whole blood – is it safe? Plasma levels of free haemoglobin and potassium. *NATA Symposium Lisbon, Portugal.* 2008 Apr.

Steinitz, D. Harvey, EJ. Leighton, RK. & Petrie, DP. Is homologous blood transfusion a risk factor for infection after hip replacement? *Can J Surg.* 2001;44(5):355-8.

Sukeik, M. Alshryda, S. Haddad, FS. & Mason, JM. Systematic review and meta-analysis of the use of tranexamic acid in total hip replacement. *J Bone Joint Surg Br.* 2011;93(1):39-46.

Vamvakas, EC. & Pineda, AA. Autologous transfusion and other approaches to reduce allogeneic blood exposure. *Baillieres Best Pract Res Clin Haematol.* 2000;13(4):533-47.

Van de Watering, LMG. Hermans, J. Houbiers, JGA. Van den Broek, PJ. Bouter, H. Boer, F. Harvey, MS. Huysmans, HA. & Brand, A. Beneficial Effects of Leukocyte Depletion of Transfused Blood on Postoperative Complications in Patients Undergoing Cardiac Surgery: A Randomized Clinical Trial. *Circulation.* 1998;97:562-568 doi: 10.1161/01.CIR.97.6.562.

Van den Boom, LGH. & Van Erve, RHGP. A prospective cohortstudy with 3 different retreansfusion systems after Total hip and Total knee arthroplasty [Een prospectieve cohortstudie met 3 verschillende retransfusiesystemen na totale heup-en knie arthroplastiek], *nonpublished data.*

Van Erve, RHGP. Results of a blood management program introduced in an orthopaedic practice, reduction of blood products, hospital time, and choice of system. *Transfusion.* 2008;48:2034 SABM abstracts #710.

Van Erve, RHGP. Wippert, I. Six Dijkstra, WMC. & Oosterveld, FGJ. Is ASA class a predictor for longer hospital stay in short track programs for elective total hip arthroplasties? [Is de ASA classificatie een voorspellende factor voor een verlenging van de ligduur in een short track programma voor electieve totale heup arthroplastieken?] (Dutch) *Presentation for the annual congress of the Dutch Orthopedic Society;* 22 Jan 2010 Abstract in *NTvO* 2010;17(1):55-56.

Van Rhenen, DJ. Haas, FJLM. & De Vries, RRP. In: *TRANSFUSIEGIDS samengesteld op basis van de CBO Richtlijn Bloedtransfusie 2011*, march 2011 (Dutch).

Waters, JH. Williams, B. Yazer, MH. & Kameneva, MV. Modification of suction-induced hemolysis during cell salvage. *Anesth. Analg.* 2007;104 (3):684-7.

Weber, EW. Slappendel, R. Prins, MH. Van der Schaaf, DB. Durieux, ME. & Strümper, D. Perioperative blood transfusions and delayed wound healing after hip replacement surgery: effects on duration of hospitalization. *Anesth Analg.* 2005;100(5):1416-21.

Wiekenkamp, AC. Salden, H. Gerrits, HJ. & Van Erve, RHGP. Patient safety in two systems for intraoperative autologous blood reinfusion in elective total hip arthroplasties. *Presented at the annual congress of the Dutch Orthopedic Society 2010 jan.* Abstract in *NTvO* 2010;17(2):105-106.

Yazer, MH. Waters, JH. Elkin, KR. Rohrbaugh, ME. & Kameneva, MV. A comparison of hemolysis and red cell mechanical fragility in blood collected with different cell salvage suction devices. *Transfusion.* 2008;48(6):1188-91.

Blood Transfusion Therapy in High Risk Surgical Patients

João Manoel Silva Junior[1] and Alberto Mendonça P. Ferreira[2]

[1]*Anesthesiology and intensive care Department,*
Hospital do Servidor Público Estadual, São Paulo,
[2]*Intensive Care Department from Hospital do Servidor Público Estadual, São Paulo*
Brazil

1. Introduction

Anemia is common in surgical patients. The number of patients transfused with red blood cell (RBC) in the United States increased from 12.2 million, to more than 14 million most recently, specially in the perioperative period (Park et al. 2004). Anemia is associated with considerable morbidity and poor outcome. Equally, blood transfusion has been related to worse outcome, including in surgical patients (Sakr et al. 2010).

Transfusion is the cornerstone of treatment for serious anemia in this population, to restore oxygen carrying capacity, consequently, reducing tissue hypoxia. Vincent and colleagues reported a 37% transfusion rate in intensive care unit (ICU) patients, and directly 73% of patients who remained in the ICU more than one week received transfusion (Vincent et al. 2002). Similarly, Taylor and colleagues found 85% transfusion rate among patients who stayed in the ICU more than seven days (Taylor et al. 2002).

Blood transfusion was independently associated with organ failure, longer ICU length of stay and increased risk of death. Possible, because deleterious effects of transfusions, especially, immunosuppression that is associated with nosocomial infection and directly related to the number of packed red cells unit used (Taylor et al. 2002).

Another complication is the transfusion-related acute lung injury (TRALI). TRALI is determined as a non-cardiogenic pulmonary edema, temporary related to the transfusion (Looney et al. 2004).

Besides, there were no radical changes in transfusion practice over time. Recent study has demonstrated that mean pre-transfusion hemoglobin was about 8.0g/l. In 30% of patients hemoglobin concentrations are targeted above 9g/dl (Silva Jr et al. 2008).

Hébert and colleagues, in a randomized controlled study, investigated the impact of two different therapeutic strategies for anemia in ill critical patients (Hebert et al. 1999). A restrictive transfusion strategy (hemoglobin concentrations targeted above 7g/dl) was as effective as and maybe more efficient than a liberal strategy (hemoglobin concentrations targeted above 10g/dl). A subgroup of patients that presented unstable angina was excluded. According to this evidence, it is recommended a blood transfusion trigger of 7.0g/dl for ICU patients.

The cause of anemia in these patients is likely to be multifactorial.

Intraoperative:
Loss of blood:
Surgery, trauma
Blood sampling
Other bleeding
Postoperative:
Gastrointestinal bleeding
Less production
Lower red cells production:
Lower erythropoietin synthesis
Erythropoietin resistence
Iron shortage
Erythrocytes half life decrease
Hemolysis increase

Table 1. Factors associated with anemia in peri-operative period

2. Blood transfusion epidemiology

Because of the high anemia incidence perioperatively, many patients will receive blood transfusion at some point. Many studies have appraised the blood transfusion epidemiology.

In a Canadian study, enrolling 5298 people, 25% from patients received blood transfusion (Hebert et al. 1999). In the United Kingdom, this number escalated to 53% of 1247 patients during length of ICU stay. The ABC study, in 146 ICUs from Western Europe, covered 3534 patients and showed 37% transfusion rate in ICU. Longer length of hospital stay was associated with blood transfusion (25% with 2 days, 56% with more than 2 days and 73% with more than seven days).

In the CRIT study, 44% of the patients received one or more transfusions in ICU (Corwin et al. 2004). The recent SOAP (*Sepsis Occurrence in Acutely ill Patients*) study showed a 33% transfusion incidence (Vincent et al. 2008).

Finally, a randomized study made with patients in postoperative period for cardiac surgery demonstrated that blood transfusion with hemoglobin trigger of 7 g/dl did not result in a worst clinical evolution. Otherwise, there was better outcome (Hajjar et al. 2010).

Authors	Year when the study was made	Number of patients	Transfusion percentage	Comments
Herbert et al	1999	5298	25%	Significant institutional variation was identified in the transfusion practice
Vincent et al	1999	3534	37%	For patients with similar levels of organ dysfunction, the ones who received blood transfusion displayed high mortality rates
Rao et al	1999	1247	53%	Average pre-transfusion hemoglobin was greater than 9g/dl in 75% of the transfusions
Corvin et al	2000/2001	4892	44%	The number of transfusions was associated with a greater length hospitalization and ICU stay, and greater mortality
Walsh et al	2001	1023	39,5%	Almost half of the transfusions were not associated with signifcant bleeding
French et al	2001	1808	19,8%	The most common transfusion indication was acute bleeding. Only 3% of the transfusions were considered inappropriate
Hajjar et al	2010	512	63%	As greater number of transfusions as greater mortality within 30 days. The restrictive strategy resulted in less complications

Table 2. Recent important studies assessing transfusion periodicity

3. Oxygen transportation

Hemoglobin (Hb) is essential to oxygen transportation. Human Hb is composed of 2 α and 2 β chains of polypeptides. One heme group transport one molecule of oxygen (1 g of Hb ties 1.39 mL of O2) and changes in hemoglobin affinity for oxygen correlates with change in red cell 2,3- Diphosphoglycerate (2,3-DPG) content, carbon dioxide, pH and body temperature.

The 2,3-DPG molecule binds to one of the b-chains of Hb favouring deoxygenation, reducing hemoglobin oxygen affinity. Thereby, low 2,3-DPG concentrations increases the Hb affinity to O2, dislocating the oxyhemoglobin dissociation curve to the left, described as P50 (PO2 at which the hemoglobin becomes 50% saturated with oxygen). P50 in adults is 26.3 mmHg (Moore et al. 2005).

The blood concentration of hydrogen ion or carbon dioxide reduces hemoglobin oxygen affinity, the Bohr effect. Otherwise, the Haldane effect states that deoxygenated Hb has a greater affinity for CO2 than does oxyHb. Only 10% of the carbon dioxide is removed from the tissues as carboxyhemoglobin, 80% is removed as bicarbonate and 10% remaining as physical solution.

In addition, low body temperature and high blood pH increases the Hb affinity to O2 and reduces P50.

4. Blood transfusion risks and benefits

Blood transfusion is safer today, however adverse are events still clinically relevant. The expected benefit is to improve the oxygen demand, preventing cellular injury. However, it is difficult to demonstrate these benefits in current clinical studies.

Risks related to blood transfusion are divided in infectious and noninfectious. Infectious risks include HIV transmission, estimated in 1:676,000 transfusions in the USA and transmission of A, B and C hepatitis virus, estimated in 1:1,000,000, 1:63,000 and 1:103,000, respectively (Goodnough et al. 2003).

Other viral infections related to transfusions are the human T-lymphotropic virus (HTLV) types I and II, the parvovirus B19 and the Creutzfeldt-Jacob disease, caused by a prion, causing encephalopathy with fast evolution to dementia.

As viral infections, bacterial infections are also frequent complications of transfusion. The contamination incidence is 1 per 1,000,000 transfusion units in USA. The most important bacterial infections are caused by gram-negative bacteria, such as *Yersinia enterocolitica*, *Serratia* and *Pseudomonas*, which have the ability to grow even between 1 and 6 °C. The contamination rate is associated with the blood packed storage time (Shorra et al. 2005).

Immunosupression is a noninfectious complication, that increase the risk of infection. Other noninfectious risks are related to acute lung injury and human error, when there is an incorrect identification of the patients or the red blood cell package. In this case, it can cause hemolytic reactions.

The transfusion related acute lung injury (TRALI) is one of the most serious complications by noninfectious causes and is defined as acute respiratory disease that happens within the first 4 hours after the transfusion. TRALI is distinguished by dyspnea and hypoxia due to noncardiogenic pulmonary edema. The incidence is about 1 to 5000 transfusions. The treatment is just support.

		Incidence frequency per a million units (for current unit)
Infectious		
Virus		
	Hepatitis B	4 (1/220,000)
	Hepatitis C	1 (1/800,000–1/1.6 X10^6)
	HIV	1 (1/1.4–2.4 X10^6)
Bacteria		
	Red blood cells	2 (1/500,000)
	Platelets	500 (1/2,000)
Acute hemolytic transfusion reaction		1 to 4 (1/250,000–1,000,000)
Delayed hemolytic transfusion reaction		1000 (1/1,000)
TRALI		125 (1/8,000)

Adapted from Goodnough LT, et al. *New Engl J Med* 1999; 340:438–447.

Table 3. Risk estimates for blood transfusions.

Silva Jr. and colleagues reported a 57.5% incidence of post-operative complications in ICU patients. Mostly frequent, up to 28 days after the blood transfusion, and included infections (36.3%), changes in the markers of tissue hypoperfusion (30.0%), shock (22.5%), Acute Renal Failure (ARF) (12.5%), cognitive changes (11.33%), fistulas of the digestive tract (6.3%), and ARDS (5.0%) (Silva Jr et al. 2008).

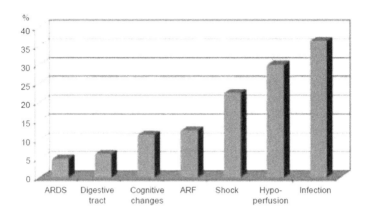

Fig. 1. Postoperative complications. Columns indicate the percentage of postoperative complications.

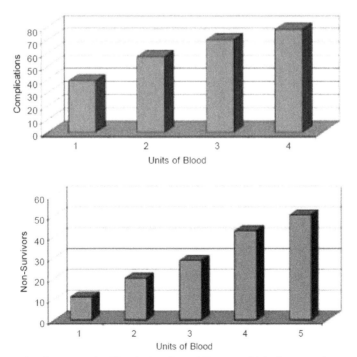

Fig. 2. Relationship between the Blood Number of Units and Morbi-mortality

In addition, the number of units of blood transfused was directly related to the incidence of these complications and mortality, i.e., the greater the number of units transfused intraoperatively, it was higher the chances of complications and death in the postoperative period. (Silva Jr et al. 2008)

5. Blood transfusion necessity assessment

The optimal transfusion trigger in ICU patients has been a matter of controversy. The ongoing debate about risks and benefits regarding blood transfusions is based on a individual assessment, considering diagnosis and comorbidities to help therapeutic aproach.

Serum concentrations of hemoglobin would be an easy reference and were used for years as a guide to start transfusions, but the optimal hemoglobin concentration varies considerably in each patient, according to several characteristics as age, preexisting chronic diseases (coronariopathy), current diagnosis and the cause of anemia.

Using the simple hemoglobin level, below which all patients should be transfused, and specific values for certain groups, are also rigid. The concept of critical hemoglobin level, defined as the minimal hemoglobin concentration while there is no pathological O2 supply dependency, seems to be a reasonable indication for blood transfusion.

There are some parameters to evaluate tissue hypoxia in clinical practice, like blood lactate, but this parameter indicates that the hypoperfusion is already in place and may be too late to indicate the point to start transfusion. However, a recent study in surgical patients demonstrated that transfused patients with high venous oxygen saturation had worse outcomes in the postoperative period (Silva JM et al. 2009).

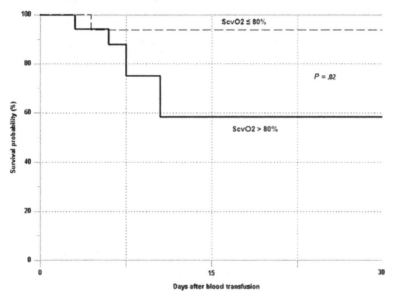

Fig. 3. Kaplan-Meier curve of transfused patients with ScvO2 80% or less and ScvO2 greater than 80%: (Silva JM et al. 2009).

Hébert and colleagues (Hebert et al. 2001) demonstrated in their study that, in critically ill patients, hemoglobin levels between 7 g/dl and 9 g/dl are safe (except in patients with myocardial infarction and unstable angina). Hajjar and colleagues (Hajjar et al. 2010) have also demonstrated that in postoperative cardiac patient hemoglobin level of 7 g/dl is safe and blood transfusion was associated with higher rates of complication.

Today the recommendations for septic hemodinamically stable or unstable patients are to maintain hemoglobin levels around 7g/dl before indicate transfusion. Besides, a study in health volunteers with isovolumetric hemodilution and hemoglobin concentration ≤ 5.0 g/dl, did not result in clear anaerobic metabolism (Weiskopf et a. 1998). Moreover, studies made with Jehovah's Witnesses patients showed that survival is possible even with lower hemoglobin levels. In a case report, a patient presenting hemoglobin level of 1.8 g/dL, had a acceptable evolution (Howell et al. 1998).

6. Strategies to avoid blood transfusion risks

There are several techniques to prevent blood transfusion, but they are summarized in blood loss optimization, blood cells production increasing and auto transfusion.

Several evidences show that the most effective way to increase blood production is the use of erythropoietin in preoperative period, but the time to reach recommended hemoglobin values is very long, making the process very slow and not useful.

Among the self-transfusion modes, there is the self preoperative donation (removing the blood before the surgery and, if needed, using it in the intraoperative or postoperative). This method is recommended only for patients above 20 kg . Besides that, this technique may be accompanied by hemodilution, allowed for patients with hematocrit above 35%. The blood is replaced, using crystalloid fluids to lower hematocrit to 25%, recommended for patients above 1 year old, because of the presence of fetal hemoglobin in neonates. Thus, this technique can be used shortly before surgery.

During the intraoperative, the self-transfusion can be performed using machines that reutilize the lost blood on surgery. In cardiac surgeries, the blood from the extracorporeal circulation circuit is returned. The same technique is difficult to be performed in children, because the lost blood is too small to be replaced.

In an attempt to prevent intraoperative blood losses, there are some measures such as desmopressin 0.3 ug/kg, which stimulates the release of von Willebrand factor, needed for platelets adhesiveness for damaged tissues, which does not apply to pediatric patients, and antifibrinolytics, preventing fibrinolysis and stabilizing clot formation. This last, in spite of reducing bleeding, it showed some harm potential, because it can cause thrombi, leading to myocardial ischemia and renal failure. Finally, the recombinant activated factor seven (rFVIIa) has shown positive evidence in patients with trauma and heavy bleeding.

Another way to avoid the transfusion risks is the minimal exposure to transfusion, in other words, transfusion from a single donnor and permissive hypotension, in an attempt to prevent blood losses. But we must consider the risks and benefits, being contraindicated in children under 2 years and patients with systemic diseases, showing vital organs damages.

The transfusion reactions risks can also be minimized by the using of the leukoreduction of blood, which means to remove leukocytes in transfused blood, resulting in less immunological effects because of the transfusion, such as alloimmunization to leukocyte antigens, febrile reactions and TRALI.

7. Massive transfusion

Massive transfusion defined as a whole blood volume changed within 24 hours, a replacement greater than 10 units of RBC packages within 24 hours, greater than 4 units of RBC packages within 1 hour or a 50% replacement of total blood volume within 3 hours.

So, the strategy used in intense and uncontrollable bleeding is to prevent the overuse of isotonic crystalloid solutions and to associate massive transfusions to early administration of products that help hemostasis (plasma, platelets and cryoprecipitate) in proportion to the blood transfusion, in other words, 1 erythrocytes concentrate: 1 plasma: 1 platelet, measure that has brought great benefits in patients requiring large transfusions.

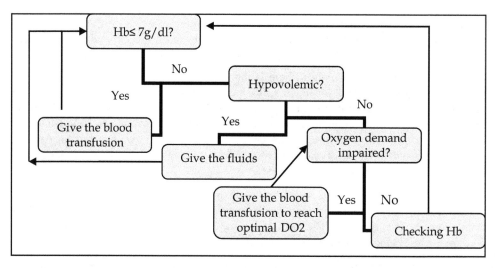

Fig. 4. Transfusion therapy summary in surgical patients.

8. Conclusion

Anemia is common in surgical patients and results in numerous blood transfusions. There are few evidences showing that blood transfusions are benefic to surgical patients. For those patients without active bleeding or acute cardiovascular disease, 7g/dl hemoglobin is well within tolerable limits. Besides hypoperfusion associated with low hemoglobin level appears to be an important indicator to be taken into consideration to decide for blood transfusion. Strategies to avoid blood losses and increase blood production may as well be an important tool for those patients.

9. References

[1] Carson JL, Duff A, Poses RM, et al. Effect of anaemia and cardiovascular disease on surgical mortality and morbidity. *Lancet* 1996;348:1055-60.

[2] Chernow B: Blood conservation in critical care—The evidence accumulates. 1993; 21: 481–482.

[3] Corwin HL, Gettinger A, Pearl RG, et al: The CRIT Study: Anemia and blood transfusion in the critically ill—Current clinical practice in the United States. *Crit Care Med* 2004; 32: 39–52.

[4] Dellinger RP, Carlet JM, Masur H, et al: Surviving sepsis campaign guidelines for management of severe sepsis and septic shock. *Crit Care Med* 2004; 32:858–873.

[5] French CJ, Bellomo R, Finfer SR, et al: Appropriateness of red blood cell transfusion in Australasian intensive care practice. *Med J Aust* 2002; 177:548–551.

[6] Foulke GE, Harlow DJ: Effective measures for reducing blood loss from diagnostic laboratory tests in intensive care unit patients. *Crit Care Med* 1989; 1143–1145.

[7] Goodnough LT: Risks of blood transfusion. *Crit Care Med* 2003; 31(2): S678-S686.

[8] Hajjar LA.; Vincent JL; Galas FRBG.; et al. Transfusion Requirements After Cardiac Surgery: The TRACS Randomized Controlled Trial. *JAMA*. 2010;304(14):1559-1567

[9] Hebert PC, Wells G, Tweeddale M, et al. Does transfusion practice affect mortality in critically ill patients? Am J Respir Crit Care Med 1997; 155:1618-23.

[10] Hebert PC, Wells G, Blajchman MA, et al: A multicenter, randomized, controlled clinical trial of transfusion requirements in critical care. *N Engl J Med* 1999; 340:409–417

[11] Hebert PC, Wells G, Martin C, et al: Variation in red cell transfusion practice in the intensive care unit: A multicentre cohort study. *Crit Care* 1999; 3:57–63.

[12] Hebert PC, Yetisir E, Martin C, et al: Is a low transfusion threshold safe in critically ill patients with cardiovascular diseases? *Crit Care Med* 2001; 29:227–234.

[13] Howell PJ, Bamber PA: Severe acute anaemia in a Jehovah's Witness. Survival without blood transfusion. *Anaesthesia* 1987; 42: 44–48.

[14] Looney MR, et al. Transfusion-Related Acute Lung Injury. A Review. CHEST 2004; 126:249-258.

[15] Madjdpour C, Spahn DR, Weiskopf RB: Anemia and perioperative red blood cell transfusion: A matter of tolerance. Crit Care Med 2006; 34 (5): 102S-108S.

[16] Moore EE., Johnson JL., Cheng AM., et al: Insights from studies of blood substitutes in trauma. *Shock* 2005; 24(3): 197–205

[17] Park KW. Chandhok D. Transfusion-associated complications. *International Anesthesiology Clinics*. 42(3):11-26, 2004.

[18] Rao MP, Boralessa H, Morgan C, et al: Blood component use in critically ill patients. *Anaesthesia* 2002; 57:530–534.

[19] Robinson WP III, Ahn J, Stiffler A, et al. Blood transfusion is an independent predictor of increased mortality in nonoperatively managed blunt hepatic and splenic injuries. *J Trauma* 2005;58:437-44.

[20] Russell JA, Phang PT. The oxygen delivery/consumption controversy: an approach to management of the critically ill. *Am J Respir Crit Care Med* 1994;149:533-7.

[21] Sakr Y, Lobo S, Knuepfer S, Esser E, Bauer M, Settmacher U, Barz D, Reinhart K. Anemia and blood transfusion in a surgical intensive care unit. *Crit Care*. 2010; 14(3): R92.

[22] Shorra AF, Jacksonb WL: Transfusion practice and nosocomial infection: assessing the evidence. *Current Opinion in Critical Care* 2005; 11:468-472.

[23] Silliman CC, et al. Transfusion-Related Acute Lung Injury. Review Article. *Blood* 2005; 105:2266-2273.

[24] Silva JM Jr, Toledo DO, Magalhães DD, Pinto MA, Gulinelli A, Sousa JM, da Silva IF, Rezende E, Pontes-Arruda A. Influence of tissue perfusion on the outcome of surgical patients who need blood transfusion. *J Crit Care.* 2009;24(3):426-34.

[25] Silva Jr João Manoel, Cezario T Abreu, Toledo Diogo O, Magalhães D Dourado, Pinto M Aurélio Cícero, Victoria L Gustavo F. Complications and prognosis of intraoperative blood transfusion. *Rev. Bras. Anestesiol.* 2008; 58(5): 447-46.

[26] Taylor RW, Manganaro L, O'Brien J, Trottier SJ, Parkar N, Veremakis C. Impact of allogenic packed red blood cell transfusion on nosocomial infection rates in the critically ill patient. *Crit Care Med* 2002;30:2249-54.

[27] Vincent JL, Baron JF, Reinhart K, et al: Anemia and blood transfusion in critically ill patients. *JAMA* 2002; 288:1499-1507.

[28] Vincent JL, Piagnerelli M. Transfusion in the intensive care unit. *Crit Care Med* 2006; 34, No. 5 (Suppl.): S96-S101.

[29] Vincent JL, Sakr Y, Sprung C, Harboe S, Damas P: Are blood transfusions associated with greater mortality rates? Results of the Sepsis Occurrence in Acutely Ill Patients study. *Anesthesiology* 2008, 108: 31-39.

[30] Walsh TS, Garrioch M, Maciver C, et al: Red cell requirements for intensive care units adhering to evidence-based transfusion guidelines. *Transfusion* 2004; 44:1405-1411.

[31] Weiskopf RB, Viele MK, Feiner J, et al: Human cardiovascular and metabolic response to acute, severe isovolemic anemia. *JAMA* 1998; 279:217-221.

5

Scope of Blood Transfusion in Obstetrics

Subhayu Bandyopadhyay
Ninewells Hospital, Dundee,
UK

1. Introduction

Obstetrics is one of the major areas in medicine requiring blood transfusion. In the UK about 4000 cases of severe obstetric haemorrhage take place each year, of which most of the patients need blood transfusion (RCOG Green top guideline no. 47). On one hand maternal morbidity and even mortality depends on availability of blood and blood products and on the other hand injudicious use of blood and blood products can cause infection, allergic reaction or antibody production in the mother which can have major impact on the present or future pregnancies (Blood transfusion in obstetrics , RCOG Green top guideline no. 47). The most common complication of blood transfusion is error in transfusion. In the UK, SHOT (Serious Hazard Of Transfusion) is informed about all the complications of transfusion. The largest category of untoward incidents reported to SHOT is 'incorrect blood component transfused' (71%) and the incidence is on the rise (SHOT in Obstetrics: 2005 Annual Report). In this chapter we will discuss the main indication for blood transfusion in obstetric practice in developed world and the ways to prevent blood transfusion.

In modern day obstetric practice, the complications of blood transfusion is well-recognised and in many hospitals in the UK, protocols are in place to boost pre-delivery haemoglobin, so that blood transfusion can be avoided in case of postpartum haemorrhage. If the mother has low haemoglobin in the antenatal period then oral iron supplement (Ferrous Sulphate or Ferrous Fumerate) should be given. Intravenous iron is indicated when there is poor tolerance to oral iron or a quick response is needed. There are two main preparations: iron-dextran and iron sucrose. There is evidence that intravenous iron therapy replenishes iron stores faster and more efficiently than oral iron therapy (Singh et al 1998). Recombinant human erythropoietin is used when anaemia is caused by renal disease. It is safe to use in pregnancy and there is no reported cases of teratogenicity (Braga et al 1996).

There are two main indications for blood transfusion in obstetrics: Ante Partum Hemorrhage (APH) and Post Partum Hemorrhage (PPH). The other important and common indication for blood transfusion in pregnancy is ectopic pregnancy, which like miscarriage may be considered as a gynaecological cause in most units. In the developing world obstetric haemorrhage is the most important cause for maternal morbidity and sometimes mortality (Saving Mothers' Lives: CEMACH Report 2003-2005). In view of all the complications of the blood transfusion, it is only prudent to use blood and blood products with caution and when appropriate. All the other pharmacological agents should be used first. The newer techniques of management of PPH (Intrauterine balloon, use of cell salvage and recombinant factor seven) have revolutionised management of PPH in developed world.

Anaemia in pregnancy: It is hard to determine the prevalence of anaemia in pregnancy in both developing and developed world due to the difference in definition of anaemia worldwide. In the developing world it is found in most severe form whereas in the developed world it is mild. In a comprehensive report on prevalence of anaemia worldwide by WHO (WHO Global Database on Anaemia), the prevalence of anaemia in Afghanistan was highest (61%). In the developed world prevalence of severe anaemia is uncommon (USA 5.7 % of pregnant women and UK 15.2%) .However, in the developed world it is seldom an indication for blood transfusion by itself, when there is no ongoing bleeding or haematological disorder has not been incriminated as the cause for the anaemia.

2. Early pregnancy complications

There are two main types of early pregnancy complications may need blood transfusion - Miscarriage and ectopic pregnancy.

There are different types of miscarriages:

a. Threatened miscarriage
b. Incomplete miscarriage
c. Complete miscarriage
d. Inevitable miscarriage
e. Missed miscarriage

Patients classically presents with heavy vaginal bleeding and cramp like lower abdominal pain in most of the types. Missed Miscarriage may remain asymptomatic and sometimes an incidental finding during routine ultrasound examination. Speculum examination may reveal open cervical os in case of incomplete and inevitable miscarriage. Bleeding can be heavy and sometimes clinically underestimated. Careful assessment of bleeding and timely decision of operative management can prevent unnecessary blood transfusion and prolonged hospital stay.

2.1 Ectopic pregnancy

Ectopic pregnancy is defined as implantation of blastocyst at a site other than uterine cavity. It may develop in the fallopian tube (most common), ovaries or even peritoneum.

The main complication of ectopic pregnancy is rupture and if prompt medical attention is not given, it can even be fatal due to intraperitoneal bleeding from the ruptured fallopian tube. It is a common and important cause of maternal morbidity and mortality worldwide, especially in developing countries, where prompt medical care and facilities for blood transfusion is not available. Even in developed countries like UK, the morbidity and mortality can be high. There were 13 maternal deaths deaths from ruptured ectopic pregnancy in 1997-1999 (CEMACH report 2001)

2.1.1 Risk factors for ectopic pregnancy

Idiopathic
Salpingitis - Possibility of sexually transmitted infection should be excluded (Ankum et al 1996)
Previous ectopic pregnancy (Bouyer et al 1996)

Failure of sterilisation
History of infertility
Increased Maternal age

2.1.2 Presentation

The patient typically presents with pain in one of the iliac fosse which may or may not be associated with vaginal bleeding. The pain and bleeding can be of varying severity. Sometimes the patient may pass decidual cast with vaginal bleeding which can be confused with product of conception.

2.1.3 Diagnosis

Ectopic pregnancy is difficult to diagnose clinically as most of the time the patient compensates for bleeding and not tachycardic or hypotensive unless significant intraperitoneal bleeding has taken place. Speculum examination of the cervix may be helpful in excluding miscarriage where the cervical os is open. Vaginal examination may show cervical excitation which, if positive, points towards ectopic pregnancy. However it is not a specific test for ectopic. Ultrasound scan is the investigation of choice. Also, in asymptomatic patients, serial BHCG can be checked to exclude ectopic pregnancy.

2.1.4 Management

There are two main treatment options- Surgical and Medical. An expectant approach may be taken in some selective asymptomatic patients with variable success.

Surgical: Laparoscopic salpingectomy is the surgical method of choice in hemodynamically stable patients. Compared to laparotomy, it is associated with less intraoperative blood loss, shorter operative time and shorter hospital stay (Murphy et al 1992 and Gray et al 1995)

If the patient is not hemodynamically stable, management should be by quickest method, which in most cases is by laparotomy. However, it does depend on surgeon's expertise (RCOG Guideline no 21). Crossmatched blood should be available prior to operation as it is difficult to predict the degree of haemorrhage.

If the contralateral tube is not healthy, a salpingotomy can be considered instead of salpingectomy to increase the chance of intrauterine pregnancy in future (Silva et al 1993)

Medical Management: Methotrexate is used for the management of ectopic pregnancy in a stable patient. The patient should always be counselled about the possibility of rupture. Lipscomb et al. (1998) has shown methotraxate to be as effective as surgery in suitable patients.

All mothers with Rh negative blood group should receive Anti D immunoglobulin (RCOG Guideline no 21).

3. Antepartum Haemorrhage

Antepartum Hemorrhage (APH) classically is described as any bleeding from the genital tract after 24 weeks of pregnancy. Spotting or minimal bleeding is common in pregnancy and cervical cause, such as ectropion should be ruled out first. If the patient is having regular contraction, heavy show (which is a sign of labour) should be ruled out as well.

There are two major causes of APH -Placenta previa & Placental Abruption which might need blood transfusion.

3.1 Risk assessment for APH

(RCOG. Green top Guideline No. 27 & National Collaborating Centre for Women's and Children's Health. Antenatal care: Clinical Guideline. 2003).

- During the anomaly/detailed ultrasound scan at 18-22 weeks:placental localisation should be done.
- Further scans after 30 weeks to confirm low-lying placenta,if placenta was found to be low in the earlier scans.
- Anaemia, if present to be corrected during antenatal period
- If previous caesarean section: exclude placenta accreta exclude placenta accreta in the third trimester
- In case of placental abruption: Remember that there might be concealed bleeding and not all of the bleeding is apparent.

3.2 Diagnosis of placenta previa

Placenta previa is defined as when the placenta covers the internal os of the cervix partly or fully in such a way as to prevent the baby's head to deliver vaginally. It is one of the most important causes for maternal morbidity in obstetrics and contributes not only to Antepartum haemorrhage, but also post partum haemorrhage (Onwere et al 2011). It is divided into two categories by ultrasound scan: Major, when the placenta covers the internal os fully and minor, when it is close to internal os but does not cover it fully. Transvaginal ultrasound scan is vital in diagnosing placenta previa, especially when it is posterior (RCOG. Green top Guideline No. 27 & Leerentveld RA 1990).

Clinical Signs/symptoms
1. Recurrent painless vaginal bleeding in third trimester
2. Persistent malpresentation such as transverse lie, breech, oblique lie.
3. High presenting part in labour
Ultrasound Scan:
1. Suspect at anomaly scan (second trimester)
2. If placenta is low-lying in second trimester scan, confirm placental position in third trimester
3. Ultrasound scan if sufficient degree of suspicion ,even when the placenta is not noted to be low-lying in second trimester
4. Transvaginal ultrasound is safe and particularly useful in posterior placenta previa
5. Possible to diagnose placenta accreta or percreta by ultrasound scan.
MRI Scan: Reserved for suspected placenta accreta, percreta and increta

Table 1. Diagnosis of Placenta Previa.

3.3 Placental abruption

Abruption on the other hand is the separation of the placenta from the uterine wall. The bleeding resulting from the separation can be fully or partly revealed or sometimes can be concealed. The problem of concealed bleeding is that a major internal haemorrhage can take place before the patient becomes symptomatic. Hence, it can be difficult to diagnose and manage. The patient typically presents in third trimester with severe abdominal pain and vaginal bleeding with or without intra-uterine fetal death. The uterus has classically been described as woody hard. Sheiner et al showed that the perinatal morbidity and mortality is significantly higher in placental abruption (OR = 30.0, 95% CI 19.7-45.6; p < 0.001). Common causes of placental abruption are mentioned in table 2.

3.3.1 Diagnosis of placental abruption

Diagnosis of placental abruption is mainly clinical. The patient commonly presents with abdominal pain and vaginal bleeding. Bleeding is generally less severe than placenta previa. It is important to rule out concealed bleeding. In case of significant abruption the CTG may show fetal distress or even intrauterine fetal death. The condition is sometimes complicated by disseminated intravascular coagulopathy. Management is by delivery of the baby if there is evidence of fetal distress. If there is intrauterine death, vaginal delivery can be considered after correction of coagulopathy. Management plan should be discussed with the anaesthetist, haematologist and paediatrician- if there is fetal distress or preterm delivery.

• Pregnancy induced hypertension: pre-eclampsia and eclampsia (Ananth et al 1997)
• Polyhydramnios or oligohydramnios (Hung et al 2007)
• Cocaine misuse (Mbah et al 2011)
• Trauma (OR = 10.0; 95% CI 3.9-25.5; P < 0.001) (Weintraub 2006)
• Maternal diabetes (Dafallah & Babikir 2004)

Table 2. Common causes of abruption of placenta

3.4 Management of major antepartum haemorrhage

3.4.1 Management of placenta previa

Management of placenta previa depends on different factors. The first and foremost is the bleeding. If the mother is symptomatic, i.e. presents with severe vaginal bleeding, delivery is indicated. At this stage fetal maturity is irrelevant and delivery should be considered in the maternal interest. If the mother is in labour with known major degree placenta previa a prompt caesarean section is indicated. In this situation, senior help should be sought urgently and blood should be crossmatched. The mother should be counselled about possibility of caesarean hysterectomy beforehand. If the mother is asymptomatic and the fetus is still premature, conservative management is reasonable with or without hospital admission. If the mother is asymptomatic and fetus is matured, delivery by elective (planned) caesarean section is indicated.

Vaginal bleeding in case of placenta previa is sudden and can be moderate to severe. Usually it is preceded by repeated 'warning' bleeds. The CTG of the fetus usually does not show any abnormality.

Elective caesarean section is the method of choice for the delivery of the fetus, but many patients need emergency caesarean section for moderate to severe unexpected bleeding. In case of major placenta previa, when an anterior placenta covers the whole lower segment, caesarean section can be technically difficult and complicated by severe haemorrhage; hence it should be performed electively by a senior obstetrician with senior anaesthetist caring for the woman and senior paediatrician caring for the baby. The risk of massive haemorrhage and possibility of hysterectomy should be discussed with the patient prior to the operation if time permits and should be documented in the consent as both the risks are considerably higher (about 12 times more chance of blood transfusion and about one third might need hysterectomy). Delivery should be considered in asymptomatic placenta previa around 38 weeks of gestation. Some units offer in patient management from third trimester in cases of major placenta previa. In these cases two units of cross matched blood should be kept in fridge which should be replaced by newly crossmatched blood every week (British Committee for Standards in Haematology. Blood Transfusion Task Force 2004). The decision for delivery should be made by the consultant obstetrician and proper evaluation of each case is required.

Management of symptomatic Placenta previa (The MOET course Manual): Communication is the key to proper management. It is easy to underestimate bleeding, hence weighing of the sheets will be more accurate indicator of the amount of blood loss. The management of acute bleeding has been outlined in table 3.

• Manage Airway, Breathing, Circulation • Assessment of the bleeding • Intravenous access: 2 large bore (16 gauge) cannulae • Blood for Full Blood count, coagulation profile, Crossmatch • Indwelling catheter to monitor urine output • Fluid resuscitation • Crossmatch bloods and availability of blood products: alert Blood Transfusion that more blood may be needed • Alert: Senior-most Obstetrician, Anaesthetist, Paediatrician, Hematologist, Blood Transfusion Service • If life threatening bleeding – consider group specific or O negative blood • Decision for delivery/conservative management: Senior Obstetrician should be involved.

Table 3. Management of symptomatic Antepartum haemorrhage

3.4.2 Management of major placental abruption

In case of suspected significant abruption, delivery is indicated in both maternal and fetal interest. In severe placental abruption, delivery by caesarean section is indicated. If the mother presents with signs of abruption with a viable fetus which is distressed, prompt delivery improves outcome (Kayani et al 2003). If the mother is symptomatic and the fetus is already dead, artificial rupture of membrane can be performed and a trial for a vaginal delivery can be undertaken. However, if the bleeding is severe, then caesarean section might be the appropriate mode of delivery in maternal interest irrespective of the status of the fetus.

4. Postpartum Haemorrhage (PPH)

4.1 Introduction

It is one of the most common causes for maternal mortality and morbidity worldwide. In Scotland, the rate of life-threatening haemorrhage is about 3.7/1000 (Brace, Kernaghan & Penney 2007). Life threatening haemorrhage includes bleeding more than 2.5 litres or the patients who need treatment to correct coagulopathy or where more than five units of blood have been transfused.

The WHO has defined postpartum haemorrhage as any bleeding from the genital tract over 500mls.after the delivery of the baby. In the developed world, most mothers show no sign of hypovolumia till 1000 mls of blood is lost (Drife 1997). Hemorrhage within 24 hours of delivery is termed as primary and a haemorrhage after 24 hour is termed as secondary.

Common causes of PPH are uterine atony, vaginal or cervical trauma, retained placental tissue or membranes and Disseminated Intravascular Coagulopathy (DIC), out of which the commonest being uterine atony (70%), where the uterus fails to contract after delivery. This is a situation where urgent action is life-saving and may require transfusion of multiple units of blood and blood products. The clotting factors are exhausted quickly and unless they are replenished as part of resuscitation, there is little chance that bleeding will be controlled by simply blood transfusion. However, prompt action and transfusion of blood and blood products can save life and even preserve uterus in cases of massive haemorrhage.

4.2 Strategies to prevent major Post Partum Haemorrhage

It is possible to prevent major obstetric haemorrhage and subsequent blood transfusion in majority of the anticipated cases.All the factors mentioned in table 4 have been identified as risk factors for PPH and if the patient is at higher risk ,it should be clearly documented in the notes and communicated to the relevant health professionals. In four cochrane reviews active management of third stage of labour has been found superior to physiological third stage (Prendiville 2000). Active management of third stage include early cord clamping, controlled cord traction and early uterotonic drugs such as syntocinon,ergometrine or syntometrine as per local protocol. Proper risk assessment in the antenatal period and individualisation of cases are the vital steps which must be taken in order to prevent blood transfusion.

• Parity: Primiparity or Grand Multiparity • Prior Caesarean section (Kramer et al 2011) • Placenta previa or low-lying placenta, marginal umbilical cord insertion in the placenta • Past history of PPH • Placenta previa or accreta in previous pregnancy	• Labour induction and augmentation (Kramer et al 2011) • Prolonged labour • Uterine or cervical trauma at delivery • Transverse lie • Gestational age < 32 weeks • Birth weight ≥ 4500 g. • Multiple pregnancy

Table 4. Risk factors for PPH

4.3 Management of major Post Partum Haemorrhage

Most of the time PPH is unpredictable and pose major health concern when they are severe. If PPH is anticipated proper steps should be taken to reduce the likelihood of blood transfusion and maternal morbidity. These steps include use of cell salvage if available, support from senior obstetrician, senior anaesthetist and other health professionals.

Uterus should be rubbed up for a contraction should be the first step and sometimes this is enough to reduce blood loss. Pharmacological agents such as oxytocin, ergometrine and prostaglandins (intramuscular or Intramyometrial) injections remain the mainstay of management. Effective communication between the health professionals is important as resuscitation should run side by side to the definitive management.

If bleeding is uncontrollable with pharmacological agents, surgical measures such as Brace sutures, Examination under anaesthesia (EUA) and repair of cervical or uterine injury are undertaken. Intrauterine Balloon is one of the most common and effective method of controlling moderate to severe PPH.

If facilities permit, Interventional radiologist and haematologist should be involved early as often the PPH can lead to DIC and will be requiring expert input. The interventional radiologist will play a key role if the bleeding is from any branch of internal or external iliac artery. If this facility is not available either hysterectomy or transfer of the patient to a tertiary referral centre after stabilisation should be considered.

• Assessment of Bleeding • Indwelling Catheter • Rubbing up a contraction • Ask for help • Multidisciplinary approach, including Senior obstetrician, senior anaesthetist, Senior midwives, • Airway, Breathing and circulation • 2 large bore cannulae • Frequent monitoring of BP, Pulse, oxygen saturation, urine output and vaginal bleeding
Medical Management: • Oxytocin bolus • Oxytocin infusion • Ergometrine • Prostaglandin: Intramuscular, Intramyometrial, Per-rectal
Surgical Management: • Brace sutures • Intrauterine Balloon • Internal Iliac artery ligation • Hysterectomy
Interventional Radiology
Recombinant factor VII concentrate: Not licensed for use in the UK for treatment of PPH

Table 5. Summary of Management of PPH

Recombinant Factor VII concentrate (rFVIIa): Not licensed for use for obstetric haemorrhage, but can be used when benefit outweighs risk. Senior haematologist should always be involved in the decision making. Franchini, Lippi & Franchi, in a review of published data of 65 women treated with rFVIIa for PPH, suggested that rFVIIa reduced bleeding.

Hysterectomy should be considered as a last resort. A timely hysterectomy can save life.

5. Blood transfusion in APH & PPH

Ideally, fully cross matched blood is preferable in case of major obstetric haemorrhage. However, obstetric haemorrhage is extremely unpredictable and it is not always possible to wait for fully cross matched blood. Generally volume replacement should start with up to 2 litres of crystalloid. Plasma expanders should follow until the blood is available (The MOET course Manual). If the haemorrhage is life-threatening, O negative or type specific blood should be used. In most hospitals O negative blood is readily available either in the labour suite or at the on-site blood bank. Patients, who are at higher risk of haemorrhage, should be admitted and delivered in a unit where blood and blood products are readily available (CEMACH Sixth Report, 2004).

6. Risk management

Availability of blood does not always guarantee best standard of care to the patients. Standard of care depends on the team-work and competence of the healthcare professionals. Two strategies can be employed to improve these factors. The doctors and other healthcare professionals should attend appropriate course to maintain their skills and update their knowledge of both resuscitation and managing obstetric emergencies to improve health professionals' knowledge. The other important step is to organise regular obstetric emergency drills (commonly known as obstetric fire drills in the UK).

A local protocol should be in place to manage major obstetric haemorrhage and regular audit of practice and analysis of cases with major blood loss should be carried out. This is vital as lessons are to be learned from every mistake made to improve patient care in future. Also, emphasis should be given to the importance of appropriate and detailed documentation including the timings of steps of medical and surgical management.

7. Morbidly adherent placenta

The Royal College of Obstetricians and Gynaecologists (UK) have brought out an excellent guideline (Green top Guideline No. 27) on the management of morbidly adherent placenta (placenta accreta, increta and percreta). From the guideline and searching other literature, the salient points are:

- The incidence of placenta previa accreta is on the rise as the incidence of caesarean section is rising
- The patient should be reviewed by the consultant obstetrician and consultant anaesthetist in the antenatal period and a proper plan should be documented.
- The consent form should include discussion about Interventional Radiology, Cell salvage, Recombinant Factor VII concentrate and hysterectomy.

- Interventional Radiology can be safely and effectively used for an elective caesarean section (Jung et al 2011). Intra-arterial balloon can be inserted before the procedure.
- At caesarean section the uterus should be opened distal to the placenta so that the baby can be delivered undisturbed and to have the option of conservative management.
- If the placenta is covering the whole anterior lower segment, a midline skin incision will not be unreasonable.
- If the placenta fails to separate at caesarean section and bleeding is minimal, it can be left in situ. Attempting placental separation risks hysterectomy in up to 100% of cases (Eller et al 2009).If there is major haemorrhage, the uterine wound should be closed and a subtotal or total hysterectomy can be performed
- If the placenta is left behind serial ultrasound scan and beta HCG monitoring should be performed. Post operative antibiotics should be given to minimise the risk of infection and close monitoring is needed to diagnose infection early.

8. Interventional radiology in anticipated intrapartum and postpartum haemorrhage

In case of major placenta previa or known morbidly adherent placenta, interventional radiology can be used to minimise the risk of potential PPH. The Radiologist may insert the balloons preoperatively either in the uterine artery or in the anterior division of internal iliac artery which can be inflated preoperatively to minimise in case of uncontrollable haemorrhage or even can be used for embolisation. The overall success rate of interventional radiology in controlling bleeding and avoidance in hysterectomy rate has been quoted around 71-97% (Dildy GA 3rd 2002 &. Hong et al 2004)

In a large study (involving sixty six women, who have undergone embolisation) in Boston, USA, Ganguly et al suggested that the 'threshold for Uterine Artery Embolisation in women with PPH should be low, as it is associated with a high clinical effectiveness rate and a low complication rate'.

9. Cell salvage

Cell salvage is an effective way of reducing blood transfusion rate in women where the anticipated blood loss is more than 1.5 litres (RCOG Green top guideline no. 47). Prior consent is necessary for this procedure. In intra-operative cell salvage blood is collected usually after the liquor is drained then collected in a reservoir centrifuged, washed and processed for transfusion. In a case series in a large maternity unit in the UK, introduction of cell saver has been a major factor in reducing heterologous blood transfusion from 10.2% to 7.9% (King et al 2009) The main problem with this process is that there is no available filter to filter out fetal cells. Hence, a Kleihauer test is necessary after its use.

10. Management of patients refusing blood transfusion on religious/ethical belief

Some women, mostly due to their religious belief, decline blood or blood products transfusion. Most common of these groups are Jehovah's witnesses and transfusing them under any circumstances without their consent may be considered as to assault, hence should not be undertaken even if it is indicated. In UK, legally a woman can decline treatment even if it might prove fatal. But this is a decision, only a competent patient can make and no one else. Also, if she has declined transfusion, no one else can make a decision on her behalf to transfuse her.

A detailed discussion regarding the risks should take place at first or second trimester. The discussion should also include possibility of hysterectomy, morbidity and possibility of death. Two large case series in UK (Massiah et al 2007) and USA (Singla et al 2001) looked into the obstetric outcome of the labour and deliveries in Jehovah's witnesses. The reported mortality rate is 65 fold higher in the UK and 44 fold higher in USA.

A written consent should be taken during the antenatal period after a detailed discussion about pros and cons of the decision. Anaemia should be corrected aggressively before delivery, if necessary with intravenous iron therapy. Prior consent about cell salvage should be taken if the patient is due to have elective caesarean section or even in emergency caesarean section if time and facilities permit. This cell salvage should run in continuous loop without disconnection till the end of the procedure (Currie et al 2010). In these patients prompt decision making about prevention of PPH and using all the relevant uterotonics and surgical methods (intrauterine compression balloon, brace sutures, interventional radiology) are vital and if necessary hysterectomy should be undertaken sooner rather than later. The patient's wishes should be respected and it is not legally and ethically justified to transfuse her against her wishes. Senior input from the obstetric and anaesthetic consultants should be sought early.

11. Acknowledgement

Dr. Pauline Lynch, Consultant Obstetrician and Dr. Antony Nicoll, Consultant Obstetrician Ninewells Hospital for their whole hearted support. Royal College of Obstetricians and Gynaecologists for their guidelines on Placenta Previa (no.27), Blood Transfusion in pregnancy (no.47) and Post partum Haemorrhage (no.52)

12. References

Ananth CV, Savitz DA, Bowes WA Jr, Luther ER. Influence of hypertensive disorders and cigarette smoking on placental abruption and uterine bleeding during pregnancy. Br J Obstet Gynaecol. 1997 May; 104(5):572-8.

Ankum WM, Mol BWJ, Van der Veen F& Bossuyt PMM; Risk factors for ectopic pregnancy –a meta analysis. Fertility & Sterility 1996, vol 65, 1093-1099

Blood transfusion in obstetrics, RCOG Green top guideline no. 47:2007;

Bouyer J, Job-Spira N & Pouly JL et al; Fertility after ectopic pregnancy-results of the first three years of the Auvergne register. 1996, Contracept Fertil Sex 24,475-81

Brace V, Kernaghan D, Penney G. Learning from adverse clinical outcomes: major obstetric haemorrhage in Scotland, 2003–05.*BJOG* 2007; 114:1388–96.

Braga J, Marques R, Branco A, Gonçalves J, Lobato L, Pimentel JP,et al. Maternal and perinatal implications of the use of human recombinant erythropoietin. Acta Obstet Gynecol Scand , 1996;75:449–53.

British Committee for Standards in Haematology. Blood Transfusion Task Force. Guidelines for compatibility procedures in blood trans-fusion laboratories. Working Party of the British Committee for Standards in Haematology. Blood Transfusion Task Force. Transfusion Medicine 2004; 14:59–73.

Confidential Enquiry into Maternal and Child Health. Why Mothers Die 2000–2002. Sixth Report on Confidential Enquiries into Maternal Deaths in the United Kingdom. London: RCOG Press; 2004

Crofts JF, Ellis D, Draycott TJ, Winter C, Hunt LP, Akande VA;Change in knowledge of midwives and obstetricians following obstetric emergency training: a randomised controlled trial of local hospital, simulation centre and teamwork training. BJOG 2007;114:1534–41.

Dafallah SE, Babikir HE.'Risk factors predisposing to abruptio placentae. Maternal and fetal outcome. Saudi Med J. 2004 Sep;25(9):1237-40.

Dildy GA 3rd. Postpartum haemorrhage: new management options.Clin Obstet Gynecol 2002;45:330–44.

Drife J. Management of primary postpartum haemorrhage. Br J Obstet Gynaecol 1997;104:275-7

Eller AG, Porter TF, Soisson P, Silver RM. Optimal management strategies for placenta accreta. BJOG 2009; 116:648–54.

Franchini M, Lippi G, Franchi M. The use of recombinant activated factor VII in obstetric and gynaecological haemorrhage.BJOG 2007;114:8–15.

Ganguli S, Stecker MS, Pyne D, Baum RA, Fan CM.;Uterine artery embolization in the treatment of postpartum uterine hemorrhage. . J Vasc Interv Radiol. 2011 Feb;22(2):169-76. Epub 2010 Dec 22.

Gray D, Thorburn J, Lundorff P, Strandell A, Lindblom B. A cost-effectiveness study of a randomised trial of laparoscopy versus laparotomy for ectopic pregnancy. Lancet 1995;345:1139–43.

Hong TM,Tseng HS, Lee RC,Wang JH, Chang CY.Uterine artery embolization: an effective treatment for intractable obstetric haemorrhage.Clin Radiol 2004;59:96–101.

Hung TH, Hsieh CC, Hsu JJ, Lo LM, Chiu TH, Hsieh TT.; Risk factors for placental abruption in an Asian population. Reprod Sci. 2007 Jan;14(1):59-65

Jane Currie, Matthew Hogg, Nandini Patel, Karen Madgwick, Wai Yoong; Management of women who decline blood and blood products in pregnancy, The Obstetrician & Gynaecologist, http://onlinetog.org 2010;12:13–20

Jung HN, Shin SW, Choi SJ, Cho SK, Park KB, Park HS, Kang M, Choo SW, Do YS, Choo IW.; Uterine artery embolization for emergent management of postpartum hemorrhage associated with placenta accreta; Acta Radiol. 2011 Jul 1;52(6):638-42.

Kayani SI,Walkinshaw SA,Preston C: Pregnancy outcome in severe placental abruption. British Journal Of Obstetrics and Gynaecology 110:679,2003

King M, Wrench I, Galimberti A, Spray R.,Introduction of cell salvage to a large obstetric unit: the first six months; . Int J Obstet Anesth. 2009 Apr;18(2):111-7. Epub 2009 Jan 13.

Kramer MS, Dahhou M, Vallerand D, Liston R, Joseph KS; Risk factors for postpartum hemorrhage: can we explain the recent temporal increase?, J Obstet Gynaecol Can. 2011 Aug;33(8):810-9.

Le Ray C, Fraser W, Rozenberg P, Langer B, Subtil D, Goffinet F; for the PREMODA Study Group.; Duration of passive and active phases of the second stage of labour and risk of severe postpartum haemorrhage in low-risk nulliparous women. Eur J Obstet Gynecol Reprod Biol. 2011 Oct;158(2):167-172.

Leerentveld RA, Gilberts EC, Arnold MJ, Wladimiroff JW. Accuracy and safety of transvaginal sonographic placental localisation. *Obstet Gynecol* 1990;76: 759–62.

Lewis G, Drife J, editors. Why Mothers Die 1997–1999. The Fifth Report of the Confidential Enquiries into Maternal Deaths in the United Kingdom. London: RCOG Press; 2001.

Lipscomb G, Bran D, McCord M, Portera J, Ling F. Analysis of three hundred fifteen ectopic pregnancies treated with single-dose methotrexate. Am J Obstet Gynecol 1998; 178:1354–8.

Lundorff P, Thorburn J, Lindblom B. Fertility outcome after conservative surgical treatment of ectopic pregnancy evaluated in a randomized trial. Fertil Steril 1992; 57:998–1002.

Massiah N, Athimulam S, Loo C, Okolo S, Yoong W. Obstetric care of Jehovah's Witnesses: a 14-year observational study. Arch Gynecol Obstet 2007;276:339–43. doi:10.1007/s00404-007-0346-0

Mbah AK, Alio AP, Fombo DW, Bruder K, Dagne G, Salihu HM'. Association between cocaine abuse in pregnancy and placenta-associated syndromes using propensity score matching approach; Early Hum Dev. 2011 Oct 3.

Murphy AA, Nager CW, Wujek JJ, Kettel LM, Torp VA, Chin HG. Operative laparoscopy versus laparotomy for the management of ectopic pregnancy. Fertil Steril 1992;57:1180–5.

National Collaborating Centre for Women's and Children's Health. Antenatal care: routine care for the healthy pregnant woman. Clinical Guideline. London: RCOG Press; 2003.

Onwere C, Gurol-Urganci I, Cromwell DA, Mahmood TA, Templeton A, van der Meulen JH., Maternal morbidity associated with placenta praevia among women who had elective caesarean section, Eur J Obstet Gynecol Reprod Biol. 2011 Aug 9.

Paterson-Brown S, Singh C. Developing a care bundle for the management of suspected placenta accreta. The Obstetrician & *Gynaecologist* 2010; 12:21–7.

Prendiville WJP, Elbourne D, McDonald SJ. Active versus expected management in the third stage of labour. Cochrane Database Syst Rev 2000;(3):CD000007.

Royal College of Obstetricians and Gynaecologists Green top Guideline: The management of Tubal Pregnancy : Guideline No. 21 ,May 2004,Reviewed 2010

Royal College of Obstetricians and Gynaecologists. Green–top Guideline No.52: Prevention and management of postpartum haemorrhage. London: RCOG; 2009.

Royal College of Obstetricians and Gynaecologists. Placenta Praevia and Placenta Praevia Accreta: Diagnosis and Management. Green top Guideline No. 27. London: RCOG; 2005.

Saving Mothers' Lives: Reviewing maternal deaths to make motherhood safer -2003-2005

Sheiner E, Shoham-Vardi I, Hallak M, Hadar A, Gortzak-Uzan L, Katz M, Mazor M, Placental abruption in term pregnancies: clinical significance and obstetric risk factors, J Matern Fetal Neonatal Med. 2003 Jan;13(1):45-9.

SHOT in Obstetrics: 2005 Annual Report (www.shotuk.org)

Silva P, Schaper A, Rooney B. Reproductive outcome after 143 laparoscopic procedures for ectopic pregnancy. Fertil Steril 1993;81:710–5.

Singh K, Fong Y, Kuperan P.; A comparison between intravenous iron polymatose complex (Ferrum Hausmann) and oral ferrous fumerate in the treatment of iron deficiency anaemia in pregnancy. European Journal of Haematology. 1998;60(2):119-24

Singla A, Lapinski R, Berkowitz R, Saphier C. Are women who are Jehovah's Witnesses at risk of maternal death? Am J Obstet Gynecol 2001;185:893–5. doi:10.1067/mob.2001.117357

The MOET course Manual, edited by Kate Grady, Charlott Howell and Charles Cox, Second edition, page 174-175

Vermesh M, Silva P, Rosen G, Stein AL, Fossum GT, Sauer MV. Management of unruptured ectopic gestation by linear salpingostomy: a prospective, randomized clinical trial of laparoscopy versus laparotomy. Obstet Gynecol 1989;73:400–4.

Weintraub AY, Levy A, Holcberg G, Sheiner E.,The outcome of blunt abdominal trauma preceding birth. Int J Fertil Womens Med. 2006 Nov-Dec;51(6):275-9.

World Health Organization. The Prevention and Management of Postpartum Haemorrhage. Report of a Technical Working Group. Geneva:WHO;1990.

Worldwide prevalence of anaemia 1993–2005 ;WHO Global Database on Anaemia

6

Uterine Atony: Management Strategies

Pei Shan Lim*
*Universiti Kebangsaan Malaysia Medical Center,
Universiti Kebangsaan Malaysia
Malaysia*

1. Introduction

It is estimated about 529,000 mothers die every year (World Health Organisation [WHO] 2005). Postpartum haemorrhage (PPH), a life-threatening condition, remains the major cause of maternal mortality worldwide (Pahlavan et al., 2001). Majority of these mortalities are from Asia (48%) and Africa (47.5%) with only the minority (less than 1%) from developed countries.(Ramanathan & Arulkumaran, 2006) In Malaysia, the Confidential Enquiry into Maternal Deaths (CEMD) from 1991 to 2005 revealed that PPH attributed 13-27% of all reported deaths(Division of Family Health Development, Ministry of Health, 1994; Division of Family Health Development, Ministry of Health, 1996; Division of Family Health Development, Ministry of Health, 2000; Division of Family Health Development, Ministry of Health, 2005).

Although PPH is no longer the leading cause of maternal mortality in the developed countries, it still remains as one of the most important causes of maternal morbidity. Recently, two reports from Canada and United States (Joseph et al. 2007; Callaghan, Kuklina & Berg 2010) reported a 23-26% increase in the rate of PPH. Despite reports of an increasing rate, maternal mortality in these two countries remained low indicating the effective management of PPH. Nevertheless, in developing countries, PPH related maternal mortality remains a serious concern due to limited health care facilities, underdeveloped management strategies and deprivation of trained health care personnel.

Disastrously massive PPH can lead to coagulopathy, pituitary ischaemia, cardiovascular insufficiency, and multi-organ failure. It is also associated with an increased need for blood and blood products transfusion, intensive care admission, peri-partum hysterectomy and its related intra- or post-operative complications. Even in a milder form of haemorrhage, anaemia itself would interfere with bonding and care for the newborn (Devine, 2009).

Uterine atony is identified as the main cause of PPH accounting for about 90% in most reports (Bateman et al., 2010; Carroli et al., 2008; Combs et al., 1991; Doran et al, 1955). In developing countries like Malaysia, uterine atony contributed 37.5% to 67.7% of PPH

---
* Mohamad Nasir Shafiee, Nirmala Chandralega Kampan, Aqmar Suraya Sulaiman,
Nur Azurah Abdul Ghani, NorAzlin Mohamed Ismail, Choon Yee Lee,
Mohd Hashim Omar and Muhammad Abdul Jamil Mohammad Yassin
Universiti Kebangsaan Malaysia Medical Center, Universiti Kebangsaan Malaysia, Malaysia

associated mortality between 1994-2005 (Division of Family Health Development, Ministry of Health, 1994; Division of Family Health Development, Ministry of Health, 1996; Division of Family Health Development, Ministry of Health, 2000; Division of Family Health Development, Ministry of Health, 2005).

2. Definition

2.1 Postpartum haemorrhage

Postpartum haemorrhage is defined as blood loss of 500ml or more from genital tract in the first 24 hours of delivery. Massive PPH is defined as blood loss of 1000ml or more (Carroli et al., 2008).

Conventionally, PPH is classified according to the timing of its occurrence. Bleeding within 24 hours of delivery is defined as the primary postpartum haemorrhage. Secondary postpartum haemorrhage is defined as bleeding that occurs after 24 hours until six weeks postpartum.

Assessment of blood loss during delivery is commonly performed using visual estimation. This is often inaccurate and underestimated (Prasertcharoensuk et al., 2000). The traditional assumption of transfusing a pint of red blood cells in a patient who has bled 500 ml blood will increase the haemoglobin to 1 gm is only accurate if not actively bleeding. Estimation of blood loss as well as amount to be transfused is impossible to gauge in an ongoing PPH (Gutierrez et al., 2004). Some centres advocate PPH to be significant with a 10% drop in haematocrit from antenatal to postpartum. Nevertheless this requires laboratory facilities which impose delay in the diagnosis and further management of PPH.

The ability of women coping with haemorrhage largely depends on their health status as well as the severity of bleeding. Most healthy pregnant women can tolerate blood loss up to 1500ml as the result of blood volume increment during pregnancy (Bonnar, 2000). However, in the presence of pre-existing anaemia or hypovolaemia, compensatory mechanism will be jeopardised. Individual responses towards blood loss limit the use of clinical signs and symptoms in defining PPH and determining its severity.

2.2 Uterine atony

Uterine atony is defined as failure of myometrium to contract and retract following delivery (Cunningham et al., 2005). Powerful and effective myometrial contractions are vital to arrest bleeding. Uterine atony in contrary, the uterus is soft and 'boggy' with presence of excessive bleeding from genital tract. A prompt recognition followed by uterine massage and administration of uterotonic agents often arrest the bleeding. However, in the presence of already well contracted uterus, any persistent bleeding should prompt exploration for other causes of postpartum haemorrhage such as retained placental fragments or genital tract injuries.

3. Risk factors for uterine atony

Identification of women at risk of uterine atony is of utmost importance to allow optimisation and preventive measures to be taken. Hence, a well-arranged delivery plan and appropriate referral to a well-equipped centre should be done. The recognised risk factors that are associated with uterine atony are listed in Table 1.

Factors associated with uterine over distension
•   Multiple pregnancy
•   Polyhydramnios
•   Fetal macrosomia
Labour related factors
•   Induction of labour
•   Prolonged labour
•   Precipitate labour
•   Oxytocin augmentation
•   Manual removal of placenta
Use of uterine relaxants
•   Deep anaesthesia
•   Magnesium sulphate
Intrinsic factors
•   Previous postpartum haemorrhage
•   Antepartum haemorrhage
•   Obesity
•   Age > 35 years

Table 1. Risk factors for uterine atony. (Breathnach & Geary, 2006)

Multiple pregnancies, polyhydramnios and fetal macrosomia cause uterine over-distension. The odds ratio to develop PPH from fetal macrosomia and multiple pregnancies are 1.8 (95% CI 1.4 to 2.3) and 2.2 (95% CI 1.5 to 3.2) respectively (Magann et al., 2005). In the presence of twin-twin transfusion syndrome, the odds ratio increases to 5.1 (95% CI 1.5 to 15.7) (Magann et al., 2005). On contrary, Carroli et al. did not find any relationship between multiple pregnancies with occurrence of uterine atony (Carroli et al., 2008). A study based data obtained from Nationwide Inpatient Sample (NIS), a large public use administrative dataset in the United States, had reported an association of polyhydramnios with uterine atony requiring blood transfusion in the odds ratio of 1.9 (95% CI 1.2-3.1) (Bateman et al., 2010).

Intrapartum factors such as induction of labour, prolonged labour, oxytocin exposure and abnormal third stage are also recognised to associate with uterine atony. Induction of labour had an odds ratio of 1.5 (95% CI 1.2 to 1.7) (Magann et al., 2005) and was the cause of 17% of uterine atony requiring blood transfusion (Bateman et al., 2010) .

Prolonged usage of oxytocin in labour contributes to uterine atony. Grotegut et al. had demonstrated that massive PPH secondary to uterine atony was significantly higher in women who were exposed to oxytocin (Grotegut et al., 2011). The authors proposed that persistent oxytocin administration causes desensitisation of oxytocin receptors which further contributed into uterine atony.

The presence of uterine fibroids or connective tissue disorders may hinder the myometrium contractility thus leading to uterine atony. However, the existing data are conflicting with regards to relationship between uterine fibroids and uterine atony (Hasan et al., 1991;

Qidwai et al., 2006; Roberts et al., 1999; Vergani et al., 1994). Patients with connective tissue disorders are at a higher risk of PPH as compared to the general population (Kominiarek & Kilpatrick, 2007) which is explained by poor connective tissue support. Hence, uterotonic agents would be the first-line treatment for these conditions.

Though identification of risk factors is essential, they have only moderate positive predictive value (Callaghan et al., 2010) as uterine atony can happen in any women with no apparent risk factor. Therefore, although early detection is important, timely and appropriate management is also crucial.

4. Management strategies

4.1 Prevention of PPH

Post-partum haemorrhage is preventable in many ways. Prevention begins early in high-risk women, as early as in preconception period. Prevention and optimisation of anaemia allows better tolerability to variable severity of PPH. Induction and augmentation of labour should be made with clear indications, performed judiciously by skilled birth attendants. Women at high-risk of PPH should be delivered at tertiary centres with well-equipped operation theatre, intensive care unit and blood transfusion services. The International Federation of Gynaecology and Obstetrics (FIGO) promotes active management of the third stage of labour (AMTSL) in all women in order to reduce the incidence of postpartum haemorrhage (Leduc et al., 2009).

4.1.1 Family planning

Low contraceptive prevalence rate leads to high fertility among women. In 2007, based on the United Nation Statistics Division report, contraceptive prevalence rate among married Malaysian women (aged 15 to 49 years old) was at 54% (Department of Economic and Social Affairs, United Nations Statistics Division, United Nation, 2010). In the Malaysian CEMD report from 2001 to 2005, up to 70% of maternal deaths were recognised in women who did not practise contraception. This reflects high parity contributing to more than half of maternal deaths was due to PPH during the same period (Division of Family Health Development, Ministry of Health, 2005).

4.1.2 Risk assessment and stratification

Uterine atony, the commonest cause of PPH, is best prevented by ensuring that immediate haemostasis is achieved by effective myometrial contractility (Mukherjee & Arulkumaran, 2009). Uterine blood vessels supplying the placental bed pass through the myometrium. However, in uterine atony, there is failure of myometrial contractions leading to impaired vasoconstriction of these blood vessels, resulting in excessive blood loss.

Nevertheless up to 60% of women with PPH have no identified risk factors (Mukherjee & Arulkumaran, 2009). Thus, constant awareness, early detection, timely resuscitation and management skills are necessary to overcome this problem.

4.1.2.1 Colour coding system

Colour coding system which was initially introduced by the Ministry of Health of Malaysia in 1989 is a risk stratification method used among women receiving antenatal care. (Table 2)

Prenatal assessment is applied in determining the level and place of antenatal care. Four colour codes are used: red indicates immediate hospital referral or admission, yellow indicates antenatal review by a doctor, green indicates antenatal care can be rendered by a senior nurse and white indicates women with no or low risk who may receive antenatal care in local clinics and can deliver in a low risk birthing centres (Ravindran et al., 2003). These codes are attached to the women's antenatal card using coloured sticker. Women with PPH in previous pregnancies have an increased risk of haemorrhage by 2 to 4 folds when compared to women with no previous history (Waterstone et al., 2001).They are coded red.

Colour codes	Associated risk factors
WHITE	primigravida, age <18 or >40,gravida 6 and above, spacing < 2years or >5years, short stature <145cm, single mother
YELLOW	Mothers with HIV positive or Hepatitis B positive, blood pressure >140/90 and <160/110mmHg with no proteinuria,diabetes, gestation >EDD+7 days.
GREEN	Rhesus negative, pre-pregnancy weight <45kg,medical problem excluding diabetes and hypertension,previous gynaecological surgery, drug/tobacco/alcohol addiction, unsure of last menstrual period, recurrent miscarriage, previous obstetrics history (previous caesarean section, gestational hypertension, diabetes, intrauterine death, baby <2.5 or >4kg, third degree perineal tear, retained placenta.
RED	eclampsia, pre-eclampsia, heart disease, breathlessness on exertion, uncontrolled diabetes, antepartum haemorrhage,symptomatic anaemia, prelabour rupture of membrane, preterm contractions, abnormal fetal heart rate <110/min after 26 weeks and >160/min after 34 weeks

Table 2. Colour coding system based on risk factors, used in antenatal clinics in Malaysia as cited by Ravindran et al. in 2003 (Ravindran et al., 2003)

Although used extensively, the actual value in predicting outcomes is not reflected in clinical practice as reported in the CEMD 2001 to 2005. Maternal deaths in women whom were tagged green actually increased from 13.5% in 2001 to 28.8% in 2005. This is in contrast to deaths among women tagged yellow which decreased from 45.3% in 2001 to 16% in 2005. This was probably due related to these codes (green and white) were considered to be 'low risk' leading to lesser attention given (Division of Family Health Development, Ministry of Health, 2005). Limitation to the colour coding system is that occasionally when the newly onset current problems are overlooked and could have added risks later in pregnancy, e.g. polyhydramnios leading to PPH.

Reliability of colour coding system in Malaysia needs to be reviewed as recommended by Ravichandran et al in 2003. The author reported that the accuracy of the codes in predicting morbidity and mortality were only about 50% in a retrospective cohort of 1122 among 8388 women from several districts in peninsular Malaysia (Ravindran et al., 2003).

4.1.3 Optimisation prior to onset of labour

4.1.3.1 Treatment of anaemia

World Health Organisation defined anaemia in pregnancy as haemoglobin level below 11g/dL (WHO, 1992; WHO, 2007). Iron deficiency anaemia is the commonest cause of anaemia in pregnancy, being in mild, moderate or severe forms. In developing countries, anaemia is usually associated with malnutrition and concurrent medical disorders which may potentially reduce women's tolerance to PPH (WHO, 1992). Despite its association with serious morbidity and mortality, there is a paucity of data assessing clinical outcomes of mothers and neonates with anaemia. Treatment with oral iron reduces the incidence of anaemia (RR 0.38; 95%CI 0.26-0.55) (Reveiz et al., 2007). Haemoglobin optimisation antenatally is important in an attempt for safe delivery. Women with optimal haemoglobin level are able to tolerate blood loss. The MMR of women with haemoglobin of less than 5g/dL was reported to be increased by 8 to 10 fold (Kalaivani, 2009).

4.1.4 Safe delivery

4.1.4.1 Judicious oxytocin usage

Prolonged usage of oxytocin paradoxically causes uterine atony and PPH (Grotegut et al., 2011). Judicious use of oxytocin during induction and augmentation of labour may prevent uterine atony. A correct diagnosis of labour is of utmost importance in avoiding unnecessary and prolonged exposure to oxytocin. A clear guideline should be drawn for indications of induction of labour.

4.1.4.2 Active management of the third stage of labour

Active management of the third stage of labour is the crucial step in avoiding PPH secondary to uterine atony. AMTSL reduces the incidence of PPH compared to women who were managed expectantly (RR 0.34; 95%CI 0.14-0.87) (Begley et al., 2010) .

The definition of AMTSL varies from use of uterotonic agents immediately after baby is delivered, delivery of the placenta by controlled cord traction (CCT) and early cord clamping and cutting (Prendiville et al., 2000). The International Federation of Obstetrics and Gynaecology (FIGO) and International Confederation of Midwives (ICM) recommended similar approach followed by uterine massage without early cord clamping (ICM and FIGO, 2003). Previous studies have recommended that active versus expectant management which showed significant reduction in the incidence of PPH. Prendiville et al. concluded that expectant management in comparison with AMTSL is three times more likely to result in PPH (OR 3.1; 95%CI2.3-4.2) (Prendiville et al., 1988). Prophylactic administration of uterotonic agents as part of AMTSL has significantly reduced the amount of blood loss (RR 0.5; 95%CI 0.43-0.59) with less requirement of therapeutic oxytocin   (RR 0.5; 95%CI 0.39-0.64) (Elbourne et al., 2001).

4.1.5 Skilled birth attendants

Presence of skilled birth attendants in dealing with PPH proved to reduce maternal morbidity and mortality up to 30% (Carlough & McCall, 2005). WHO defines skilled birth attendants to be those with the minimum knowledge and skills to manage normal childbirth and provide basic (first line) emergency obstetric care (Carlough & McCall, 2005). They should be familiar with early identification of uterine atony and are able to initiate basic intervention such as uterine massage and administration of intramuscular/intravascular oxytocin. Prefilled oxytocin (Uniject™) with easy administration is available in low resource countries and is recommended to be in the bags of birth attendants.

Based on the Safe Motherhood Initiative report from 1987 to 2005, the number of deliveries in developing countries attended by skilled birth attendants has increased significantly from 41 to 57% (Safe Motherhood Initiative, 2005). In low resourced settings, skilled birth attendants' knowledge in PPH however was found to be at an average of 60% and less than one- third of them were able to perform bimanual uterine compression (Harvey et al., 2007). Hence, further training, regular drills and audits are needed to enhance their skills and knowledge.

4.1.6 Training

Suboptimal obstetric care has been shown to cause maternal death from PPH. Delay in establishing diagnosis, failure to carry out appropriate intervention and lack of team effort had been associated with poor maternal outcomes (Siassakos et al., 2009). Lombard et al. reported PPH related deaths among women in South Africa from 2002 to 2006 with 2.25 errors per death as compared to 0.61 errors per death in the near missed group (Lombaard & Pattinson, 2009).

Implementation of the training programme has been shown to reduce in the incidence of substandard care (Hofmeyr et al., 2009). Training includes in-service training and drills. In-service training programme involves induction training for all new staffs inclusive of labour ward management. Regular training in the form of continuous medical education sessions (CME), lectures and scientific meetings will ensure updates the knowledge of all staffs.

In obstetrics drills, staffs are trained to be familiar with simulated obstetrics emergency scenarios. Clinical algorithm and action plans are practised either individually or as a team activity. Accurate blood loss estimation enables early recognition of PPH. Ability to perform initial fluid resuscitation, measures on initial ways to stop bleeding such as bimanual uterine and aortic compression, prevent women from further developing hypovolaemic shock.

However, a Bristol based study analysing a cohort of midwives who had undergone training in Practical Obstetrics Multi professional training (PROMPT) revealed a significant reduction in Apgar score of less than 6 at 5 minutes and neonatal encephalopathy (Draycott et al., 2006). However, there is no available published data on the outcome of staff training to reduction of PPH. In Malaysia, joint efforts between the Obstetrics and Gynaecology Society Malaysia, Ministry of Health and Royal College of Obstetricians and Gynaecologists have successfully delivered several obstetrics emergency and live saving courses since 2008. This programme has expanded throughout the whole country as far as invitation to train personnel in Myanmar. A study on the effectiveness of this training programme is currently ongoing.

4.1.7 Facilities

4.1.7.1 Maternal child health clinic

Since introduction of the Maternal and Child Health (MCH) services in 1957, extensive development towards improving access and quality of care had been well established in Malaysia. Majority of women in Malaysia are able to have easy access to healthcare facilities, family planning services and upgraded essential care in obstetrics service. In developing countries, recent estimation of MMR has seen a reduction by 34% from 1990 to 2008, from 440 deaths to 290 deaths per 100,000 live births (Department of Economic and Social Affairs, United Nations Statistics Division, United Nation, 2011). Over the past two decades, improvement in maternal health is reflected by reduction in the trend of MMR from 47.8 in 1991 to 26.6 per 100,100 live birth in 2005 (Department of Economic and Social Affairs, United Nations Statistics Division, United Nation, 2010). MCH services in Malaysia are inclusive of antenatal care, postnatal home visits, family planning consultation, nutrition support, and immunisation programmes.

4.1.7.2 Red alert system

A designated system to respond to emergency situations allows prompt mobilisation of health personnel to institute timely and optimal patient management. (Gosman et al., 2008). The emergency team is alerted via a paging system simultaneously. In dire emergency such as massive PPH, this system has successfully delivered early interventions hence improving maternal outcomes (Gosman et al., 2008). A delay in intervention of 20 minutes or more had led to a poorer outcome. (Korhonen & Kariniemi, 1994) All the major hospitals in Malaysia with obstetrics unit are equipped with the red alert system.

4.1.8 Risk management and monitoring system

Risk management includes incidence reporting, clinical practice guidelines review, near miss audits and CEMD. Standardised practice among all healthcare personnel is achievable by complying the clinical practice guidelines and hospital protocols. Incidences reporting involving a retrospective detailed documentation of adverse events are done by staffs. The whole document is reviewed by the risk management team to determine any preventable or substandard care. This is followed by a series of event including audit, re-audit, staff-education and training to improve in subsequent care.

Obstetrics near miss events are inclusive of massive PPH and peri-partum hysterectomy (Upadhyay & Scholefield, 2008). Audits of these events allow risk identification and implementation of preventive measures. Brace et al. reported that massive PPH was the major maternal morbidity in Scotland from 2003 to 2005 with the incidence of 3.7 per 1000 births (Brace et al., 2007). Up to 40% of near missed events received suboptimal care (Upadhyay & Scholefield, 2008).

Implementation of CEMD has allowed access of information with regards to the cause of death, areas of substandard care and identification of high risk women (Neilson, 2009). Each maternal death is studied and analysed in detail followed by expert's recommendation. Malaysia CEMD was introduced back in 1991. To date there has been several published reports over the past two decades. This allows identification of deficiency in the health care system. The MOH had put tremendous efforts and resources allocation into improvising the health care system. This is evident by a marked reduction in MMR in recent years (Division of Family Health Development, Ministry of Health, 2005).

4.2 Non-pharmacological/ Mechanical strategies

Varatharajan et al. evaluated the outcome of management for massive PPH using the algorithm `HAEMOSTASIS' (Help; Assess and resuscitate; Established diagnosis; Massage of uterus; Oxytocin infusion and prostaglandins; Shift to operation theatre; Tamponade test; Apply compression sutures; Systematic pelvic devascularisation; Interventional radiology and Subtotal/total hysterectomy) (Varatharajan et al., 2011). The algorithm was found to provide a logical management pathway to reduce blood transfusions, hysterectomy, admissions to intensive care units and also maternal deaths (Varatharajan et al., 2011).

4.2.1 Uterine massage

Uterine massage is performed by rubbing or stimulating the fundus of the uterus. It is hypothesised that massage releases local prostaglandins that promote uterine contractility hence reduces bleeding (Abdel-Aleem et al., 2010). Systematic review has shown that uterine massage is effective in preventing PPH. Abdel-Aleem et al. conducted a randomised controlled trial involving 200 women who were allocated to either uterine massage or no uterine massage following active management of third stage (Abdel-Aleem et al., 2006). Women who received uterine massage had lesser amount of bleeding and requirement for additional uterotonic agents (Abdel-Aleem et al., 2006).

In another randomised trial by Abdel-Aleem et al., 1964 women were randomised into 3 groups; intramuscular oxytocin after delivery of the anterior shoulder, sustained uterine massage for 30 minutes followed by delayed oxytocin or received oxytocin and uterine massage immediately after delivery (Abdel-Aleem et al., 2010). It was found that oxytocin was more superior in controlling haemostasis as compared to sustained uterine massage. Uterine massage performed immediately after administration of oxytocin did not show significant additional benefit as compared to oxytocin alone (Abdel-Aleem et al., 2010). The limitation of this trial was that, it was unable to demonstrate the effect of uterine massage on the amount of blood loss in the absence of oxytocin as this was non-ethical.

4.2.2 Aortic compression

Aortic compression can assist in controlling the amount of blood loss by decreasing the blood flow at the distal end including uterine artery (Riley & Burgess, 1994). Aortic compression is achieved via applying pressure with the flat surface of the knuckles above the contracted uterus and slightly to the left (Figure 1). Absence of femoral pulse indicates correct and complete occlusion of the aorta. It is crucial to release and re-apply the pressure every 30 minutes to allow intermittent blood flow to the lower limbs. Aortic compression is a simple intervention that can be used while preparing for a definitive management or during the transfer of patient from a district hospital to another tertiary hospital.

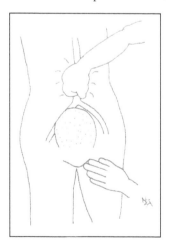

Fig. 1. Aortic compression

External aortic compression devices have been described by several authors (Winter, 1939; Soltan et al., 2009). These have been shown to be effective in reducing the resuscitation time and also the amount of blood being transfused with minimal side-effects reported. However, these devices are not readily available in Malaysia. There is a potential use of this device in our setting especially in district hospital setting. According to CEMD report in the year 2000, 6.6% of PPH mortality had occurred during transfer of patients. Such simple device can be applied by any health care provider (with minimal training) would be of great value in reducing maternal morbidity and mortality.

4.2.3 Bimanual compression

Bimanual compression is performed by inserting the right hand into vagina at anterior surface of the uterus and the left hand is on abdomen at the fundus towards the posterior surface of uterus. The uterus is compressed between the two hands to minimise bleeding (Figure 2). This technique can be used as a temporary measure while patient is being stabilised for definitive treatment.

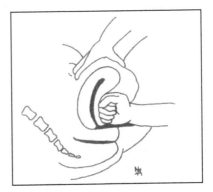

Fig. 2. Bimanual compression

4.2.4 Uterine tamponade

In the past, sterile roller gauze had been used to pack the uterine cavity to reduce blood loss during massive PPH caused by uterine atony (Douglass, 1955). Despite its effectiveness, the popularity of uterine packing has dramatically declined with the wide availability of uterotonic agents (Douglass, 1955).

Nowadays, balloon devices have been recognised as an effective adjuvant strategy for achieving haemostasis in massive PPH in uterine atony. It was hypothesised that intra-uterine balloon exert hydrostatic pressure on the uterine arteries resulting in reduced blood loss (Georgiou, 2009). The most commonly described balloon devices are Bakri balloon, Rusch catheter, Sengstaken-Blackmore catheter, Foley catheter and Condom catheter (Airede & Nnadi, 2008; Keriakos & Mukhopadhyay, 2006; Marcovici & Scoccia, 1999; Majumdar et al., 2010; Vitthala et al., 2009).

Bakri balloon is the only device that is specifically designed for uterine tamponade in massive PPH. It is equipped with large drainage channel that allow drainage of blood from the uterine cavity (Georgiou, 2009). Although both Sengstaken-Blackmore and Foley catheter have drainage channel, they are small in size thus prone to blockage by blood clots. In addition, the distal tip of Sengstaken-Blackmore catheter would deter the contact between the balloon surface and the fundus of uterus. The other two catheters (Rusch and Condom catheter) do not have drainage channel and thus result in difficulty in drainage of blood from the uterine cavity (Georgiou, 2009).

The capacity of balloon insufflations differs between various types of balloons. Rusch catheter has the largest capacity of 1500 ml of fluid (Keriakos & Mukhopadhyay, 2006) followed by Bakri balloon with 500 ml (Georgiou, 2009) while both Sengstaken-Blackmore catheter and Condom catheter have the capacity to accommodate 300 ml (Georgiou, 2009). Foleys catheter has the smallest capacity with 30 ml and the use of multiple Foley catheters have been described (Marcovici & Scoccia, 1999).

Tamponade test' is used to determine the success of controlling the haemostasis in atonic PPH. A negative `tamponade test' indicate inadequate control of bleeding thus require additional strategies such as applying compressive sutures, systematic pelvic devascularisation or hysterectomy.

The use of concomitant uterotonic agents such as oxytocin and Carbetocin while the balloon is still in-situ is recommended to maintain the tamponade effect (Georgiou, 2009). Antibiotic therapy is also recommended to reduce ascending infection during balloon placement (Keriakos & Mukhopadhyay, 2006). However, there is no consensus on duration of its usage. Most authors remove the balloon within 48 hours. However, variations in the rate of deflation have been reported (Georgiou, 2009).

The adverse effects of the balloon devices reported so far were mainly due to over-distension of the balloon which includes pressure necrosis and uterine rupture. Other reported complications were uterine perforation and air embolism especially if air was used to inflate the balloon. Due to this risk, insufflation of balloon with air is not recommended. With regards to subsequent fertility, successful pregnancies have been reported following the use of these balloon devices (Georgiou, 2009).

As uterine atony is a significant contributing factor in PPH, balloon tamponade devices may play a major role in pre-hospital emergency management prior to safe transfer to tertiary centre in reducing blood loss, hence lowering morbidity and mortality. However, to date there is paucity of data in addressing this issue.

4.3 Pharmacological strategies

Effective uterine contractions are crucial to ensure adequate haemostasis following delivery. Several uterotonic agents have been described to be effective in promoting myometrium contractility hence avoiding the need for surgical intervention.

4.3.1 Oxytocin

Oxytocin is the first line therapy for uterine atony. It acts by stimulating rhythmic uterine contraction particularly in the upper segment. It is administered intramuscularly or intravenously; however the onset of action is delayed if given intramuscularly (3-7minutes) as compared to immediate onset if given by intravenous route. Furthermore, due to its short plasma half-life of 3minutes, continuous intravenous infusion is preferred (Breathnach & Geary 2009).

Most centres use the regime of 20 IU oxytocin in 500 ml of crystalloid solution (Breathnach & Geary, 2009; Rajan & Wing, 2010). In Malaysia, 40 IU oxytocin in 500 ml of crystalloid solution is given over the duration of 6 hours. In certain circumstances, 80 IU oxytocin in 500 ml of crystalloid solution has been used effectively.

Adverse effects of oxytocin infusion were mainly related to its anti-diuretic properties resulting in water intoxication, manifesting as headache, vomiting, drowsiness and convulsions (Breathnach & Geary, 2009b). In cases where fluid restriction is indicated, concentrated oxytocin via infusion pump is recommended.

4.3.2 Ergometrine

As opposed to oxytocin, ergometrine results in sustained myometrial contraction. As it also acts on the vascular smooth muscle, it is not suitable for those with hypertension, migraine, heart disease and peripheral vascular disease such as Raynaund's syndrome. It is given as 0.25 mg intramuscularly or intravenously with rapid clinical effect within 2 to 5 minutes that can persist up to 3 hours. Ergometrine is metabolised in the liver and has a plasma half-life of 30 minutes. A repeat dose of ergometrine can be given after 5 minutes if the uterus is still not well contracted. Nausea, vomiting and dizziness are commonly reported side-effects (Breathnach & Geary 2009b).

Syntometrine consists of 5 IU oxytocin and 0.5 mg ergometrine in a single preparation. This preparation results in a rapid onset of uterine contraction due to its oxytocic properties and sustained contractility from the ergometrine component (Rajan & Wing, 2010).

4.3.3 Carbetocin

Carbetocin is a long-acting synthetic oxytocin analogue that is administered via intramuscular or intravenous route. The recommended dose is 100 µg. Carbetocin has the advantage of rapid onset of action, within 2 minutes, similar to oxytocin with additional benefit of longer duration of action. These actions do not differ by the route of administration. However, intramuscular Carbetocin (120 minutes) had been reported to give a longer uterine contraction as compared to intravenous route (60 minutes) (Rath, 2009).

Side effects of carbetocin include headache, hypotension, tremor, flushing, abdominal pain and nausea. Rarely, it was associated with dizziness, chest pain, dyspnoea, metallic taste, vomiting, back pain and chills (Rath, 2009).

Randomised controlled trials have found Carbetocin to be associated with lesser requirement for additional uterotonic agents and uterine massage in high risk patients after caesarean deliveries (Su et al., 2007). However, there was no significant difference in the amount of blood loss and rate of PPH between Carbetocin and oxytocin in these women. Furthermore, a single dose of Carbetocin was found to be more convenient than oxytocin infusion that require intravenous line and is time-consuming (Su et al., 2007).

There are three randomised controlled trials assessing the use of Carbetocin following vaginal delivery. Boucher et al. compared Carbetocin with 2-hour 10 IU oxytocin infusion in 160 women with at least one risk factor for PPH (Boucher et al., 2004). The number of women requiring uterotonic intervention (either additional uterotonic agents or uterine massage) was significantly lower in the Carbetocin group (Boucher et al., 2004). Leung et al. randomised 329 women to intramuscular Carbetocin and intramuscular syntometrine and found no difference in the decline of haemoglobin two days after delivery (Leung et al., 2006). Although the rate of PPH was lower in the Carbetocin group, it was not statistically significant (Leung et al., 2006). About 120 women were randomised to Carbetocin and Syntometrine groups had showed lower haemoglobin drop in the Carbetocin group (Nirmala et al., 2009). All three studies had shown Carbetocin to be associated with lower incidence of adverse effects.

Carbetocin is not widely available in developing countries. In Malaysia, though it is available, its use is restricted to high risk cases due to its higher cost.

4.3.4 Misoprostol

Misoprostol is a synthetic analogue of prostaglandin E_1 that has uterotonic properties (Hofmeyr & Gulmezoglu, 2008). Although it has been used widely as uterotonic agents in certain developed country misoprostol has only been registered for therapeutic use in refractory gastro-duodenal ulcers, and has not been made legally available for pregnancy in view of safety concerns in pregnancy (Health Technology Assessment Unit, Ministry of Health Malaysia, 2003).

Misoprostol is a cheap and effective uterotonic agent that can be administered via oral, sublingual, vaginal or rectally. The onset of action is slower if given rectally with more favourable side effects. Adverse effects of misoprostol are dose-related and commonly reported are diarrhoea, shivering and pyrexia (Breathnach & Geary, 2009).

A Cochrane review has concluded that misoprostal administered at a dose of 600 mcg was effective in reducing blood loss after compared to placebo (Gulmezoglu et al., 2007). However, it was found to be less superior to oxytocin in preventing PPH. More recent trials have challenged the superiority of oxytocin. Several studies have shown that there were no difference in the amount of blood loss between misoprostol and oxytocin (Hofmeyr & Gulmezoglu, 2008; Parsons et al., 2006). In fact, Parsons et al. found that those who received misoprostol required less additional uterotonic (Parsons et al, 2006).

Due to its cost and easy storage, misoprostol may indeed be of value to prevent PPH in low resource setting where oxytocin may not be readily available (Mobeen et al., 2011; Nasreen et al., 2011).

4.3.5 Carboprost/Haemabate

In Malaysia, carboprost is used as second-line therapy for uterine atony-related PPH that has failed to respond to either oxytocin or syntometrine. It is an analogue of PG $F_{2\alpha}$ and acts on smooth muscle resulting in myometrial contractions. The recommended dose is 0.25 mg and it can be given as intramuscular or intramyometrial injection. Intramyometrial administration can be performed trans-abdominally or under direct vision during caesarean deliveries (Breathnach & Geary, 2009).

The clinical effect is faster if given intramyometrial (peak within 5 minutes) as compared to intramuscularly (peak within 15 minutes). A maximum dose of 2mg (8 doses) can be given at 15 minutes interval (Breathnach & Geary, 2009).

Commonly reported adverse effects are nausea, vomiting, diarrhoea, pyrexia, bronchospasm and systemic hypertension. Therefore contraindication to its usage would be those with cardiac and pulmonary disease (Breathnach & Geary, 2009).

4.4 Surgical intervention

In most cases, the use of non pharmacological approach and uterotonic agents are able to curb massive bleeding due to uterine atony. Those who are not responding to these interventions may require surgical interventions. Multidisciplinary support involving anaesthetists and haematologists expertise is essential to ensure an optimal outcome.

4.4.1 B-Lynch compression sutures

In the atonic uterus, the vessels especially at the placental bed are unable to contract to secure bleeding. B-Lynch suture, which was first reported in 1997, comprises of vertical compression suture on the uterine vascular system. The reported success rate was 91.7% (95% CI 84.9%-95.5%) (Doumouchtsis et al., 2007). It is a simple, quick and life-saving procedure to combat bleeding from a lax uterus.

Before performing this procedure, its efficacy should be predicted by doing manual compression of the uterus. The surgeon's left hand is placed behind the uterus while the right hand compresses the lower segment of the uterus just above the bladder reflection. If the amount of bleeding reduces, the compression suture is likely to be effective.

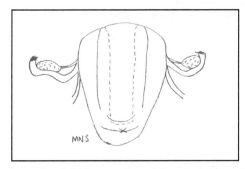

Fig. 3. A puncture 3 cm from the right lower edge of the uterine incision and 3 cm from right lateral border made and threaded through the uterine cavity to emerge at the upper incision margin 3 cm above and its lateral border. Then, the suture is looped over the uterine fundus 3-4 cm from the right border before it being pulled downward vertically to enter the posterior uterine wall at the same level of the first puncture site. The suture is passed through the cavity and emerged on the left uterine border horizontally before it is brought up to the fundus and looped anteriorly. After the needle has passed through the uterine cavity and brought out 3 cm anteriorly and below the incision margin on the left, the two lengths of catgut are pulled tight, while the assistant continuously compressed on the uterus. A knot applied anteriorly to secure the tension.

Lloyd-Davis position is preferred when performing this procedure as the vaginal bleeding can be assessed simultaneously. B-Lynch suture is performed by using absorbable sutures with round bodied needle. The technique B-Lynch suture application is described in Figure 3. B-Lynch surgical technique is relatively safe and allows fertility preservation. Two uterine necroses were reported. (Joshi & Shrivastava M, 2004; Treloar et al., 2006) However, these two cases had received numerous comments and queries regarding the suturing techniques. In one of the comments, B-Lynch had stated among 948 successful cases of B-Lynch sutures worldwide only seven cases failed. (B-Lynch, 2005) Allam et al reviewed 10 case reports involving a total of 38 women who underwent B-Lynch surgical technique for massive PPH. There were 36 successful cases with 2 failures reported. Till date, no known post-operative mortality reported (Allam & B-Lynch, 2005).

4.4.2 Hayman suture

Hayman uterine compression suture (Figure 4) is another method which has been described to arrest bleeding in uterine atony. This technique does not require lower segment hysterotomy therefore it is a good option when PPH occurs following vaginal delivery (Hayman et al., 2002). It is faster, easier and less traumatic to the uterus. The success rate of this procedure is approximately 93.75% (Nanda & Singhal, 2011). However, it may entrap blood within the uterine cavity and subsequently induces haematometra, pyometra and uterine necrosis (B-Lynch, 2005)

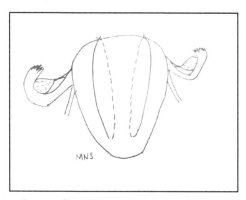

Fig. 4. This procedure involves making two stitches approaching from below the bladder reflection anteriorly to the posterior wall of the uterus at the same level. The knots are placed at the fundus while the uterus is being compressed by an assistant simultaneously.

4.4.3 Vascular ligation/ Occlusion

Currently there is no evidence or consensus regarding the superiority of one treatment to another in massive PPH. The limitations are depending on the availability and experience of surgeons, facilities, and local policies. In the past, laparotomy has been advocated to facilitate devascularisation. Vascular ligation is advocated following failure of compression sutures before resorting to hysterectomy is considered, especially when fertility is of concern. However with recent advancement of less invasive radiological intervention, it has become a viable alternative to vascular ligation.

4.4.3.1 Bilateral uterine artery ligation

This easier technique with fewer complications was first described by Waters in 1952 (Waters, 1952). It involves a low abdominal approach like in Pfannenstiel incision. The uterus is exteriorised and pulled upward to facilitate identification of uterine vessels. An absorbable suture is placed 2 cm below the bladder reflection on both sides of the uterus avoiding the ureters. This technique occludes the ascending branch of uterine vessels, with reported success rate of 80-96% (Morel et al., 2011). This procedure is technically safe other than possible risk of ureteric injury.

4.4.3.2 Bilateral internal iliac (hypogastric artery) ligation

This is one of the oldest surgical technique (Figure 5) introduced as early as 1960's (Sziller et al., 2007). It requires a good knowledge of anatomy to avoid inadvertent injuries to the external iliac vessels and ureters. The success rate of internal iliac artery ligation varies between 42-93% (Morel et al., 2011). Incorrect ligation entails high risks of limbs ischaemia, gluteal claudication, further bleeding and possible ureteric and nerve injury.

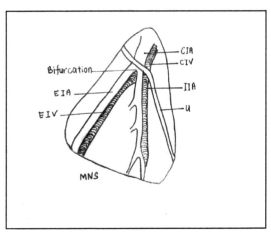

(EIA: external iliac artery; EIV: external iliac vein; CIA: common iliac artery; CIV: common iliac vein; IIA: internal iliac artery; U: ureter)

Fig. 5. The broad ligament is opened and traced upward until at the level of bifurcation of common iliac artery parallel to the sacroiliac curvature. The ureter is commonly on the medial leaf of the broad ligament after crossing the bifurcation of common iliac artery. The vascular sheath needs to be cleared for better visualisation and recognition, minimising inadvertent ligature and venous injury. The internal iliac is a branch of medio-inferior after the bifurcation of common iliac artery. By using a right angle forceps to isolate this vessel, an absorbable ligature is placed 1 to 2 cm below the bifurcation. Following this, a distal pulse at femoral artery is checked to ensure its patency. The same procedure is repeated to the contra-lateral side (Given et al., 1964).

4.4.3.3 Other type of vascular ligation

Many other vascular ligation techniques had been described. For example, triple ligations (Tsirulnikov, 1979) and stepwise sequential ligation (AbdRabbo, 1994).

4.4.4 Embolisation

Uterine artery embolisation is relatively a new technology in managing PPH. It is only available in tertiary hospitals and it requires an interventional radiologist with the attending obstetrician. This procedure requires haemodynamic stability. Ideally, anticipation of its role is best done pre-operatively example in morbidly adherent placenta. However, uterine atony related PPH often unpredictable hence its use is limited. In cases where balloon tamponade has partially reduced bleeding, concurrent use of uterine artery embolisation may be of value to avoid hysterectomy for conserving fertility.

The success rate of emergency uterine artery embolisation for refractory uterine atony ranges from 70 to 100% (Soncini et al., 2007). As pelvic vasculature is very rich in anastomosis, both sides of uterine artery occlusion are required to ensure its effectiveness.

Possible complications include procedure failure with persistent bleeding, infection, vascular injury, postoperative pain and fever. The overall risk is approximately 5% (Soncini et al., 2007). However the reproductive function following this procedure is maintained (Soncini et al., 2007) but may be associated with malpresentation, preterm delivery and PPH.

4.4.5 Hysterectomy

Peri-partum hysterectomy for PPH is a difficult decision to make but a life saving definitive procedure. Although this is usually the last resort however early consideration should be given in selected cases especially when fertility is of less concern and in morbidly adherent placenta. The incidence varies up to 8 per 1,000 deliveries (Lone et al., 2010).

Peri-partum hysterectomy has a morbidity rate of 30-40% (Christopoulos et al., 2011). Complications include ureteric and bladder injury, persistent bleeding requiring re-exploration, pneumonia, and urinary fistula (Christopoulos et al., 2011).

Peri-partum hysterectomy can be performed either as total or subtotal hysterectomy. A total hysterectomy reduces risk of cervical stump malignancy (El-Jallad et al., 2004), but requires longer operating time and has higher rate of urinary tract injuries. A subtotal hysterectomy is faster and safer (Rahman et al., 2008) but regular cervical screening is mandatory.

5. Role of intensive care management

5.1 Intensive care unit (ICU)

Critical care management is an essential component in the management of PPH. A timely management with early involvement of a multidisciplinary team is likely to result in a better maternal outcome by arresting the progression to multi-organ failure, hence lowered morbidity and mortality (Demirkiran et al., 2003; Price et al., 2008; Price et al., 2009).

Postpartum haemorrhage, which contributed to 15% of maternal deaths, has been reported in CEMACH as preventable death or morbidity in some cases. Only a third of mothers who died had received some form of intensive care management (Wong, 2011).

For deaths attributable to PPH, which occurred outside the ICU, the main contributory factors were:

1. Failure to recognise the severity of PPH.
2. Delay in referral to anaesthetist and ICU.
3. Sub-optimal management of PPH while awaiting ICU transfer.

In contrast to the obstetric management of PPH, the critical care management is likely independent of its cause. The majority of obstetric patients who require ICU admission suffer from complications of PPH, sepsis and hypertensive disorders (Naylor & Olson, 2003; Williams et al., 2008).

5.2 High dependency unit (HDU)

The HDU is a specific area in a hospital that provides either a 'step-up' or 'step-down' care as compared to a general ward or ICU respectively. It provides an intermediate care for invasive monitoring and support for patients at risk of developing organ failure. Patients who require mechanical ventilation or suffer multiple organ failure or dysfunction are best managed in ICU (Price et al., 2009).

Early involvement of the anaesthetist at this stage allows assessment to determine if there is a need to 'step-up' to ICU care. Indications for ICU transfer in PPH are shown in Table 3.

Indications for transfer to ICU	
Respiratory	Need for mechanical ventilation Severe respiratory acidosis (uncorrected) Airway protection
Cardiovascular	Inotrope support Pulmonary oedema
Renal	Renal replacement therapy Severe metabolic acidosis (uncorrected)
Neurological	Deteriorating / Poor Glasgow coma scale (GCS)
Others	Multi-organ failure Hypothermia

Table 3. Indications for transfer to ICU

5.3 Transport of the critically ill

When transfer is needed in severely ill patients, it should be done without any delay. This is to ensure closer or more intensive monitoring, rapid resuscitation and more detailed assessment and therapy. A pre-planned and well-prepared transfer reduces the morbidity of patient and allows rapid and safe transfer. Sufficient notice is necessary to the recipient unit to allow adequate time for assembly of equipment and monitors as well as allocation of staff and presence of intensivist on site for rapid assessment upon arrival. In an unstable patient, the minimum team for transfer should consist of a trained and skilled doctor who is able to re-intubate a ventilated patient and to detect any change in condition, a nurse and two assistants to manoeuvre the bed (Guise & Segel, 2008; Haupt et al., 2003; Price et al., 2009; Price et al., 2008).

5.4 Staffing for critical care management team

Early multidisciplinary involvement and planning for critical care is crucial in the management of PPH. This should involve the obstetricians, midwives, physicians, intensivists, anaesthetists, haematologists, blood bank technicians, nursing and other allied health professionals. The role of each of the main personnel in ICU is defined below.

Early combined care of high-risk patients with intensivist/anaesthetist, as early as antenatal period, is prudent in reducing morbidity. Intensivist/anaesthetist plays a key role in the critical care management. This enables immediate detection and early management of complications, hence, may prevent or lower morbidity and mortality. (Guise & Segel, 2008; Martin & Foley 2006; Plaat & Wray, 2008)

Nursing the critically ill is a complex job. Their main role is to provide continuous close monitoring of the patient. They are able to analyze patient's clinical changes, anticipate possible complications leading to shorter recovery period and better emotional support for both the patient and family members. (Price et al., 2008; Simpson & Barker, 2008; Guise & Segel 2008)

Physiotherapist plays an important role in reducing overall morbidity of the patient. Post-operative physiotherapy enables a faster recovery phase, lower risk of ventilation-associated sepsis or pneumonia, and a shorter ICU stay. (Daber & Jackson 1987; Skinner et al., 2008; Thomas et al., 2006)

5.5 Blood bank

Blood bank facilities in a hospital are essential for immediate provision of blood in cases of massive PPH. Adherence to blood bank policies and guidelines is necessary to avoid injudicious use of blood and blood products. Liaison with haematologist will go a long way to ensure appropriate handling and usage of blood and blood products.

5.6 Haemodynamic monitoring

Acute circulatory failure or shock is a condition in which there is inadequate tissue perfusion. The main aim of management is to restore perfusion to the compromised areas in order to provide adequate oxygenation to the affected tissue. In situations where the diagnosis is in doubt, resuscitation is initiated to improve the patient's haemodynamic status before appropriate definitive therapy is rendered (Wise & Clark 2010b).

Identification of patients who require resuscitation, and assessment of its adequacy thereof, is essential in critical management. Clinical assessment of patient's haemodynamic status is easy to perform and rapidly informative. This includes clinical parameters such as conscious level (Glasgow Coma Scale), pulse rate, respiratory rate, capillary refill and urine output (Pearse & Rhodes, 2004; Price et al., 2008).

Monitoring equipment provides additional information to assess adequacy of resuscitation efforts. This can be broadly categorised into non-invasive and invasive types of monitoring. The former includes continuous electrocardiography, non-invasive blood pressure monitoring, pulse oximetry and capnography, while the latter includes direct measurements of intra-arterial blood pressure, central venous pressure, pulmonary artery pressure, central venous oxygen saturation, and cardiac output. In massive obstetric haemorrhage, invasive monitoring may be crucial to allow continuous assessment of the haemodynamic status until clinical improvement occurs. However, not all sophisticated monitoring equipment may be available in every hospital, in which case management decisions may need to be based on clinical assessment (Martin & Foley, 2006; Moore & Chandraharan, 2010; Pearse & Rhodes, 2004).

5.7 Haemodynamic management

Cardiovascular support may be required in women with PPH to maintain an adequate cardiac output and blood pressure. This includes fluid administration, treatment of abnormal heart rate and rhythm, use of vasoactive agents, thrombolysis, ventilatory support and uncommonly other mechanical devices, such as pacemaker, ventricular assist devices, or extracorporeal membrane oxygenator (Pearse & Rhodes, 2004; Price et al., 2008).

Rapid intravenous infusion is the key to initial resuscitation. The aim is to improve microvascular blood flow to provide tissue oxygenation by expanding the intravascular volume and improving cardiac output. The type and amount of fluid used is dependent on the underlying aetiology of circulatory insufficiency, and to a lesser extent the availability of any particular fluids. The choice between crystalloid and colloid during resuscitation remains a debate. Excessive use of normal saline has been reported to result in hyperchloraemic acidosis. The composition of Ringer lactate solution closely resembles that in the plasma and is considered to be one of the most "physiological" cystalloids available for use. In contrast to crystalloid, colloid remains longer in the intravascular compartment and therefore may be more effective in severe hypovolaemia (Bauer et al., 2009; Shoemaker & Kram, 1988).

A useful guide is to infuse an initial amount of 10 ml/kg of colloid or 20 ml/kg of crystalloid followed by clinical and haemodynamic assessment of the response. More fluids should be administered if the patient remains hypovolaemic. Approximately three times the volume of crystalloid is required to achieve blood volume expansion to the same degree as colloid. Large volumes of intravenous fluids may have to be administered while awaiting the availability of cross-matched blood (Price et al., 2008; Shoemaker & Kram, 1988).

Coagulopathy may ensue during massive blood loss or as a result of massive blood transfusion. Correction of hypothermia is essential to prevent exacerbation of coagulopathy. Severe acidosis may warrant correction with sodium bicarbonate to prevent acidosis-induced myocardial depression, provided ventilation is not compromised (Bauer et al., 2009; Price et al., 2009).

Patients who have no prior cardiac disease usually respond to volume resuscitation with intravenous fluids, blood and blood products. However, a small percentage of patients, especially those with pre-existing cardiovascular compromise, may require vasoactive agents to improve cardiac function and peripheral circulation. Cardiac failure secondary to coronary artery insufficiency may require vasodilator therapy using glyceryl trinitrate. Loop diuretics may be needed to reduce pulmonary congestion in acute pulmonary oedema associated with left ventricular failure. Infusion of a positive inotrope (e.g. epinephrine, dobutamine) and/or a vasoconstrictor (e.g. norepinephrine) should be considered to provide circulatory support and maintain adequate renal perfusion. Mechanical devices such as ventricular assist devices and intra-aortic balloon pumps to improve cardiac output have been advocated in critically ill patients unresponsive to pharmacologic therapy. (Pearse & Rhodes, 2004; Price et al., 2008).

5.8 Respiratory management

Acute respiratory distress syndrome is one of the complications of massive haemorrhage, which may require ventilatory support. The aim of respiratory management is to maintain adequate gas exchange by ensuring a patent airway, sufficient oxygen therapy and sustainable ventilation. Airway management is a challenge in pregnant women due to a combination of factors such as weight gain, fluid retention, and enlarged breasts resulting in difficult laryngoscopy. The patient may rarely present with stridor, and difficult endotracheal intubation may complicate airway management. (Price et al. 2009)

5.9 Renal management

Acute renal failure is one of the main causative factors of maternal deaths following massive PPH. The mainstay of treatment is aimed at providing support by minimising damage to the surviving nephrons till the kidneys recover. Restoration of circulation by fluid or blood together with the judicious use of vasopressors will improve perfusion pressure and maintain adequate urine output (> 0.5-1 ml/kg/hour). Electrolyte derangement, especially involving potassium, needs to be corrected. Severe acidosis may require sodium bicarbonate therapy. Renal replacement therapy, if indicated, should be started without delay following early nephrology consultation. (Demirkiran et al., 2003; Anthony & Johanson, 1996)

5.10 Others

Prevention of venous thrombo-embolism is necessary in view of the hypercoagulable state during post-partum period. This can be achieved with compression stockings, adequate hydration, thromboprophylactic agents, limb physiotherapy and early mobilisation (Price et al., 2009).

6. Transfusion of blood & blood products

According to British Committee for Standards in Haematology, the therapeutic aim for management of massive blood loss is to maintain:

- Haemoglobin ≥ 8.0 g/dl
- Platelet count ≥ 75 x 10^9/l
- Prothrombin time ≤ 1.5 mean control
- Activated prothrombin time ≤ 1.5 mean control
- Fibrinogen ≥ 1.0 g/l

Massive PPH would require blood and blood products to replace the clotting factors, fibrinogen and platelets. There are various definitions on massive blood transfusion. These include replacement of the full circulating volume within 24 hours, loss of 50% of circulating blood volume within 3 hours, estimated blood loss of more than 5000 ml, or transfusion of more than 4 units of blood in an hour with ongoing blood loss (Moore & Chandraharan, 2010; Wise & Clark, 2010a).

Massive transfusion may be complicated by citrate toxicity, acid-base and electrolyte disturbances, and hypothermia. Other risks of transfusion include haemolytic reactions, anaphylactic reactions, febrile non-haemolytic reactions, transmission of infectious disease, and alloimmunisation (Moore & Chandraharan, 2010; Padmanabhan et al., 2009).

6.1 Red cell transfusion

Concentrated red blood cells (RBC) is the first line therapy in massive PPH. The aim is to improve oxygenation in the peripheral tissues. Each unit of concentrated RBC improve haemoglobin by 1.0 g/dl as well as haematocrit by 3%. Commencement of blood transfusion should be guided by clinical assessment rather than result of full blood count (Bolan & Klein, 2007; Klein, 2006; Padmanabhan et al., 2009).

6.2 Management of coagulopathy

Management of transfusion-associated coagulopathy entails anticipation, prompt recognition and early initiation of therapy. Late detection of disseminated intravascular coagulation (DIVC) results in systemic bleeding which may lead to multi-organ failure and poor prognosis. Hence, it is not necessary to wait for laboratory results if coagulopathy is suspected and clinical bleeding is present. The management of coagulopathy should be in liaison with the haematologist. Blood components that are required in management of DIVC include fresh frozen plasma, cryoprecipitate and platelet (Bolan & Klein, 2007; Chandraharan & Arulkumaran, 2007; Klein, 2006; Moore & Chandraharan, 2010;).

Fresh frozen plasma (FFP) is derived from whole blood. It contains all the coagulation factors, main inhibitors, anti-thrombin III and protein C. A prothrombin time (PT) and APTT ratios of >1.5 are significantly associated with an increased risk of clinical coagulopathy. About 5 to 10 units of cryoprecipitate (containing Factor VIII, fibrinogen, factor XIII and fibronectin) should be infused following FFP used to correct hypofibrinogenaemia. Platelet transfusion is required when the count is lower than 50 x10^9/l in the context of persistent bleeding (Key & Negrier, 2007; Klein, 2006).

Recombinant Factor VIIa (rFVIIa) is an activated form of Factor VII. It is licensed for use in haemophilia but not in massive PPH due to paucity of data on its use. There are currently no guidelines for its use in obstetric haemorrhage, although proposals for guidelines are starting to appear. However, it may have a role in the management of massive PPH refractory to conventional treatment. Recombinant Factor VIIa was found to be effective in a review of 65 case studies of women with massive PPH. There are limitations to its use, including limited information about safety when used in obstetric patients, cost and non-response in a minority of patients. Further evaluation is required (Haynes et al., 2007; Karalapillai & Popham, 2007; Searle et al., 2008).

6.3 Jehovah witness

It is important to identify women who refuse blood and blood products, e.g. Jehovah's Witnesses. These patients will not accept either the whole blood or its other main components i.e. packed red cells, white blood cells, platelets, or plasma. Consent or advanced directive' should be obtained with regards to the acceptability of types of blood products or other recombinant factors. (Moore & Chandraharan, 2010; Wise & Clark, 2010a). Various strategies have been employed to prevent PPH and requirement of blood transfusion in these high-risk patients.

Correction of anaemia prior to delivery is of utmost importance. Use of iron supplementation and good nutrition with appropriate dietician referral are usually employed. In selected cases, erythropoietin may be given after discussion with haematologist.

The use of Carbetocin as the first line uterotonic agent at AMTSL had been shown to be associated to lesser blood loss (Nirmala et al., 2009); In the event of uterine atony, early involvement of senior personnel and a more aggressive approach to definitive treatment i.e. hysterectomy; in cases with retained placenta, intra-umbilical oxytocin injection instead of manual removal of placenta has been shown to reduce the amount of blood loss though not at a significant level (Lim et al., 2011). These intra-partum strategies will reduce the risk of massive blood loss and hence reducing the need for transfusion.

When operative intervention is needed, certain steps to minimise bleeding may be employed. The use of diathermy or blunt dissection to open the layers of abdominal wall will reduce bleeding as compared sharp dissection. Appropriate autologous blood transfusion techniques, such as normovolaemic haemodilution, pre-operative autologous blood donation, intra-operative red cell salvage, should be considered in this group of women to avoid blood transfusion (Moore & Chandraharan, 2010; Wise & Clark, 2010a; Heard & Quinn, 2010). However, these services are not readily available in all centres. Hence these women should have their deliveries in centres that provide this particular service.

The use of cell salvage may be acceptable by Jehovah's Witness as the blood remained in continuity with their body circulation (King, 2009; Remmers & Speer, 2006). However, its use in obstetric cases due to PPH is still viewed negatively for the potential fear of amniotic fluid embolism due to fetal cells, fat or faecal matter contamination. This potential risk has to be communicated to the patient.

Acute normovolaemic haemodilution may be used by the anaesthetist intra-operatively during either elective or emergency cases. Following anaesthesia, a total of 15 to 20 ml/kg of blood is withdrawn from the patient and is replaced by either crystalloid or colloid. The blood is kept and re-transfused after completion of operation. The re-transfused blood will contain clotting factors and platelets. This procedure is also acceptable to the Jehovah's Witness as the replaced blood is in continuity with body circulation. However, this procedure is not without complication as it may cause cardiovascular instability (Remmers & Speer, 2006).

Pre-operative autologous blood donation involves repeated donation of blood by the patient at least 4 to 6 weeks prior to the delivery or operation. The blood is kept and transfused if necessary. Though this method can reduce risk of transfusion related infection and reaction, it is not acceptable among Jehovah's Witness. This is in view of discontinuity of blood from their circulation (Heard & Quinn, 2010; Remmers & Speer, 2006).

Other methods acceptable to Jehovah's Witness include the use of antifibrinolytics (aprotinin and tranexamic acid) and Perfluorocarbon-based or haemoglobin-based oxygen-carrying compounds (Hemopure, Oxygent or PolyHeme). These products have been shown to reduce the risk of re-laparotomy for bleeding and the need for blood transfusion (Heard & Quinn, 2010).

7. Conclusion

PPH is a major cause of maternal deaths worldwide and uterine atony is the main attributor. In order to reduce maternal mortality, one of the strategies should be towards primary, secondary and tertiary prevention of uterine atony. Close relationship with ancillary support i.e. blood bank facilities, intensivists and ICU care completes the team in management of atonic PPH.

8. References

Abdel-Aleem, H.; Hofmeyr, G.J.; Shokry, M. & El-Sonoosy, E. (2006). Uterine massage and postpartum blood loss, *International journal of gynaecology and obstetrics: the official organ of the International Federation of Gynaecology and Obstetrics*, Vol. 93, No. 3, pp. 238-239.

Abdel-Aleem, H.; Singata, M.; Abdel-Aleem, M.; Mshweshwe, N.; Williams, X. & Hofmeyr, G.J. (2010). Uterine massage to reduce postpartum hemorrhage after vaginal delivery, *International journal of gynaecology and obstetrics: the official organ of the International Federation of Gynaecology and Obstetrics*, Vol. 111, No. 1, pp. 32-36.

AbdRabbo, S.A. (1994). Stepwise uterine devascularization: a novel technique for management of uncontrolled postpartum hemorrhage with preservation of the uterus, *American Journal of Obstetrics and Gynecology*, Vol. 171, No. 3, pp. 694-700.

Airede, L.R. & Nnadi, D.C. (2008). The use of the condom-catheter for the treatment of postpartum haemorrhage - the Sokoto experience, *Tropical doctor*, Vol. 38, No. 2, pp. 84-86.

Allam, M.S. & B-Lynch, C. (2005). The B-Lynch and other uterine compression suture techniques, *International journal of gynaecology and obstetrics: the official organ of the International Federation of Gynaecology and Obstetrics*, Vol. 89, No. 3, pp. 236-241.

Anthony, J. & Johanson, R.B. (1996). Critical care in pregnancy, *Current Obstetrics & Gynaecology*, Vol. 6, No. 2, pp. 98-104.

Bateman, B.T.; Berman, M.F.; Riley, L.E. & Leffert, L.R. (2010) The epidemiology of postpartum hemorrhage in a large, nationwide sample of deliveries, *Anesthesia and Analgesia*, Vol. 110, No. 5, pp. 1368-1373.

Bauer, W.O.; Monti, G.; Cecconi, M. & Rhodes, A. (2009) Management of the circulation on ICU, *Surgery (Oxford)*, Vol. 27, No. 11, pp. 486-491.

Begley, C.M.; Gyte, G.M.; Murphy, D.J.; Devane, D.; McDonald, S.J. & McGuire, W. (2010) Active versus expectant management for women in the third stage of labour, *Cochrane database of systematic reviews (Online)*, Vol. 7, No. 7, pp. CD007412.

B-Lynch, C. (2005). Partial ischemic necrosis of the uterus following a uterine brace compression suture, *BJOG : an international journal of obstetrics and gynaecology*, Vol. 112, No. 1, pp. 126-127.

Bolan, C.D. & Klein, H.G. (2007) Blood Component and Pharmacologic Therapy of Hemostatic Disorders in *Consultative Hemostasis and Thrombosis (Second Edition)* W.B. Saunders, Philadelphia, pp. 461-490.

Bonnar, J. (2000). Massive obstetric haemorrhage, *Bailliere's best practice & research.Clinical obstetrics & gynaecology*, Vol. 14, No. 1, pp. 1-18.

Boucher, M.; Nimrod, C.A.; Tawagi, G.F.; Meeker, T.A.; Rennicks White, R.E. & Varin, J. (2004). Comparison of carbetocin and oxytocin for the prevention of postpartum hemorrhage following vaginal delivery:a double-blind randomized trial, *Journal d'obstetrique et gynecologie du Canada : JOGC*, Vol. 26, No. 5, pp. 481-488.

Brace, V.; Kernaghan D & Penney G. (2007). Learning from adverse clinical outcomes: major obstetric haemorrhage in Scotland, 2003–2005. *British Journal of Obstetrics & Gynaecology*, Vol.114, pp. 1388–1396

Breathnach, F. & Geary, M. (2006). Standard Medical Therapy in *A Textbook of Postpartum Hemorrhage*, eds. C. B-Lynch, L.G. Keith, A.B. Lalonde & M. Karoshi, Sapiens Publishing, United Kingdom, pp. 256.

Breathnach, F. & Geary, M. (2009). Uterine atony: definition, prevention, nonsurgical management, and uterine tamponade, *Seminars in perinatology*, Vol. 33, No. 2, pp. 82-87.

Callaghan, W.M.; Kuklina, E.V. & Berg, C.J. (2010). Trends in postpartum hemorrhage: United States, 1994-2006, *American Journal of Obstetrics and Gynecology*, Vol. 202, No. 4, pp. 353.e1-353.e6.

Carlough, M. & McCall, M. (2005). Skilled birth attendance: what does it mean and how can it be measured? A clinical skills assessment of maternal and child health workers in Nepal, *International journal of gynaecology and obstetrics: the official organ of the International Federation of Gynaecology and Obstetrics*, Vol. 89, No. 2, pp. 200-208.

Carroli, G.; Cuesta, C.; Abalos, E. & Gulmezoglu, A.M. (2008). Epidemiology of postpartum haemorrhage: a systematic review, *Best practice & research.Clinical obstetrics & gynaecology*, Vol. 22, No. 6, pp. 999-1012.

Chandraharan, E. & Arulkumaran, S. (2007). Massive postpartum haemorrhage and management of coagulopathy, *Obstetrics, Gynaecology & Reproductive Medicine*, Vol. 17, No. 4, pp. 119-122.

Christopoulos, P.; Hassiakos, D.; Tsitoura, A.; Panoulis, K.; Papadias, K. & Vitoratos, N. (2011). Obstetric hysterectomy: a review of cases over 16 years, *Journal of obstetrics and gynaecology : the journal of the Institute of Obstetrics and Gynaecology*, Vol. 31, No. 2, pp. 139-141.

Combs, C.A.; Murphy, E.L. & Laros, R.K.,Jr (1991). Factors associated with postpartum hemorrhage with vaginal birth, *Obstetrics and gynecology*, Vol. 77, No. 1, pp. 69-76.

Cunningham, F.G.; Leveno, K.J.; Bloom, S.L.; Hauth, J.C.; Gilstrap, L. & Wenstrom, K.D. (2005). *Williams Obstetrics*, 22nd edn, MacGraw-Hill, USA.

Daber, S.E. & Jackson, S.E. (1987). Role of the physiotherapist in the intensive care unit, *Intensive care nursing*, Vol. 3, No. 4, pp. 165-171.

Demirkiran, O.; Dikmen, Y.; Utku, T. & Urkmez, S. (2003). Critically ill obstetric patients in the intensive care unit, *International Journal of Obstetric Anesthesia*, Vol. 12, No. 4, pp. 266-270.

Department of Economic and Social Affairs, United Nations Statistics Division, United Nation (2011). *Millennium Development Goals report 2011*.

Department of Economic and Social Affairs, United Nations Statistics Division, United Nation (2010). *Millennium Development Goals Indicators*. Available: http://mdgs.un.org/unsd/Data.aspx, 30.07.2010

Devine, P.C. (2009). Obstetric hemorrhage, *Seminars in perinatology*, Vol. 33, No. 2, pp. 76-81.

Division of Family Health Development, Ministry of Health (2005). *Report on the confidential enquiries into maternal deaths in Malaysia 2001-2005*, pp. 1-24.

Division of Family Health Development, Ministry of Health (2000). *Report on the confidential enquiries into maternal deaths in Malaysia 1997-2000.*

Division of Family Health Development, Ministry of Health (1996). *Report on the confidential enquiries into maternal deaths in Malaysia 1995-1996.*

Division of Family Health Development, Ministry of Health (1994) *Report on the confidential enquiries into maternal deaths in Malaysia 1994,* pp. 31-40.

Doran, J.R.; O'Brien, S.A.,Jr & Randall, J.H. (1955). Repeated postpartum hemorrhage, *Obstetrics and gynecology,* Vol. 5, No. 2, pp. 186-192.

Douglass, L.H. (1955). The passing of the pack, *Bulletin of the School of Medicine (Baltimore, Md.),* Vol. 40, No. 2, pp. 38-39.

Doumouchtsis, S.K.; Papageorghiou, A.T. & Arulkumaran, S. (2007) Systematic review of conservative management of postpartum hemorrhage: what to do when medical treatment fails, *Obstetrical & gynecological survey,* Vol. 62, No. 8, pp. 540-547.

Draycott, T.; Sibanda, T.; Owen, L.; Akande, V.; Winter, C.; Reading, S. & Whitelaw, A. (2006). Does training in obstetric emergencies improve neonatal outcome?, *BJOG : an international journal of obstetrics and gynaecology,* Vol. 113, No. 2, pp. 177-182.

Elbourne, D.R.; Prendiville, W.J.; Carroli, G.; Wood, J. & McDonald, S. (2001). Prophylactic use of oxytocin in the third stage of labour, *Cochrane database of systematic reviews (Online),* Vol. (4), No. 4, pp. CD001808.

El-Jallad, M.F.; Zayed, F. & Al-Rimawi, H.S. (2004). Emergency peripartum hysterectomy in Northern Jordan: indications and obstetric outcome (an 8-year review), *Archives of Gynecology and Obstetrics,* Vol. 270, No. 4, pp. 271-273.

Georgiou, C. (2009). Balloon tamponade in the management of postpartum haemorrhage: a review, *BJOG : an international journal of obstetrics and gynaecology,* Vol. 116, No. 6, pp. 748-757.

Given, F.T.,Jr; Gates, H.S. & Morgan, B.E. (1964). Pregnancy Following Bilateral Ligation of the Internal Iliac (Hypogastric) Arteries, *American Journal of Obstetrics and Gynecology,* Vol. 89, pp. 1078-1079.

Gosman, G.G.; Baldisseri, M.R.; Stein, K.L.; Nelson, T.A.; Pedaline, S.H.; Waters, J.H. & Simhan, H.N. (2008). Introduction of an obstetric-specific medical emergency team for obstetric crises: implementation and experience, *American Journal of Obstetrics and Gynecology,* Vol. 198, No. 4, pp. 367.e1-367.e7.

Grotegut, C.A.; Paglia, M.J.; Johnson, L.N.; Thames, B. & James, A.H. (2011). Oxytocin exposure during labor among women with postpartum hemorrhage secondary to uterine atony, *American Journal of Obstetrics and Gynecology,* Vol. 204, No. 1, pp. 56.e1-56.e6.

Guise, J. & Segel, S. (2008). Teamwork in obstetric critical care, *Best Practice & Research Clinical Obstetrics & Gynaecology,* Vol. 22, No. 5, pp. 937-951.

Gulmezoglu, A.M.; Forna, F.; Villar, J. & Hofmeyr, G.J. (2007). Prostaglandins for preventing postpartum haemorrhage, *Cochrane database of systematic reviews (Online),* Vol. (3), No. 3, pp. CD000494.

Gutierrez, G.; Reines, H.D. & Wulf-Gutierrez, M.E. (2004). Clinical review: hemorrhagic shock, *Critical Care (London, England),* Vol. 8, No. 5, pp. 373-381.

Harvey, S.A.; Blandon, Y.C.; McCaw-Binns, A.; Sandino, I.; Urbina, L.; Rodriguez, C.; Gomez, I.; Ayabaca, P.; Djibrina, S. & Nicaraguan Maternal and Neonatal Health Quality Improvement Group (2007). Are skilled birth attendants really skilled? A measurement method, some disturbing results and a potential way forward, *Bulletin of the World Health Organization,* Vol. 85, No. 10, pp. 783-790.

Hasan, F.; Arumugam, K. & Sivanesaratnam, V. (1991). Uterine leiomyomata in pregnancy, *International journal of gynaecology and obstetrics: the official organ of the International Federation of Gynaecology and Obstetrics,* Vol. 34, No. 1, pp. 45-48.

Haupt, M.T.; Bekes, C.E.; Brilli, R.J.; Carl, L.C.; Gray, A.W.; Jastremski, M.S.; Naylor, D.F.; PharmD, M.R., Md, A.S; Wedel, S.K., Md, M.H. & Task Force of the American College of Critical Care Medicine, Society of Critical Care Medicine (2003). Guidelines on critical care services and personnel: Recommendations based on a system of categorization of three levels of care, *Critical Care Medicine,* Vol. 31, No. 11, pp. 2677-2683.

Hayman, R.G.; Arulkumaran, S. & Steer, P.J. (2002). Uterine compression sutures: surgical management of postpartum hemorrhage, *Obstetrics and gynecology,* Vol. 99, No. 3, pp. 502-506.

Haynes, J.; Laffan, M. & Plaat, F. (2007). Use of recombinant activated factor VII in massive obstetric haemorrhage, *International Journal of Obstetric Anesthesia,* Vol. 16, No. 1, pp. 40-49.

Health Technology Assessment Unit, Ministry of Health Malaysia (2003), *Misoprostol in Pregnancy.*

Heard, J.S.; Quinn, A.C. (2010). Jehovah's Witnesses – surgical and anaesthetic management options, *Anaesthesia & intensive care medicine,*Vol. 11, No. 2, pp. 62-64.

Hofmeyr, G.J. & Gulmezoglu, A.M. (2008). Misoprostol for the prevention and treatment of postpartum haemorrhage, *Best practice & research.Clinical obstetrics & gynaecology,* Vol. 22, No. 6, pp. 1025-1041.

Hofmeyr, G.J.; Haws, R.A.; Bergstrom, S.; Lee, A.C.; Okong, P.; Darmstadt, G.L.; Mullany, L.C.; Oo, E.K. & Lawn, J.E. (2009). Obstetric care in low-resource settings: what, who, and how to overcome challenges to scale up?, *International journal of gynaecology and obstetrics,* Vol. 107 Suppl 1, pp. S21-44, S44-5.

International Confederation of Midwives (ICM) and International Federation of Gynaecologists and Obstetricians (FIGO) (2003). Management of the Third Stage of Labour to Prevent Post-partum Haemorrhage (Joint statement). Available: http://www.pphprevention.org/files/ICM_FIGO_Joint_Statement.pdf

Joseph, K.S.; Rouleau, J.; Kramer, M.S.; Young, D.C.; Liston, R.M.; Baskett, T.F. & Maternal Health Study Group of the Canadian Perinatal Surveillance System (2007). Investigation of an increase in postpartum haemorrhage in Canada, *British Journal of Obstetrics & Gynaecology,* Vol. 114, No. 6, pp. 751-759.

Joshi, V.M.; Shrivastava, M. (2004). Partial ischemic necrosis of the uterus following a uterine brace compression suture, *British Journal of Obstetrics & Gynaecology,* Vol. 111, pp. 279-280.

Kalaivani, K. (2009). Prevalence & consequences of anaemia in pregnancy, *The Indian journal of medical research,* Vol. 130, No. 5, pp. 627-633.

Karalapillai, D. & Popham, P. (2007). Recombinant factor VIIa in massive postpartum haemorrhage, *International Journal of Obstetric Anesthesia,* Vol. 16, No. 1, pp. 29-34.

Keriakos, R. & Mukhopadhyay, A. (2006). The use of the Rusch balloon for management of severe postpartum haemorrhage, *Journal of obstetrics and gynaecology : the journal of the Institute of Obstetrics and Gynaecology,* Vol. 26, No. 4, pp. 335-338.

Key, N.S. & Negrier, C. (2007). Coagulation factor concentrates: past, present, and future", *The Lancet*, Vol. 370, No. 9585, pp. 439-448.

King, M.; Wrench, I.; Galimberti, A.; Spray, R. (2009). Introduction of cell salvage to a large obstetric unit: the first six months, *International Journal of Obstetric Anesthesia*, Vol. 18, No. 2, pp. 111-117.

Klein, H.G. (2006). Transfusion Medicine in *Blood Substitutes*, eds. Robert M. Winslow & MD, Academic Press, Oxford, pp. 17-33.

Kominiarek, M.A. & Kilpatrick, S.J. (2007). Postpartum hemorrhage: a recurring pregnancy complication, *Seminars in perinatology*, Vol. 31, No. 3, pp. 159-166.

Korhonen, J. & Kariniemi, V. (1994). Emergency cesarean section: the effect of delay on umbilical arterial gas balance and Apgar scores, *Acta Obstetricia et Gynecologica Scandinavica*, Vol. 73, No. 10, pp. 782-786.

Leduc, D.; Senikas, V.; Lalonde, A.B.; Ballerman, C.; Biringer, A.,;Delaney, M.; Duperron, L.; Girard, I.; Jones, D.; Lee, L.S.; Shepherd, D.; Wilson, K.; Clinical Practice Obstetrics Committee & Society of Obstetricians and Gynaecologists of Canada (2009). Active management of the third stage of labour: prevention and treatment of postpartum hemorrhage, *Journal of obstetrics and gynaecology Canada: JOGC = Journal d'obstetrique et gynecologie du Canada : JOGC*, Vol. 31, No. 10, pp. 980-993.

Leung, S.W.; Ng, P.S.; Wong, W.Y. & Cheung, T.H. (2006) A randomised trial of carbetocin versus syntometrine in the management of the third stage of labour, *BJOG : an international journal of obstetrics and gynaecology*, Vol. 113, No. 12, pp. 1459-1464.

Lim, P.S.; Singh, S.; Lee, A.; Muhammad Yassin, M.A. (2011) Umbilical vein oxytocin in the management of retained placenta: an alternative to manual removal of placenta? Archives Gynecology and Obstetrics, Vol. 284, No. 5, pp. 1073-1079. doi: 10.1007/s00404-010-1785-6

Lombaard, H. & Pattinson, R.C. (2009). Common errors and remedies in managing postpartum haemorrhage, *Best practice & research.Clinical obstetrics & gynaecology*, Vol. 23, No. 3, pp. 317-326.

Lone, F.; Sultan, A.H.; Thakar, R. & Beggs, A. (2010). Risk factors and management patterns for emergency obstetric hysterectomy over 2 decades, *International journal of gynaecology and obstetrics: the official organ of the International Federation of Gynaecology and Obstetrics*, Vol. 109, No. 1, pp. 12-15.

Magann, E.F.; Evans, S.; Hutchinson, M.; Collins, R.; Howard, B.C. & Morrison, J.C. (2005). Postpartum hemorrhage after vaginal birth: an analysis of risk factors, *Southern medical journal*, Vol. 98, No. 4, pp. 419-422.

Majumdar, A.; Saleh, S.; Davis, M.; Hassan, I. & Thompson, P.J. (2010). Use of balloon catheter tamponade for massive postpartum haemorrhage, *Journal of obstetrics and gynaecology : the journal of the Institute of Obstetrics and Gynaecology*, Vol. 30, No. 6, pp. 586-593.

Marcovici, I. & Scoccia, B. (1999). Postpartum hemorrhage and intrauterine balloon tamponade. A report of three cases, *The Journal of reproductive medicine*, Vol. 44, No. 2, pp. 122-126.

Martin, S.R. & Foley, M.R. (2006). Intensive care in obstetrics: An evidence-based review, *American Journal of Obstetrics and Gynecology*, Vol. 195, No. 3, pp. 673-689.

Mobeen, N.; Durocher, J.; Zuberi, N.; Jahan, N.; Blum, J.; Wasim, S.; Walraven, G. & Hatcher, J. (2011). Administration of misoprostol by trained traditional birth attendants to prevent postpartum haemorrhage in homebirths in Pakistan: a randomised placebo-controlled trial, *BJOG : an international journal of obstetrics and gynaecology,* Vol. 118, No. 3, pp. 353-361.

Moore, J. & Chandraharan, E. (2010). Management of massive postpartum haemorrhage and coagulopathy, *Obstetrics, Gynaecology & Reproductive Medicine,* Vol. 20, No. 6, pp. 174-180.

Morel, O.; Malartic, C.; Muhlstein, J.; Gayat, E.; Judlin, P.; Soyer, P. & Barranger, E. (2011). Pelvic arterial ligations for severe post-partum hemorrhage. Indications and techniques, *Journal of Visceral Surgery,* Vol. 148, No. 2, pp. e95-e102.

Mukherjee, S. & Arulkumaran, S. (2009). Post-partum haemorrhage, *Obstetrics, Gynaecology & Reproductive Medicine,* Vol. 19, No. 5, pp. 121-126.

Nanda, S. & Singhal, S.R. (2011). Hayman uterine compression stitch for arresting atonic postpartum hemorrhage: 5 years experience, *Taiwanese journal of obstetrics & gynecology,* Vol. 50, No. 2, pp. 179-181.

Nasreen, H.E.; Nahar, S.; Al Mamun, M.; Afsana, K. & Byass, P. (2011). Oral misoprostol for preventing postpartum haemorrhage in home births in rural Bangladesh: how effective is it?, *Global health action,* Vol. 4, pp. 10.3402/gha.v4i0.7017. Epub 2011 Aug 10.

Naylor, D.F. & Olson, M.M. (2003). Critical care obstetrics and gynecology, *Critical Care Clinics,* Vol. 19, No. 1, pp. 127-149.

Neilson, J.P. (2009). Maternal mortality, *Obstetrics, Gynaecology & Reproductive Medicine,* Vol. 19, No. 2, pp. 33-36.

Nirmala, K.; Zainuddin, A.A.; Ghani, N.A.; Zulkifli, S. & Jamil, M.A. (2009). Carbetocin versus syntometrine in prevention of post-partum hemorrhage following vaginal delivery, *The journal of obstetrics and gynaecology research,* Vol. 35, No. 1, pp. 48-54.

Padmanabhan, A.; Schwartz, J. & Spitalnik, S.L. (2009). Transfusion Therapy in Postpartum Hemorrhage, *Seminars in perinatology,* Vol. 33, No. 2, pp. 124-127.

Pahlavan, P.; Nezhat, C. & Nezhat, C. (2001). Hemorrhage in obstetrics and gynecology, *Current opinion in obstetrics & gynecology,* Vol. 13, No. 4, pp. 419-424.

Parsons, S.M.; Walley, R.L.; Crane, J.M.; Matthews, K. & Hutchens, D. (2006). Oral misoprostol versus oxytocin in the management of the third stage of labour, *Journal of obstetrics and gynaecology Canada : JOGC = Journal d'obstetrique et gynecologie du Canada : JOGC,* Vol. 28, No. 1, pp. 20-26.

Pearse, R.M. & Rhodes, A. (2004). Haemodynamic monitoring and management of the circulation in intensive care, *Surgery (Oxford),* Vol. 22, No. 4, pp. 88-93.

Plaat, F. & Wray, S. (2008). Role of the anaesthetist in obstetric critical care, *Best Practice & Research Clinical Obstetrics & Gynaecology,* Vol. 22, No. 5, pp. 917-935.

Prasertcharoensuk, W.; Swadpanich, U. & Lumbiganon, P. (2000). Accuracy of the blood loss estimation in the third stage of labor, *International journal of gynaecology and obstetrics: the official organ of the International Federation of Gynaecology and Obstetrics,* Vol. 71, No. 1, pp. 69-70.

Prendiville, W.J.; Harding, J.E.; Elbourne, D.R. & Stirrat, G.M. (1988). The Bristol third stage trial: active versus physiological management of third stage of labour, *BMJ (Clinical research ed.),* Vol. 297, No. 6659, pp. 1295-1300.

Prendiville WJ, Elbourne D, McDonald S. (2000). Active vs. expectant management in the third stage of labour. In: *The Cochrane Library.*

Price, L.C.; Germain, S.; Wyncoll, D. & Nelson-Piercy, C. (2009). Management of the critically ill obstetric patient, *Obstetrics, Gynaecology & Reproductive Medicine*, Vol. 19, No. 12, pp. 350-358.

Price, L.C.; Slack, A. & Nelson-Piercy, C. (2008). Aims of obstetric critical care management, *Best Practice & Research Clinical Obstetrics & Gynaecology*, Vol. 22, No. 5, pp. 775-799.

Qidwai, G.I.; Caughey, A.B. & Jacoby, A.F. (2006). Obstetric outcomes in women with sonographically identified uterine leiomyomata, *Obstetrics and gynecology*, Vol. 107, No. 2 Pt 1, pp. 376-382.

Rahman, J.; Al-Ali, M.; Qutub, H.O.; Al-Suleiman, S.S.; Al-Jama, F.E. & Rahman, M.S. (2008), Emergency obstetric hysterectomy in a university hospital: A 25-year review, *Journal of obstetrics and gynaecology : the journal of the Institute of Obstetrics and Gynaecology*, Vol. 28, No. 1, pp. 69-72.

Rajan, P.V. & Wing, D.A. (2010). Postpartum hemorrhage: evidence-based medical interventions for prevention and treatment, *Clinical obstetrics and gynecology*, Vol. 53, No. 1, pp. 165-181.

Ramanathan, G. & Arulkumaran, S. (2006). Postpartum hemorrhage, *Journal of obstetrics and gynaecology Canada : JOGC = Journal d'obstetrique et gynecologie du Canada : JOGC*, Vol. 28, No. 11, pp. 967-973.

Rath, W. (2009). Prevention of postpartum haemorrhage with the oxytocin analogue carbetocin, *European journal of obstetrics, gynecology, and reproductive biology*, Vol. 147, No. 1, pp. 15-20.

Ravindran, J.; Shamsuddin, K. & Selvaraju, S. (2003). Did we do it right?--an evaluation of the colour coding system for antenatal care in Malaysia, *The Medical journal of Malaysia*, Vol. 58, No. 1, pp. 37-53.

Remmers, P.A.; Speer, A.J. (2006). Clinical Strategies in the Medical Care of Jehovah's Witnesses, *The American Journal of Medicine*, Vol. 119, No. 12, pp. 1013-1018.

Reveiz, L.; Gyte, G.M. & Cuervo, L.G. (2007). Treatments for iron-deficiency anaemia in pregnancy, *Cochrane database of systematic reviews (Online)*, Vol. 2, No. 2, pp. CD003094.

Riley, D.P. & Burgess, R.W. (1994). External abdominal aortic compression: a study of a resuscitation manoeuvre for postpartum haemorrhage, *Anaesthesia and Intensive Care*, Vol. 22, No. 5, pp. 571-575.

Roberts, W.E.; Fulp, K.S.; Morrison, J.C. & Martin, J.N.,Jr (1999). The impact of leiomyomas on pregnancy, *The Australian & New Zealand Journal of Obstetrics & Gynaecology*, Vol. 39, No. 1, pp. 43-47.

Safe Motherhood Initiative (2005). *Safe motherhood review 1987-2005*.

Searle, E.; Pavord, S. & Alfirevic, Z. (2008). Recombinant factor VIIa and other pro-haemostatic therapies in primary postpartum haemorrhage, *Best Practice & Research Clinical Obstetrics & Gynaecology*, Vol. 22, No. 6, pp. 1075-1088.

Shoemaker, W.C. & Kram, H.B. (1988). Crystalloid and colloid fluid therapy in resuscitation and subsequent ICU management, *Baillière's Clinical Anaesthesiology*, Vol. 2, No. 3, pp. 509-544.

Siassakos, D.; Crofts, J.F.; Winter, C.; Weiner, C.P. & Draycott, T.J. (2009). The active components of effective training in obstetric emergencies, *BJOG : an international journal of obstetrics and gynaecology*, Vol. 116, No. 8, pp. 1028-1032.

Simpson, H. & Barker, D. (2008). Role of the midwife and the obstetrician in obstetric critical care – a case study from the James Cook University Hospital, *Best Practice & Research Clinical Obstetrics & Gynaecology*, Vol. 22, No. 5, pp. 899-916.

Skinner, E.H.; Berney, S.; Warrillow, S. & Denehy, L. (2008). Rehabilitation and exercise prescription in Australian intensive care units, *Physiotherapy*, Vol. 94, No. 3, pp. 220-229.

Soltan, M.H.; Faragallah, M.F.; Mosabah, M.H. & Al-Adawy, A.R. (2009). External aortic compression device: the first aid for postpartum hemorrhage control, *The journal of obstetrics and gynaecology research*, Vol. 35, No. 3, pp. 453-458.

Soncini, E.; Pelicelli, A.; Larini, P.; Marcato, C.; Monaco, D. & Grignaffini, A. (2007). Uterine artery embolization in the treatment and prevention of postpartum hemorrhage, *International journal of gynaecology and obstetrics: the official organ of the International Federation of Gynaecology and Obstetrics*, Vol. 96, No. 3, pp. 181-185.

Su, L.L.; Chong, Y.S. & Samuel, M. (2007). Oxytocin agonists for preventing postpartum haemorrhage, *Cochrane database of systematic reviews (Online)*, Vol. 3, No. 3, pp. CD005457.

Sziller, I.; Hupuczi, P. & Papp, Z. (2007). Hypogastric artery ligation for severe hemorrhage in obstetric patients, *Journal of perinatal medicine*, Vol. 35, No. 3, pp. 187-192.

Thomas, P.J.; Paratz, J.D.; Stanton, W.R.; Deans, R. & Lipman, J. (2006). Positioning practices for ventilated intensive care patients: current practice, indications and contraindications, *Australian Critical Care*, Vol. 19, No. 4, pp. 122-132.

Treloar, E.J.; Anderson, R.S.; Andrews, H.S.; Bailey, J.L. (2006). Uterine necrosis following B-Lynch suture for primary postpartum haemorrhage, *British Journal of Obstetrics & Gynaecology*, Vol. 113, No. 4, pp. 486-488.

Tsirulnikov, M.S. (1979). Ligation of the uterine vessels during obstetrical hemorrhages. Immediate and long-term results (author's transl), *Journal de gynecologie, obstetrique et biologie de la reproduction*, Vol. 8, No. 8, pp. 751-753.

Upadhyay, K. & Scholefield, H. (2008)., Risk management and medicolegal issues related to postpartum haemorrhage, *Best practice & research.Clinical obstetrics & gynaecology*, Vol. 22, Vo. 6, pp. 1149-1169.

Varatharajan, L.; Chandraharan, E.; Sutton, J.; Lowe, V. & Arulkumaran, S. (2011). Outcome of the management of massive postpartum hemorrhage using the algorithm "HEMOSTASIS", *International journal of gynaecology and obstetrics: the official organ of the International Federation of Gynaecology and Obstetrics*, Vol. 113, No. 2, pp. 152-154.

Vergani, P.; Ghidini, A.; Strobelt, N.; Roncaglia, N.; Locatelli, A.; Lapinski, R.H. & Mangioni, C. (1994). Do uterine leiomyomas influence pregnancy outcome?", *American Journal of Perinatology*, Vol. 11, No. 5, pp. 356-358.

Vitthala, S.; Tsoumpou, I.; Anjum, Z.K. & Aziz, N.A. (2009). Use of Bakri balloon in post-partum haemorrhage: a series of 15 cases, *The Australian & New Zealand Journal of Obstetrics & Gynaecology*, Vol. 49, No. 2, pp. 191-194.

Waters, E.G. (1952). Surgical management of postpartum hemorrhage with particular reference to ligation of uterine arteries, *American Journal of Obstetrics and Gynecology*, Vol. 64, No. 5, pp. 1143-1148.

Waterstone, M.; Bewley, S. & Wolfe, C. (2001). Incidence and predictors of severe obstetric morbidity: case-control study, *BMJ (Clinical research ed.)*, Vol. 322, No. 7294, pp. 1089-93; discussion 1093-4.

Williams, J.; Mozurkewich, E.; Chilimigras, J. & Van De Ven, C. (2008). Critical care in obstetrics: pregnancy-specific conditions, *Best Practice & Research Clinical Obstetrics & Gynaecology*, Vol. 22, No. 5, pp. 825-846.

Winter, G.H.,J. (ed) (1939), *Operazioni Ostetriche*, Societa Editrice Libraria, Milano.

Wise, A. & Clark, V. (2010a). Challenges of major obstetric haemorrhage, *Best Practice & Research Clinical Obstetrics & Gynaecology*, Vol. 24, No. 3, pp. 353-365.

Wise, A. & Clark, V. (2010b). Obstetric haemorrhage, *Anaesthesia & Intensive Care Medicine*, Vol. 11, No. 8, pp. 319-323.

Wong, C.A. (2011). Saving Mothers' Lives: the 2006-8 anaesthesia perspective, *British journal of anaesthesia*, Vol. 107, No. 2, pp. 119-122.

World Health Organization (2007). *Iron deficiency anaemia, assessment, prevention and control: a guide for programme managers.* Available: http://www.who.int/reproductive-health/docs/anaemia.pdf, 14.02.2007

World Health Organization (2005). *Make every mother and child count.*

World Health Organization (1992). *The prevalence of anaemia in women: a tabulation of available information*, Geneva.

Effects of Blood Transfusion on Retinopathy of Prematurity

Ebrahim Mikaniki, Mohammad Mikaniki
and Amir Hosein Shirzadian
Babol University of Medical Sciences
Iran

1. Introduction

Retinopathy of prematurity (ROP) is a vasoproliferative retinal disorder, which represents the main cause of visual impairment and blindness in preterm infants (Drack,1998).ROP develops in 84% of premature survivors born at <28 weeks of gestation (Palmer et al,1991). Fortunately, it resolves in most cases (80%) without visual loss from retinal detachment or scars (Palmer et al, 1991; Cryotherapy for retinopathy of prematurity cooperative group, 1994). In this study, the total ROP incidence was 0.17% overall and 15.58% for premature infants with length of stay of more than 28 days (Lad et al, 2009). The increased survival of very small premature infants has led to the resurgence of this potentially blinding disease (Kinsey et al 1977; Shohat et al 1983)The pathogenesis of ROP isn't fully known. The altered regulation of vascular endothelial growth factor from reported episodes of hyperoxia and hypoxia is an important factor in the pathogenesis of ROP (Chow et al 2003). Apparently, any severe physiologic stress may damage the developing capillaries in immature retina and in response to ischemia, new vessel (neovascular) growth resumes (Phelps, 1992).ROP appears to be a multifactorial disease. Given the multifactorial nature of ROP and close relation of the most risk factors to prematurity, it is difficult to define the specific role of any individual factor in the pathogenesis of ROP (Hesse et al 1997).

Blood transfusion has been identified as a risk factor for ROP in several studies (Shohat et al,1983;Cats& Tan KEW ,1985 ;Clark et al ,1981; Cooke et al ,1993;Sacks et al ,1981;Yu & Hookham& Nave ,1982);Some investigator, however, could not confirm this associating (Bossi et al, 1984; Brown,1987 ;Lechner& Kalina& Hodson,1977).The damaging effects of blood transfusion on the retina are mediated via an increase in free iron that may catalyze fenton reactions, which produce free hydroxyl radicals capable of damaging the retina (Sullivan, 1988).Preterm infants are particularly susceptible to iron overload because of frequent transfusions and low levels of iron – binding proteins (Sullivan, 1988).In an effort to limit the risks associated with RBC transfusion, many neonatal units have adopted more restrictive guidelines for transfusing preterm infants (Widness et al ,1996 ;Alugappan& Shattuck& Malloy ,1998;Maies et al 2000 ;Franz & Pohlandt,2001),but the safety or potential benefits of restricting transfusions have not been adequately tested.

2. Retinopathy of prematurity

2.1 History

ROP was first described by Terry in 1942 as retrolental fibroplasias (Terry, 1942) and a few years later was recognized as one of the leading causes of infant blindness (Zacharias,1952).The indiscriminate use of oxygen from the 1940s to the mid-1950s was associated with a very high incidence of ROP. After the widespread adoption of the New York city health departments recommendation to restrict supplemental O2 concentrations to 40% ,the incidence of ROP decreased dramatically (James & Lamman,1976). During the 1960s it became obvious that although ROP incidences had decreased ,the oxygen restriction appeared to be associated with a significant increase of infant morbidity and mortality from hyaline membrane disease (Avery& Oppenheimer, 1960) and brain injury (McDonald, 1963). Oxygen supplementation was therefore liberalized in the late 1960s, and incidence of ROP began to rise again.

In the late 1960s, the incidence of ROP began to rise again. This increase continued during the 1970s and 1980s, likely as a result of the improved survival rate of very low birth weight infants associated with advances in neonatal medicine (Valentine et al, 1991).However, with improved technology and new techniques in neonatal nursing care, very low birth weight infants are now surviving with decreasing morbidity, and it is possible that the recent advances, that produced this change have also had an effect on ROP incidence (Bullord et al, 1998).

2.2 Incidence and risk factors

Kinsey et al found the incidence of ROP to be 38% in infants weighing 1200 g or less (Kinsey et al 1977.The CRYO-ROP trials reported an incidence of 65.8%,Infants weighing less than 1251 g and 81.6% in those less than 1000 g (Palmer et al, 1991). Many other studies reported ROP incidence ranging from 10% to 66% in infants with low birth weights in the United States and worldwide (Shohat et al 1983;Cats& Tan KEW ,1985; Bullord et al,1998;Fledelius& Dahl ,2000;Akkoyun et al,2006;Rowlands et al 2001;Hussain&Clive& Bhandori,1999;Wright et al,1998;Custick et al 2006;Yang et al 2006).

Chiang and associates have reported that the incidences of ROP were 20.3%, 27.3% and 33.2% in infants with a length of stay of more than 28 days with birth weight of less than 1500 g, 1200 g and 1000 g respectively (Chiang et al. 2004).

More recently Lad et al. in a large retrospective study based on the national Inpatient sample from 1997 through 2005 reported ROP incidence of 15.58% for premature infants with length of stay of more than 28 days (Lad et al, 2009).

Several risk factors have been associated with ROP .The major risk factors are prematurity (low birth weight, low gestational age at delivery).An inverse relationship was found between birth weight and the incidence and severity of retinopathy of prematurity (Lad et al, 2009; Kinsey et al 1977; Shohat et al. 1983; Bossi et al, 1984; Gunn et al,1980;Hammer et al,1986;Patz,1969).This finding emphasize, that the degree of immaturity of the eye is the main predictive factor for the devolvement of ROP.

Immature and underdeveloped retinal blood vessels in premature infants may be more vulnerable to postnatal environmental influences such as hyperoxic or hypoxic tissue injury, hypercarbia, and metabolic acidosis (Quinn, 1998). Moreover, these adverse conditions have a better opportunity to affect retinal vascular development if more development is left to occur under their influence. For many years it was thought that oxygen therapy increased the risk of ROP in preterm infants, however (Reynolds et al, 1998), ROP can occur even with careful control of oxygen therapy (Akkoyun et al, 2006). In fact, the role of oxygen has been overemphasized in the past and excessive oxygen administration has not been identified as an independent risk factor(Mccolm& Fleck ,2001).A reasonable working hypothesis is that the developing retina is highly sensitive to any disturbance in its oxygen supply either hyperoxemic or hypoxemic (Lucey & Dangman,1984).

Other proposed risk factors that are under study and may not be causally linked to ROP include: metabolic acidosis (Bossi et al, 1984), metabolic alkalosis (Shohat et al 1983), hypercarbia (Bauer & Windmayer, 1981), hypocarbia (Brown,1987), transfusions (Brown,1987; Clark et al ,1981), light (Glass et al ,1985), intraventricular hemorrhages (Brown,1987), white race(Saunders et al ,1997),chronic lung disease (Biglan et al ,1984), seizures(Biglan et al ,1984),sepsis(Gunn et al,1980),xanthine administration (Hammer et al,1986), magnesium and copper deficiency (Caddell,1995), Vitamin E deficiency (Owens & Owens ,1949),selenium deficiency (Papp & Nemeth& Pelle ,1993), and multiple gestations (Bossi et al, 1984). Any change that affects the incidence or nature of one or more of these risk factors might also affect the incidence and severity of ROP.

2.3 Pathogenesis

ROP is a condition confined to the immature retinal vascular system. The likelihood of developing retinopathy is related to the degree of vascular development so that once the retina is fully vascularized the risk of developing ROP has passed. Normally, retinal vascular development progresses from the 16th week of gestation to the 40th week in a central to peripheral wave at a rate of about 0.1 mm/day (Payne& Patz, 1979).

ROP alters this normal developmental progression, which instead follows a two –staged pathophysiologic course: an initial phase of vasoconstriction and arrested vessel growth, followed by a second phase of abnormal vessel proliferation. The onset of ROP generally requires two conditions. The first is incomplete retinal vascular development.ROP incidence and severity is directly proportional to the degree of prematurity that is, ROP outcome correlates with the size of the area of retinal avascularity at onset (Kinsey et al 1977, Schaffer et al, 1993, Kalina & Kari, 1982). The second condition involves exposure of the developing retina to an abnormal environmental influence and several have been suggested (Quinn, 1998).Most prominent among these is retinal hyperoxia resulting from postnatal hyperoxemia in infants receiving supplemental oxygen to compensate for inadequate pulmonary function. This condition, alone or in combination with other as yet unidentified results, leads to cessation of retinal vessel development. The retinal vasculature then enters a quiescent phase for days or weeks, while the formation of a ridge-like structure develops, separating the central vascularized region of the retina from the peripheral avascular region. This structure, which is pathognomonic of ROP, historically consists of mesenchymal and endothelial cells. Concomitant development of retinal neurons with advancing postnatal age results in increasing oxygen requirements, which cannot be met by attenuated vessel compliment in retinal hypoxia (Weiter& Zucherman& Schepens 1982).As a result of hypoxia another as yet undefined stimulus, angiogenic growth factor induction occurs, followed by rapid growth of new vessels within the ridge .The new vessels can regress by involution and remodeling into a nearly normal vascular pattern or the growth can progress to extraretinal neovascularization (Nelson,1790). These extraretinal vessels are weak and prone to leakage. The result is vitreous hemorrhage, scarring and contraction, leading to retinal folds or detachments and vision (loss Foos, 1985).

ROP is called stage 1 when the growing vessels end abruptly at a noticeable line separating the vascular and avascular retina takes on height and width ,it becomes a ridge and casts a little shadow; the ridge is stage 2 ROP .When the bunched up vessels in a stage 2 eye erupt into the vitreous ,The ROP becomes stage 3 and can be of variable severity .The greater the amount of extraretinal neovascularization vertically, and the greater the extent of the disease's spread around the retina, the stage 3 will be more sever. If the ROP progresses further, exudative and tractional retinal detachments occur and may be partial (stage 4) or complete (stage 5) (Phelps, 1992).

In the premature infants, the developing capillaries without a basement membrane or supporting predicts completely ablate during a prolonged period of absent retinal flow .it remains in dispute whether the vascular ablation in the premature infants is due to direct oxidative injury of the growing endothelium (Chan- Ling& Gock & Stone, 1995) Or is nearly the consequence of prolonged vasoconstriction due to a disturbed auto regulatory mechanism of the retinal vessels (Ashton & Cook,1954).The level of antioxidative in the immature retina is relatively low and therefore oxygen radicals which accumulate in the preterm baby's retina may play an important role in the pathogenesis of ROP (Hesse et al, 1997).

2.4 Terminology of ROP

The severity of ROP is described by four parameters: stage, location, extent and plus disease (table 1).

2.5 Screening for ROP

Since 1988, following the demonstration by the CRYO-ROP trial, sever ROP can be successfully treated so the ophthalmologists have had a duty to screen for this condition. The focus of screening is to identify ROP that requires treatment, at the appropriate point in the disease progression. The indication for treatment which has been reported in the CRYO-ROP study is threshold ROP. The term threshold denotes the ROP stage at which spontaneous and complete resolution is unlikely and the risk of blindness is predicted to be close to 50% (Cryotherapy for retinopathy of Prematurity Cooperative Group, 1988).The CRYO-ROP study divided all the diseases of the stage 3 into two categories: pre-threshold (or moderate ROP) and threshold (or severe ROP).Any disease of the stage 3 less than threshold was considered pre-threshold. Threshold ROP was defined as stage 3 ROP in zones one and two, in the presence of plus disease. Further studies such as that published recently by the Early Treatment for Retinopathy of Prematurity Cooperative Group (ETROP) recommends treating eyes before threshold because the outcomes of some eyes treated once they have develop threshold disease has been poor (ET-ROP,1997).

Parameter	Description
Stage 1	Demarcation line at the advancing edge of the retinal blood vessels
2	Ridge
	Stage 1 and 2 are referred to as mild ROP as they often undergo spontaneous resolution and do not result in visually disabling ophthalmic sequelae
3	Ridge with Extraretinal Fibrovascular proliferation .This is the first stage of ROP that presents a significant risk of poor structural or visual outcome and thus represents serious disease.
	Shunt lesions are well developed at the demarcation line and are often associated with "plus" (posterior retinal congestion).
	Further progression is characterized by development of secondary vitreous haze which heralds the onset of vitreoretinopathy leading to more sight threatening sequelae
4	Retinal detachment and partial retinal detachment
	a) the macula is attached
	b) the macula is detached
5	Total Funnel Retinal detachment
	Stage IV and V result in some permanent visual impairment despite surgical intervention
Location Zone 1-3	This predictable pattern of retinal vascularisation was formally recognized by the international classification of retinopathy (ICROP) in 1984 and 1987, which divided the retina into progressive concentric zones. The location of ROP is described in terms of these three arbitrarily defined ICROP zones which are centered around the optic disk
Extent 1-12	This is described by clock hours by 30 degree sectors.
Plus disease	Plus disease is characterized by active progression and at a more advanced stage the iris becomes congested resulting in poor pupil dilatation. The presence of the disease is an urgent indication for treatment

Table 1. Terminology of retinopathy of prematurity (ROP)

3. Blood transfusion in preterm infants

Preterm infants, especially those with very low birth weight (VLBW) prematurity, often need multiple blood transfusions during hospitalization. Over 50-80% of VLBW preterm infants receive at least one blood transfusion during their neonatal intensive care unit (NICU) stay (Strauss, 1997). In addition to phlebotomy losses causing low hematocrit, most VLBW infants develop the anemia of prematurity (AOP) a hypopro liferative anemia marked by inadequate production of erythropoietin (EPO). Treatment of AOP include red blood cell transfusions which are given to preterm infants based on indications and guidelines (hematocrit/ hemoglobin levels, ventilation and oxygen) that are relatively non-specific (Bishara,2008).

Transfusions to VLBW premature infants could increase weight gain, improve oxygenation and decrease lactic acidosis (Ohls, 2000). The complications and potential risk of blood transfusions include blood – transmitted infection, metabolic and cardiovascular complications, graft versus host disease, iron overload and increased oxidative stress, which are thought to be related to complications in premature infants such as chronic lung disease (CLD) and retinopathy of prematurity (ROP) (Cooke et al ,1997;Saugstad ,2003;Englert et al ,2001;Wheatley et al ,2002)considering the available evidence, many neonatal units have adopted more restrictive transfusion guidelines to reduce the frequency of transfusions and donor exposure (Windes et al, 1996; Alagappan& Shattuck& Malloy,1998; Maier et al, 2000;Franz & Pohlandt ,2001)But, these changes in practice have not been accompanied by systematic examination of the safety or potential benefits of restricting transfusions. Limiting RBC transfusion in preterm infants may reduce the potential risk of transfusion, but the resulting low hemoglobin levels may result in the morbidities associated with chronic anemic hypoxemia as recommended by some studies that advocate more than liberal transfusion guidelines to prevent apnea (Ross et al, 1989), to foster weight gain (Meyer & sive & Jacobs, 1993). More recent trials have been performed to determine the safety and efficacy of more restrictive transfusion guidelines.

Bifano was the first to evaluate neonatal transfusion guideline in prospective fashion [76]. This study compared the clinical outcomes of two groups of Extremely Low Birth Weight (EBLW) infants who were randomly assigned to restrictive or liberal transfusion criteria, based on hemoglobin thresholds for transfusion. There were no differences between groups in growth, morbidities, or mortality during hospitalization. At 12 months follow up, there were no differences in overall neurodevelopmental impairment. This study suggested that a restrictive transfusion strategy was not associated with adverse outcomes.

Bell et al. conducted a randomized trial of liberal versus restrictive guidelines for bronze baby syndrome (BBS) transfusion in preterm infants and showed that restrictive transfusions may be harmful to preterm infants in the restrictive group which had a greater incidence of intraparenchymal brain hemorrhage or periventricular leukomalacia and more frequent episodes of apnea (Bell et al, 2005).

Bednorek et al. in a prospective study examined the relationships of high and low transfusion practice styles on neonatal outcomes (Bednorek et al ,1998).Multivariate analyses showed that infants cared for in the lower transfer NICU did not have an increased risk for several adverse outcomes including IVH, NEC, BPD, Lesser weight gain, and longer hospitalizations. Kirpalani et al, performed a study to determine whether extremely low birth weight infants transfused at lower hemoglobin thresholds versus higher thresholds have different rates of survival or morbidity at discharge (Kirpalani et al, 2006).These investigators concluded that, in ELBW infants, maintaining a higher hemoglobin level result in more infants receiving transfusions but confer little evidence of benefit. This study provided evidence that transfusion thresholds in ELBW infants can be moved downward at least 10g/L, without incurring a clinically important increase in the risk of death or major neonatal morbidity.

However, most of the neonatal studies published up to the present measured what infants received, regardless of actual need for red cells. Transfusion guidelines and practices would benefit from studies that identify a useful transfusion marker, preferably one that requires minimal to no blood (Ohls, 2008).

4. The effect of blood transfusion on ROP

The role of blood transfusions as a risk factor for ROP was first suggested by Shohat et al (Shohat et al 1983), and other authors subsequently confirmed this association(Shohat et al

1983; Cats& Tan KEW ,1985; Clark et al ,1981; Cooke et al ,1993; Sacks et al,(1981); Ebrahim Mikaniki et al,2010; Yu & Hookham& Nave ,1982), some investigators, however, could not confirm it(Bossi et al, 1984; Brown,1987;Cooke et al; Lechner et al, 1977). multivariate regression analysis found that only gestational age and frequency of blood transfusions are independently associated with the risk of occurrence of ROP (Cooke et al ,1993).They reported a 9% increase in the risk of ROP with each transfusion given (95% CI 1.0-1.18). But data on iron metabolism were not analyzed and no information was given about the actual volume of transfused blood. Hesse et al demonstrated by the same statistical method, that blood transfusions are an independent risk factor for ROP. In this study, the relative risk of developing ROP was 6.4 (95% CI 1.2-33.4) for infants who received 16-45 ml/kg, and 12.3 (1.6-92.5) for those who had received more than 45 ml/kg of blood (reference, 0-15 ml/kg) (Hesse et al 1997).In contrast, there was no independent relationship between ROP and any of the parameters on iron metabolism analysis. Inder et al after multivariate regression analysis, showed that an elevation of serum iron and transferring saturation at 7 days of age is associated with an increased risk of ROP: they could not demonstrate an independent role of blood transfusions as a risk factor for ROP, but demonstrated that the iron status and the amount of transfused blood are highly correlated factors (Inder et al, 1997). Boosi et al, in another study, could not confirm an independent role of blood transfusion on development of ROP (Bossi et al, 1984).

Brooks et al, through a randomized, controlled trial, found that there was no association between hemoglobin or hematocrit ratios and ROP incidence or severity and transfusion limitation policy do not import a significant different risk for ROP (Brooks et al 1999) .However in this study, the risk of ROP was related to the number and not the volume of blood transfusion, and the incidence of ROP in the studied population was so high (76%) that it seems to be difficult to decrease the occurrence of ROP only by limiting the blood transfusions. More recently,Dani et al. showed that gestational age, blood transfusion volume and iron load by transfusions are associated with the risk of occurrence of ROP in infants with a birth weight of less than 1250 g. in this study, logistic regression analysis demonstrated that transfusion volume during the first week (OR 1.16; 95% CI 1.03-1.3) and during the first 2 months of life (OR 2.93; 95% CI 1.52-5.62), and iron intake during the first week of life (OR 1.15; CI 1.01-1.32) and during the first 2 months of life (OR 2.93; 95% CI 1.52-5.62) were associated with the development of ROP[87]. Two mechanisms by which blood transfusion could contribute to the development of ROP are discussed. First, Transfusions increase oxygen carrying capacity and a decrease in oxygen affinity caused by an increase in the proportion of adult hemoglobin. Second, transfusion increase iron load.

Sullivan Pointed out that the transfusion of 10 ml of packed red blood cells will increase the premature infant's total body iron by 20%, and that packed red blood cells contain 450 times as much hemoglobin iron as the plasma total iron- binding capacity (Sullivan,JL,1988) .This, in conjunction with the reduced iron- binding capacity of preterm infants (due to their low transferring and ceruloplasmine levels) and postnatal depression of erythrocyte production, makes preterm infants who are repeatedly transfused extremely susceptible to an accumulation of increased amounts of free iron. Free iron could catalyze fenton reactions which produce highly reactive oxygen-derived free radicals and are assumed to play an important role in the pathogenesis of ROP.

5. Conclusion

The increased survival of very small premature infants in modern NICUs led to increasing the incidence of ROP (Gibson et al, 1990; Gibson et al, 1990). Since ROP may produce serious sequel of infant blindness, all efforts must be made to prevent the development of advanced ROP. Identification of ROP risk factors will help to understand and predict ROP development in premature newborns (Akkoyun et al, 2006). One such risk factor may be multiple blood transfusions. Studies on the role of blood transfusion in ROP however have been hampered by the multifactorial nature of this disease and by the fact that most risk factors For ROP, including blood transfusions, are closely related to prematurity and are thus highly interdependent. This makes it different to define the specific role of any individual factor in the pathogenesis of ROP (Hesse et al 1997).

Using multivariate regression analysis ,which provides a helpful tool in such a situation, some studies demonstrated that blood transfusion had a strong and dose-dependent influence on the development of ROP (Hesse et al 1997; Cooke et al, 1993; Dani et al , 2001).Otherwise, some investigators reported that the limitation of blood transfusion dose not affect ROP incidence(Bossi et al, 1984;Brooks et al 1999).

The reported mechanisms by which blood transfusions could contribute to the development of ROP are (1) the increase of Oxygen delivery to the retina (James&Greenough&Naik, 1997) due to lower oxygen affinity of adult hemoglobin in pack red cell (Cooke et al, 1993), and (2) the secondary iron overload.

The reduced iron-binding capacity of preterm infants due to their low transferring levels (Scott et al, 1975) makes preterm infants who are repeatedly transfused extremely susceptible to an accumulation of increased amounts of free iron. This problem catalyze Fenton reactions which produce free hydroxyl radicals capable of damaging the retina (Wardle et al, 2002).Despite a strong and independent association between ROP and blood transfusions, parameter suggestive of increased free iron, such as low transfusion or high ferritin levels, there not found to be independently associated with ROP in the one of related studies (Hesse et al 1997). It cannot be concluded from this data that a more restrictive transfusion policy will reduce the incidence of ROP, particularly as there is evidence that low levels of tissue oxygenation, which would be expected if VLBW infants are transfused less frequently, may also be a risk for ROP (Bauer & Windmayer, 1981). Otherwise, transfusion practices may differ considerably among both institutions and individual physicians because of a lack of uniformly accepted physiologic or evidence–based transfusion criteria (Brown &Berman&Luckey, 1990).

Decisions about transfusing VLBW infants with RBCs should be based on the risks and benefits of applying various transfusions guidelines and further refining based on the clinical status of individual infants .Recent studies suggests that frequent transfusions did not offer a detectable advantage and restricted transfusion did not have an increased risk for major brain injury as reported in previous studies (Ross et al, 1989; Chen et al, 2009)

Albeit, these results must be interpreted with caution, because they may be related to other co practices in the specific NICU.

Further studies will be required to clarify whether as reduction in the number of transfusions will ultimately result in a reduced incidence of ROP without any significant difference in clinical outcome

6. References

Akkoyun, I.& et al. (2006). Risk factors in the development of mild and sever retinopathy of prematurity. *J AA, vol.*10 pp. 449-453

Alagappan, A., Shattuck, KE.& Malloy, MH. (1998).Impact of transfusion guidelines on neonatal transfusion. *J perina*tal, vol.18, pp.92-7

Alugappan, A., Shattuck, KG.& Malloy, MN. (1998). Impact of transfusion guidelines a neonatal transfusion. *J Perinatal* vol 18 pp 92-97

Ashton, N.& Cook, C.,(1954) Direct Observation of the effect of oxygen on developing vessels: Preliminary report. *Br J Ophthalmol* vol 38 pp 433-440

Avery, ME.& Oppenheimer, EH.(1960). Recent increase in mortality from hyaline membrane disease. *J Pediatr.* Vol 57 pp 553-9

Bauer, CR.& Windmayer, SM.(1981). A relationship between $PaCo_2$ and retrolental fibroplasia. *Pediatr* Res, vol. 15, pp. 649.45

Bell, EF& et al.(2005). Randomized trial of liberal versus restrictive guidelines for blood cell transfusions in preterm infants. *Pediatrics*, vol.115, pp.1685-91

Bednorek, FJ& et al.(1998). Variations in blood transfusion among newborn intensive care units. *J Pediatr,* vol.133, pp.601-7

Bifano, EN, Bode, MM.&Eugenio, DB.(2002) Prospective randomized trial of high vs. low hematocrit in ELBW infants: one-year growth and neurodevelopmental outcome. *Pediatr Res*, vol.51, pp.325A

Biglan, AW.&et al. (1984). Risk factors associated with retrolental fibroplasia. *Ophthalmology*, vol. 91,pp. 1504-1511

Bishara, N.& ohls, RK.(2008).current Controversies in the management of the anemia of prematurity. *Semin perinatal*, vol.33 pp.29-34

Bossi, E.&et al.(1984) Retinopathy of prematurity: a risk factor analysis with univariate and multivariate statistics. *Helv paediatr Acta* pp 307-317

Brooks, SE& et al.(1999).The effect of blood transfusion protocol on retinopathy of prematurity :a prospective randomized study ,pediatrics ,vol.104,p.514-518

Brown, DR.(1987) Retinopathy of prematurity. Risk factors in a live- year cohort of critically ill premature neonates. *Am J Dis child* vol 141 pp 154-160

Brown, MS.,Berman, ER.&Luckey D.(1990).prediction of need for transfusion during anemia of prematurity .J Pediatr,vol.116, pp.773-8

Bullord, SR.& et al.(1998) The decreasing incidence and severity of retinopathy of prematurity. *Journal of AAPOS* vol 3 pp 46-52

Caddell, JL.(1995). Hypothesis: the possible role of magnesium and copper deficiency in retinopathy of prematurity. *Magnes Res*, vol. 8, pp. 261-267

Cats, BP., Tan KEW.(1985) Retinopathy of prematurity: review of a four-year period. *Br J Ophthalmol* vol 69 pp 500-503

Chan- Ling, T., Gock, B.& Stone, J.(1995) The effect of oxygen on vaseformation cell division: Evidence that the physiological hypoxia is the stimulus for normal retinal vasculogenesis. *Invert Ophthalmol Vis Sci* vol 36, pp. 1201- 1214

Chen, HL& et al.(2009).Effect of blood transfusion on the outcome of very low body weight preterm infants under two different transfusion criteria.*pediatr Neonatal* ,vol.50,pp.110-116

Chiang, MF.& et al.(2004). Incidence of retinopathy of prematurity from 1996 to 2000. *Ophthalmology*, vol. 111, pp.1317-1325

Chow, LC., Wright, KW& Sola A (2003). Can changes in clinical practice decrease the incidence of sever retinopathy of prematurity in very low birth weight infants? *Pediatrics* vol 111 pp 339-345

Clark J.& et al.(1981) Blood Transfusion: a possible risk factor in retrolental fibroplasia. *Acta Pediatr Scand*. vol 70 pp 535-539

Cooke, RW.& et al.(1997). Blood transfusion and chronic lung disease in preterm infants .*Eur j Pediatr*, vol, pp.156:45-50

Cryotherapy for retinopathy of Prematurity Cooperative Group Multi Center trial of cryotherapy for retinopathy of prematurity, prelimininary results (1988). *Arch Ophthalmol, vol.106*, pp.471-479

Cryotherapy for retinopathy of prematurity cooperative group.(1994). The natural ocular outcome of premature birth and retinopathy: status at 1 year. *Arch Ophthalmol*. Vol 112: 903-912

Custick, M.& et al.(2006). Anatomical and visual results of vitreoretinal surgery for stage 5 retinopathy of prematurely. *Retina, vol*. 26, pp.729-735

Dani, C.& et al. .(2001)The role of blood transfusions and iron intake on retinopathy of prematurity. Early Human Development, vol 62, pp.57-63

Drack, AV.(1998). Preventing blindness in premature infants. *N. Engl. J. Med*. 338: 1620-1621

Early Treatment for Retinopathy of Prematurity Cooperative Group (ET-ROP).(1997).Revised indications for the treatment of retinopathy of prematurity .*Arch Ophthalmol* ,vol.121, pp.1684-1696

Englert, JA.& et al.(2001) .The effect of anemia on retinopathy of prematurity in extremely low birth weight infants. *J perinatal*, vol.21, pp.21-6

Fledelius, HC., Dahl, H.(2000). Retinopathy of prematurity, a decrease in frequency and severity. Trends over 16 years in a Danish Country. *Acta Ophthalmol Scand*, vol. 78 pp. 359-361

Foos, RY.(1985). Chronic retinopathy of prematurity. *Ophthalmology* .vol 92 pp 573- 574

Franz, AR.& Pohlandt, F.(2001). Red blood cell transfusions in very and extremely low birth weight infants under restrictive transfusion guidelines: is exogenous erythropoietin necessary? *Arch Dis child Fetal Neonatal* vol 84 pp 96-100.

Franz, AR.& Pohlandt, F .(2001).Red blood cell transfusion in very and extremely low birth weight infants under restrictive transfusion guidelines: is exogenous erythropoietin necessary? *Arch fetal neonatal, vol.84, pp.96-100*.

Gibson, DL.& et al .(1990).Retinopathy of prematurity –induced blindness: birth weight – specific survival and the new epidemic. Pediatrics, vol.86, pp.405-412.

Glass. P.& et al.(1985). Effect of bright light in the hospital nursery on the incidence of retinopathy of prematurity. *N Eng J Med*, vol. 313,pp. 410-414

Gunn, TR.& et al.(1980). Risk factors in retrolental fibroplasia. *Pediatrics* vol 65, pp. 1096-100.

Hammer, ME.& et al.(1986). Logistic analysis of risk factors in acute retinopathy of prematurity. *Am J Ophthalmol* vol. 102, pp. 1-6.

Hesse, L. et al (1997). Blood Transfusion: Iron load and retinopathy of prematurity. *Eur J Pediatr*, vol 156, pp 465-470.

Hussain, N., Clive, J.& Bhandori, V.(1999). Current incidence of retinopathy of prematurity, 1989- 1997. *Pediatrics*, vol 104, pp. 26.33.

Inder, TE .& et al.(1997).High iron status in very low birth weight infants is associated with an increased risk of retinopathy of prematurity, J Pediatr ,vol.131,pp.541-544.

James L, Greenough A, Naik S.The effect of blood transfusion on oxygenation in premature ventilated neonates, Eur.J.pediatr .1997;156:139-141.

James, LS.& Lamman, JT.(1976). History of oxygen therapy and retrolental fibroplasia. *Pediatrics* vol 57 pp 591-642.

Kalina, RE.& Kari, DJ.(1982). Retrolental Fibroplasia: experience over two decades in one institution. *Ophthalmology* vol 89 pp 91-95.

Kinsey, VE. et al.(1977). Pa O2 levels and retrolental fibroplasias: a report of the cooperative study. *Pediatrics*. Vol 60 pp 655-668.

Kirpalani, H,et al .(2006).A randomized controlled trial of a restrictive (low) versus liberal(high) transfusion threshold for extremely low birth weight infants. The PLNT study.*J Pediatr*, vol.149, pp.301-7.

Lad, EM.et al (2009). Incidence of retinopathy of prematurity in the United States: 1997 through 2005. *American Journal of ophthalmology*.vol 148, pp 451-58.

Lechner, D., Kalina, RE.& Hodson, WA.(1977). Retrolental Fibroplasia and factors influency oxygen transport. *Pediatrics*, vol 59 pp 916-91.

Lechner, D., Kokina, RE.&Hodson, WA.(1977)Retrolental fibroplasia and factors influencing oxygen transport .pediatrics, vol.59, pp.916-918.

Lucey, JF.& Dangman, B.(1984). A reexamination of the role of oxygen in retrolental fibroplasia. *Pediatrics*.vol. 73, pp. 82-96.

Maier, RF.& et al.(2000).Changing practices of red blood cell transfusion in infants with birth weight less than 1000 g .*J Pediatr*,vol.136,pp.220-4.

Maies, RF.& et al.(2000). Changing practices of red blood cell transfusions in infants with birth weight less than 1000 g. *J Pediatr* vol 136 pp 220-224.

Mccolm, JR.& Fleck, EW.(2001). Retinopathy of prematurity: Causation. *Semin Neonatal*, vol. 6, pp. 453-460.

McDonald, AO.(1963) Cerebral palsy in children of very low birth weight. *Arch Dis child*. vol 38 pp 579-88.

Meyer, J.,sive, A.&Jacobs, P. (1993) Empiric red cell transfusion in asymptomatic preterm infants .*Acta paediatr*,vol.82,pp.30-4.

Mikaniki, E., Rasoulinejad, SA.& Mikaniki M.(2010).Incidence and Risk factors of retinopathy of prematurity in Babol, North of Iran. Ophthalmic Epidemiology, vol.17, pp.166.70.

Nelson, L. (1790). Disorders of the Eye, In: *Nelson textbook of pediatrics,* Vol.15, pp. 1790, Saunders, London

Ohls, RK.(2008).why when and how should we provide red cell transfusions to neonates ,In Hematology, Immunology and infections disease, ohls R,Yoder MC,pp.44-57,Elisevir, Philadelphia

Ohls, Rk.(2000). The use of erythropoietin in neonates. *Clin perinatal*, Vol.27. pp.681-696.

Owens, WC.& Owens, EV.(1949). Retrolental Fibroplasia in premature infants: the use of alpha tocopherol acetate. *Am J Ophthalmol*, vol. 32, pp.1631-1637.

Palmer, EA, RJ, et al. (1991). Incidence and early course of retinopathy of prematurity. The cryotherapy for retinopathy of prematurity cooperative group. *Ophthalmology* vol 98 pp 1628-1640.

Papp, A., Nemeth, I.& Pelle Z.(1993). Retrospective biochemical study of the preventive property of antioxidants in retinopathy of prematurity. *Orv Hetil*, vol. 134, pp.1021-1026.

Patz, A. (1969). Retrolental fibroplasia. Surv Ophthalmol vol. 14, pp. 1-29.40

Payne, JW.& Patz, A.(1979). Current states of retrolental fibroplasias. *Ann Clin Res*, vol. 11, pp. 205-211.

Phelps DL.(1992).Retinopathy of prematurity. *Current problems in pediatrics*. pp. 349-371.

Quinn, G.(1998). Retinal development and the pathophysiology of retinopathy of prematurity. *Polin and fox fetal and neonatal physiology*. Vol 2 London: Saunders pp 2252

Reynolds, JD.& et al.(1998). Lack of efficacy of light reduction in preventing retinopathy of prematurity. Light reduction in retinopathy of prematurity (LIGHT-ROP) Cooperative group. *N Eng J Med* vol. 338, pp. 1572-6.

Ross, MP.& et al .(1989).A randomized trial to develop criteria for administering erythrocyte transfusions to anemic preterm infants 1 to 3 months of age. *J perinatal*, vol.9.pp.246-53.

Rowlands, E.& et al.(2001). Reduced incidence of retinopathy of prematurity. Br J Ophthalmol, vol. 85,pp. 933-935.

Sacks LM.& et al.(1981) Retrolental fibroplasia and blood transfusion in very low- birth-weight infants. *Pediatrics* vol 68 pp 770-774.

Saugstad, OD.(2003) Bronchopulmonary dysplasia-oxidative stress and antioxidants .*Semin Neonatal*, vol 8 ,pp.39-49.

Saunders, RA.& et al.(1997). Racial Variation in retinopathy of prematurity: the cryopathy for retinopathy of prematurity cooperative Group. Arch *Ophthalmol, vol.* 115, pp. 604-608.

Schaffer, DB.& et al.(1993). Prognostic factors in the natural course of retinopathy of prematurity. *Ophthalmology*, vol. 100, pp. 230-7

Scott, PH &et al.(1975).Effect of gestational age and intrauterine nutrition on plasma transfusion and iron in the newborn. *Arch Dis child*.vol.50 pp.796-798.

Shohat, M. et al.(1983). Retinopathy of prematurity: Incidence and risk factors. *Pediatrics*. 1983; 72: 159-163.

Strauss, RG.(1997). Practical issues in neonatal transfusion practice. *Am J Clin Pathol, vol.107.pp.557-563.*

Sullivan, JL.(1988) Iron, Plasma antioxidants, and the oxygen radical disease of prematurity. *Am J Dis Child*.vol 142 pp 1341-1344.

Terry, TL.(1942).Extreme prematurity and fibroblastic overgrowth of persistent vascular sheath behind each crystalline lens. *Am J Ophthalmol* vol 25 pp 203-204.

Valentine, PH.& Et al .(1991) Increased survival of low birth weight infants: impact on the incidence of retinopathy of prematurity. *Pediatrics* vol 84 pp 442-5.

Wardle, SP.& et al.(2002).Effect of blood transfusion lipid proxidation in preterm infants. *Arch dis child fetal neonatal*, vol.86, pp.46-8.

Weiter, JJ., Zucherman, R.& Schepens, CL.(1982). A Model for the pathogenesis of retrolental fibroplasia based on the metabolic control of blood vessel development. *Ophthalmic Surg* vol. 13 pp. 1013-1017.

Wheatley, CM.& et al.(2002). Retinopathy of prematurity: recent advances in our understanding. *Arc Dis child Fetal Neonatal*, vol.87, pp.78-82.

Widness, JA.& et al.(1996) changing patterns of red blood cell transfusion in very low birth weight infants. *J Pediatr* vol 129 pp 680-7.

Windes, JA.& et al.(1996).Changing patterns of red blood cell transfusion in very low birth weight infants ,*J Pediatr,* vol.129 ,pp.680-7.

Wright, K.& et al.(1998). Should fewer premature infants be screened for retinopathy of prematurity in the managed care era? *Pediatrics*, vol.102, pp. 31-34.

Yang, MB.& et al.(2006). Race, Gender, and clinical risk index for babies (CRIB) Score as predictors of severe retinopathy of prematurely. *J AAPOS*, vol 10 pp. 253-261.

Yu, VY.,Lim, CT.&Downe, LM.(1990).A 12-years experience of retinopathy of prematurity in infants≤28 weeks gestation or ≤1000 g birth weight. J Pediatr child health, vol.26, pp.205-208.

Yu, VYH., Hookham, DM.& Nave JRM.(1982) Retrolental fibroplasias- controlled study of 4 years' experience in a neonatal intensive care unit. *Arch Dis Child* vol 57 pp 247-252.

Zacharias, L.(1952) Retrolental fibroplasias survey. *Am J Ophthalmol*. Vol 35 pp 1427-1454.

Part 3

Preventing Transfusion Transmitted Infections

8

Implicating the Need for Serological Testing of Borna Disease Virus and Dengue Virus During Blood Transfusion

S. Gowri Sankar[1] and A. Alwin Prem Anand[2]
[1]Department of Biotechnology,
Anna University of Technology, Tiruchirappalli, Tamil Nadu,
[2]Institute of Anatomy, University of Tuebingen, Tubingen,
[1]India
[2]Germany

1. Introduction

Blood is a vital component for the living being to be alive. The composition of blood is plasma and blood cells. It helps in transport of gaseous, metabolic products, hormones, nutrients and enzymes. It helps to regulate the body temperature and body fluid electrolyte. Blood transfusion becomes a vital part during blood loss, due to severe anemic condition and during major surgeries. Despite their critical use, blood transfusion becomes risky these days by the transmission of viruses.

2. Basic information about viruses and blood transfusion

The viruses are known for its replication and functional activities inside the cells. They usually need a system to be 'alive'. Outside the cells or any living tissue, the viruses are dormant. Virus can be transmitted by various ways to human beings. The virus like hepatitis virus and its subtypes A, B, C, D, E and G, human immunodeficiency virus types 1 and 2 (HIV-1/2), human T-cell lymphotropic virus types I and II (HTLV-I/II), cytomegalovirus (CMV), Epstein-Barr virus (EBV), TT virus (TTV), human herpes virus type 6 (HHV-6), SEN virus (SEN-V), human parvovirus (HPV-B19) and West Nile Virus (WNV) has already been diagnosed and researched for its potential to cause disease via blood transfusion (Table 1). The viruses namely, Japanese encephalitis virus, WNV, Chikungunya virus, HIV, HHV, HTLV and rabies are even capable of entering into central nervous system through blood (Kristensson, 2011). However, some viruses are neither studied for their transmission through blood; because of little evidence to support their transmission and, even in some viruses the mode of transmission is not known. We would like to give more priority to Borna disease virus and Dengue virus, which has been less studied in terms of transmission and blood transfusion.

Virus	Mode of transfusion	Disease due to transmission
HBV, HCV, HIV-1/-2, HTLV-I/-II	Highly established	Yes
CMV, EBV, HAV, HPV-B19, HHV-6	Established	Only in immunocompromised state
Dengue, WNV	Rarely established	Not conclusive
HGV/GBV-C, TTV, SEN-V, HEV, HHV-8, BDV	Not well established	Not established

Table 1. Recognized mode of viral transmission and disease in human.

3. Borna disease virus

Borna disease, a fatal meningo-encephalitis was originally described in horses in Germany. The disease was named after the epidemic outbreak of equine deaths in the town Borna in Saxony, Germany in 1885 (Rott and Becht, 1995). In 1929, an infectious agent was said to the cause for Borna disease and, in 1990 the infectious agent was identified as virus (Cubitt and de la Torre, 1994). The virus was then named after the disease, Borna disease virus (BDV).

3.1 BDV genome

BDV is said to be the only non-segmented, negative sense RNA virus replicated in the nucleus and classified as a new family *Bornaviridae* under *Mononegavirales* (Briese et al., 1994; de la Torre, 2002; De La Torre et al., 1996; Ludwig et al., 1988; Ludwig et al., 1993). BDV has six open reading frames (ORF), namely nucleoprotein (N), phosphoprotein (P), matrix (M), L-polymerase (L), glycoprotein (G) and X protein (Briese et al., 1994; de la Torre, 1994). The BDV mRNA includes monocistronic, polycistronic and spliced transcripts with overlapping ORFs (Kobayashi et al., 2003). The structural proteins are nucleoprotein, matrix and glycoprotein and the functional proteins are L-polymerase, phosphoprotein and X protein. The G protein helps in entry of BDV into the host cells. The G protein is expressed as two products, 84 and 43kDa. The 84kDa protein is involved in attachment of the viral particles to the cell receptor and its cleavage product 43kDa is involved in pH-dependent fusion after internalization of the virion by endocytosis (Gonzalez-Dunia et al., 1998). The M protein observed as tetramers and octamers, helps in viral attachment to cellular membrane, essential for viral assembly and budding (Kraus et al., 2005; Stoyloff et al., 1997). The M protein is also an integral component of ribonucleoprotein complex (RNP) and, prerequisite for viral persistence in the neurons (Chase et al., 2007). The structural information on M protein, suggest that they involve in RNP formation, nucleocapsid targeting and viral maturation (Neumann et al., 2009). The L protein is involved in replication and P protein is involved in transcription of the BDV genome (Schneider, 2005). Further, the P protein interacts with other structural and functional proteins of BDV genome (Schwemmle et al., 1998). The L protein is tightly regulated by N-P stoichiometric ratio (Schneider, 2005; Schneider et al., 2005; Walker et al., 2000; Walker and Lipkin, 2002). The X protein is 10kDA protein, interacts with P protein and, acts as a negative regulator of BDV polymerase and hinders viral replication (Poenisch et al., 2004; Poenisch et al., 2007; Schwardt et al., 2005).

3.2 Behavioural effects of BDV infection in animals

Behavioural alternations during viral infection are referred as 'sickness behaviour' that include alternation in body weight, taste preferences, temperature, food and water intake and sleep pattern (Kelley et al., 2003). The 'sickness behaviour' in BDV infected rats, shows body weight stunting and abnormal salt preferences (Hornig et al., 2001), high obese rate (Herden et al., 2000) and chronic emotional abnormalities (Pletnikov et al., 2002a; Pletnikov et al., 2002b, c).

3.3 Prevalence of BDV infection in psychiatric illness

The first isolation of BDV was from a patient with mood disorder (Bode et al., 1996). There have been totally six BDV isolates and the source of isolation was blood and brain tissues from patients with psychiatric illness. The six isolates of BDV are from blood samples of two bipolar disorder patients, one obsessive-compulsive disorder, one depression, one schizophrenic patient and one from brain tissue from a patient with schizophrenia in Japan (Bode and Ludwig, 2003). In this decade, many reports have been emphasizing BDV infection in psychiatric illness. The psychiatric illness includes depression, bipolar disorder, obsessive-compulsive disorder, severe mood disorder and non-psychotic bipolar disorder (Bode, 1995; Bode et al., 1997; Bode et al., 1996; Bode et al., 1992; Bode et al., 2001; Dietrich et al., 2000; Dietrich et al., 2005; Ohlmeier et al., 2007). The infection of BDV was analysed by western blot, ELISA, immunofluorescence assay, immunoprecipitation, circulating immune complexes (CIC) from the serum of the patients with psychiatric illness, affective disorder, schizophrenia and multiple sclerosis (Hornig et al., 2003). Apart from BDV antibodies, BDV RNA was found in peripheral blood cells of psychiatric patients (Miranda et al., 2006; Sauder et al., 1996). Bode et al., (2001) reported that BDV-CIC play a major role in detection of BDV activity in contrast to the state of illness. The high amount of CIC and plasma antigen correlates with the severity of depression. It was also found in the neurophysiologic studies that brain potential amplitude varies with BDV-CIC in obsessive-compulsive disorder (Dietrich et al., 2005).

3.4 Neurotrophism or trophism for BDV infection

Neurotrophism or trophism for BDV infection is not clearly understood. BDV was found to replicate in the neurons of limbic structures especially in the regions of hippocampus (Carbone et al., 1991a; Carbone et al., 1989). Hippocampus is rich in neurotrophic growth factors like nerve growth factor (NGF) (Nieto-Sampedro and Bovolenta, 1990) as well as in kinases (Olive and Hodge, 2000).

3.4.1 Nerve growth factor (NGF) as a neurotrophic factor

Hippocampus is said to be the preferred site for replication of BDV as it is rich in growth factors (Ojika and Appel, 1984). NGF affects the replication cycle of other viruses and associated with latent HSV infection; the absence or removal of NGF is associated with recrudescence of productive HSV replication (Clements and Kennedy, 1989; Wilcox and Johnson, 1988; Wilcox et al., 1990). Carbone et al., (1993) suggested that NGF to be the neurotrophic factor influencing the replication of BDV. It was found that astrocytic cell lines were able to produce more BDV protein and RNA and suggested that astrocytic cells secrete a factor or factors that enhance the production of BDV protein and BDV RNA. It has also been found that NGF treatment was also produced the same as in astrocytic cell lines (Carbone et al., 1993).

3.4.2 Protein Kinase C (PKC) as a trophic factor

The P protein is involved in replication and also acts as a transcription factor. It has the nuclear localization signal that helps in transportation of P, L and X proteins into the nucleus (Schneider, 2005; Shoya et al., 1998; Walker et al., 2000; Walker and Lipkin, 2002). P protein is directly involved in glial cell dysfunction by reducing Brain Derived Growth Factor (BDNF) and serotonin receptor expression that results in neuropathological and neurophysiological abnormalities (Kamitani et al., 2003). The P protein is activated by phosphorylation. The kinases responsible for phosphorylation of P protein are Protein Kinase C (PKC)ε and Casein Kinase II. The major phosphorylation is through PKCε and the minor is from Casein Kinase II (Schwemmle et al., 1997). PKCε is present in higher concentrations in neuronal than in glial nuclei and are located inside the nucleus and at the nuclear envelope in brain cell nuclei (Rosenberger et al., 1995). It is found higher in the limbic structures (Olive and Hodge, 2000). BDV blocks neuronal presynaptic activity by inhibiting PKC signalling (Volmer et al., 2006), which was proved by P mutant phenotype where BDV is not able to interfere with neuronal signalling (Prat et al., 2009). The recent report indicate that PKC mediated signalling is necessary for viral spread (Schmid et al., 2010), which further proves that PKC is as tropic factor for BDV replication in hippocampal neurons.

3.5 Molecular basis of human mental disorder in virus-induced neurobehavioral disorder

Brain damage is usually observed in neurotrophic virus infection. The mechanism of virus induced neural damage occurs by direct and indirect pathways. The direct pathway involves viral replication in the nucleus leading to direct cell lysis or apoptosis. This was more commonly observed in infections with HSV, rabies virus, reovirus and alphavirus (Griffin and Hardwick, 1999). In case of BDV infection in rat models, the virus can cause neuronal cell dysfunctions in the absence of immune mediated cell destruction leading to neurological disorder (Tomonaga et al., 2002). The indirect pathway involves the modulation of host response to the viral infection. In BDV infection, the modulation occurs by the infiltrating immune cells such as CD4-positive, CD8-positive T-cells, macrophages and B cells. CD8-positive T cells represent the effector cell population exhibiting antigen specificity for the nucleoprotein (Stitz et al., 2002). Administration with anti-CD8+ results in reduction of neuronal degeneration and inhibits inflammation (Bilzer and Stitz, 1994).

Proinflammatory cytokines also play an important role in BDV infection, which alter the behaviour (Konsman et al., 2002).

3.5.1 Role of proinflammatory cytokines

Proinflammatory cytokines like IL-1α, IL-1β, IL-6 and TNF-α have a role in major depressive disorder (Licinio and Wong, 1999). The involvement of proinflammatory cytokines in experimental animals shows that the alteration in biological and behavioural abnormalities, as an analogue found in depressive patients (Konsman et al., 2002). The behavioural change mediated by cytokine seems to be regulated by multiple pathways. IL-1 is mainly involved in anxiety and sickness behaviour (Montkowski et al., 1997; Tomonaga, 2004). Likewise, in BDV infected patients, there was an increase of IL-6 was observed (personal communication). Experiments with animal model infected with BDV clearly show that there is an increase in the cytokines IL-1α, IL-6 and TNF-α (Sauder and de la Torre, 1999; Shankar et al., 1992). This may be one of the pathways of BDV in inducing psychiatric behavioural and cognitive deficits.

3.5.2 Role of serotonin system

Virus infection can directly or indirectly alter the serotonin system. Proinflammatory cytokines can also alter the expression of serotonin system (Dunn, 2000). Alteration of 5-HT (hydroxyl-tryptophan) systems leads to several mental and behavioural problems that include aggression, violence, sexual dysfunction, sleep and eating disorder in humans (Manji et al., 2001) and in rat models, reduction of 5-HT increases aggression (Nelson and Chiavegatto, 2001). In transgenic mice expressing P protein, the serotonin receptors in the hippocampus are reduced as well as these mice exhibit neurobehavioral abnormalities as in BDV infected animals (Kamitani et al., 2003). The transgenic mice also exhibit insulin-like growth factor 3 in their astrocytes, suggesting the increased vulnerability of purkinje cells in the brain (Honda et al., 2011).

3.6 Role of amantadine in BDV-infected psychiatric illness

Amantadine has been reported as an effective drug in reducing BDV replication in vitro and in vivo (Bode et al., 1997; Dietrich et al., 2000; Ferszt et al., 1999). Amantadine sulphate was used as an antiviral therapy in patients with bipolar disorder and found to be remarkable (Bode et al., 1997). All human BDV isolates are sensitive to amantadine treatment in vitro (Bode and Ludwig, 2003). Since the molecular mechanism of amantadine is unknown, here we discuss a putative mechanism based on the current understanding.

3.6.1 Amantadine in BDV infection

Astrocytes play an essential role in the homeostasis of CNS microenvironment for the proper neuronal function, where the alteration of astrocytic function leads to neuronal pathology (Benveniste, 1992, 1997). The function of astrocytes in BDV infection has been intensively studied in various aspects; the ability to uptake glucose, protein synthesis, cell viability and rate of proliferation (Billaud et al., 2000), accumulation of macrophage migratory inhibitory factor in astrocytes (Bacher et al., 2002), the expression of tissue factor, a primary cellular initiation of the coagulation protein cascades, resulting in protease thrombin by astrocytes (Gonzalez-Dunia et al., 1996), astrocytes as an antigen-presenting and target cells for virus specific CD4 lymphocytes (Richt and Stitz, 1992) and cytokine expression as a result of BDV infection resulting in neuropathology (Sauder and de la Torre, 1999; Shankar et al., 1992).

BDV infection has been reported in psychiatric illness by the presence of BDV RNA, antigen, circulating immune complex (CIC) in blood and post-mortem brain in psychiatric patients (Bode et al., 1997; Bode et al., 1995; Miranda et al., 2006; Sauder et al., 1996; Terayama et al., 2003). Amantadine is said to improve psychiatric illness such as mania and depression in bipolar disease and depressive patients (Dietrich et al., 2000; Moryl et al., 1993; Ohlmeier et al., 2007; Ohlmeier et al., 2008). Further amantadine was shown to have no role against BDV infection (Cubitt and de la Torre, 1997; Hallensleben et al., 1997; Stitz et al., 1998). Amantadine inhibits replication of BDV in cells and also prevents the infection of the naïve cells (Bode et al., 1997; Bode et al., 2001). Amantadine may not be an antiviral agent that improves psychiatric illness in BDV infected patients. Here we hypothesize the role of amantadine in improvement of psychiatric illness in patients infected with BDV.

3.6.1.1 Amantadine as a kinase inhibitor

In BDV infection, Raf/MEK/ERK signalling cascade is activated due to the infection (Planz et al., 2001) and also BDNF induced ERK1/2 phosphorylation is blocked (Hans et al., 2004). Thus BDV involves in signalling cascade that results in abnormal signalling or reduction of synaptogenesis. The MEK-specific inhibitor U0126 (1,4-diamino-2,3-dicyano-1,4-bis[2-aminophenylthio] butadiene) blocks the spread of BDV to the neighbouring cells, thereby infectious viral particle are concentrated in the nucleus. In the absence of the MEK-inhibitor, BDV regains the ability to spread in the cell culture and BDV infectious particles have been recovered from the infected cells, after the removal of MEK inhibitor. This showed that MEK inhibitor results in alteration of cellular or viral mediated process, subsequently the spreading from cell to cell, but does not interfere with the infectivity once the virus is released by cell disruption (Planz et al., 2001). Similarly amantadine was shown to prevent spreading to the naïve cells (Bode et al., 1997; Bode et al., 2001).

In influenza virus infected human bronchial epithelial cells, amantadine exhibits inhibitory effect on p38 mitogen activated protein (MAP) kinase and c-Jun-NH$_2$-terminal kinase (JNK) activity (Asai et al., 2001). Likewise, amantadine may act as a kinase inhibitor to relieve from mania or depression in BDV-infected psychiatric patients. Thus amantadine might acts as a kinase inhibitor allowing cellular changes in astrocytes.

3.6.1.2 Amantadine and IL 6

Astrocytes are one of the primary resident cells of the central nervous system with the production of cytokines. BDV-infections, neurons die both from direct viral lysis and immunopathological responses, while BDV-infected astrocytes appear to increase (Carbone et al., 1991a; Carbone et al., 1991b; Carbone et al., 1989). In rats, after intranasal infection with BDV, the proinflammatory cytokines mRNA namely interleukin (IL)-6, IL-1α and TNF-α were found to increase (Shankar et al., 1992). Similar results have been observed by Sauder and de la Torre (Sauder and de la Torre, 1999), in rats infected with BDV, the proinflammatory cytokines like IL-6, TNF-α, IL-1α, IL-1β found to be increased in the hippocampus and cerebellum in the infected rats that shows distinct behavioural and neurodevelopmental abnormalities. It is obvious that infection results in the expression of cytokines by the astrocytes.

IL-6 expression can be induced by the proinflammatory cytokines, IL-1β and TNF-α via protein kinase C (PKC) in astrocytes (Di Santo et al., 1996; Norris et al., 1994). IL-6 can also be a destructive agent during dysregulation in CNS, where over-expression leads to neuropathological conditions that include neurodegeneration, breakdown of blood-brain barrier, angiogenesis and increased expression of complement proteins (Campbell et al., 1993). The proinflammatory cytokines such as IL-6, TNF-α, IL-1α, IL-1β is known to contribute in neuropsychiatric syndromes, especially in major depression (Licinio and Wong, 1999; Tomonaga, 2004).

In BDV-infected psychiatric patients with bipolar mania or depression, after treatment with amantadine, there is a reduction in IL-6 and in BDV-CIC (personal communication). So the reduction in proinflammatory cytokine IL-6 shows that amantadine has some effects in treating BDV-infected patients. It suggests that treatment with amantadine regulates reduction of IL-6 and CIC in BDV infected patients.

In conclusion, amantadine may reduce the spread of BDV by acting as a kinase inhibitor and thereby reduce the severity by inhibiting the spreading of BDV to the neighbouring cells and also results in reduction of IL-6 by alteration of cellular mechanism in signalling pathways. Thus, amantadine can be used clinically in treating BDV-infected psychiatric patients.

3.7 Blood transfusion and BDV

Blood transfusion and BDV is least studied, because of the lack of evidence for transmission in humans and; also as a causative agent for neuropsychiatric illness in humans. In few studies, BDV has been suggested as a contributing source for neuropsychiatric illness (Chen et al., 1999), but BDV and or its viral component has been reported to present in blood of psychiatric patients (Bode et al., 1997; Bode et al., 1996; Heinrich and Adamaszek, 2010; Kitani et al., 1996; Sauder et al., 1996). In animal models, the transfusion/transfer of lymphocytes from brain of BDV-infected to immuno-compromised rats results in clinical symptoms and neuropathology of Borna disease in the recipients (Batra et al., 2003). Thus, the need for blood test for BDV has been suggested to be included during blood donation and transfusion (Alwin Prem Anand, 2010). If the viral component and/or the lymphocyte are sufficient to cause the clinical symptoms and neuropathology in recipients, blood transfusion might result in the same. Though, it is really a question whether BDV is the causative agent of neuropsychiatric illness in human. But preferably BDV infection in human beings might worsen the symptoms of any neuropsychiatric illness, if present.

4. Dengue viral disease

Dengue is the most important arthropod-borne viral infection of humans, which affects millions of people, particularly in urban and semi-urban areas. Worldwide, an estimated 2.5 billion people are at risk of infection (Gubler, 2002), with more than 100 million new infections each year. This includes 500,000 hospitalizations cases for dengue hemorrhagic fever, predominantly among children (Dussart et al., 2006). The annual average number of dengue fever/dengue hemorrhagic fever (DF/DHF) cases reported to the WHO has increased significantly in recent years. For the period 2000–2004, the annual average was 925,896 cases; almost double the figure of 479,848 cases that was reported in the period 1990–1999. Travelers' from endemic areas serve as vehicles for further spread. Dengue epidemics can have a significant economic and health toll. In endemic countries in Asia and the Americas, the burden of dengue is approximately 1,300 disability-adjusted life years per million populations, which is similar to the disease burden of other childhood and tropical diseases including tuberculosis in these regions (Gubler and Meltzer, 1999).

4.1 Dengue virus genome structure and function

Dengue viruses (DENV) belong to the genus flavivirus within the Flaviviridae family. The virus evolved in non-human primates from a common ancestor and entered the urban cycle some 500–1,000 years ago. The virus has a positive strand RNA whose genome is approximately 11kb in length. It has four antigenically distinct serotypes (Dengue virus 1-4). The RNA has a single open reading frame that encoding three structural proteins, nucleocapsid/core protein (C), membrane protein (M) and envelope protein (E) and; seven non-structural proteins (NS1, NS2A, NS2B, NS3, NS4A, NS4B and NS5) (Chambers et al., 1990). The envelope (E) and membrane proteins (M) are inserted in the lipid membrane. The glycoprotein E contains most of the antigenic determinants of the virus and essential for viral attachment and entry, while membrane protein (M) is synthesized as the precursor protein (prM), which acts as a chaperone during maturation of the viral particle. The nucleocapsid consists of capsid protein (C).

4.2 Dengue infection

Though dengue infection occurs as a mild febrile, self limiting illness i.e., Dengue fever (DF), its severe form causes Dengue hemorrhagic fever (DHF) and Dengue shock syndrome (DSS) are important public health problem because of its disease burden and high mortality rate (more than 5% in case of DHF/DSS) (Wilder-Smith et al., 2009). Infection by one serotype induces a lifelong immunity to the particular serotype and transient immunity to other serotypes, while concurrent infection by other serotype induces DHF/DSS.

4.2.1 Stages of DENV infection

In the skin, dengue viruses infect immature dendritic cells through the non-specific receptor dendritic cell specific ICAM3 grabbing non-integrin (DC-SIGN) (Wu et al., 2000). Infected dendritic cells mature and migrate to local or regional lymph nodes where they present viral antigens to T cells, initiating the cellular and humoral immune responses (Green et al., 1999). DENV also shown to replicate well in liver parenchymal cells, lymph node macrophages, liver, spleen, as well as in peripheral blood monocytes. DENVs produce several clinical syndromes, which depend up on age and immunological status of the individual. During initial stages, most infections are sub clinical (especially in children) or with mild undifferentiated febrile syndrome. In adults, primary infections with each of the four DENV serotypes, particularly with DENV-1 and -3, often results in DF. Some outbreaks of primary DENV-2 infections have been predominantly subclinical. During secondary dengue infections the pathophysiology of the disease changes dramatically. Sequential infections in which infection with DENV-1 is followed by infection with DENV-2 or DENV-3, or infection with DENV-3 is followed by infection with DENV-2 results in acute vascular permeability called as DSS (Alvarez et al., 2006). The severity of DSS is age-dependent and most severe in young children, which is due to the integrity of the capillaries (Gamble et al., 2000).

4.2.2 Genetic pre-disposition and host factors in DENV infection

Dengue infections can be life-threatening when they occur in individuals with asthma, diabetes and other chronic diseases (Lee et al., 2006). Host factors that increase the risk of severe dengue disease include sex, several human leukocyte antigen class I alleles, promoter variant of the DC-SIGN receptor gene, single-nucleotide polymorphism in the tumour necrosis factor gene and AB blood group. Host factors that reduce the risk of severe disease during a second dengue infection includes race, malnutrition, and polymorphisms in the Fcγ receptor and vitamin D receptor genes (Martina et al., 2009).

4.3 Pathogenesis of DENV infection

In adults secondary dengue infections either produces the classical DSS or severe disease complicated by hemorrhages. Most notably, in island outbreaks the severity of secondary dengue infections has been observed to increase from month-to-month (Guzman et al., 2000); and longer the interval between the first and second infection the more severe is the accompanying syndromes (Chareonsirisuthigul et al., 2007).

4.3.1 Antibody Dependent Enhancement (ADE)

Macrophages and monocytes participate in antibody dependent enhancement (ADE). Immune complexes formed between DENV antigens and non-neutralizing antibodies due to previous heterotypic dengue infections or from low concentrations of dengue antibodies of maternal origin in infant sera cross-react with Fc receptors of mononuclear phagocytes. The co-circulation of four DENV serotypes in a given population might augment the ADE phenomenon (Martina et al., 2009). One working hypothesis of dengue pathogenesis that is consistent with the available evidence is that severe disease in infants with primary infections and in older individuals with secondary infections is the result of ADE of infection of mononuclear phagocytes. Infection by an antibody–virus complex suppresses innate immune responses, increasing intracellular infection and generating inflammatory cytokines and chemokines that, collectively, result in enhanced disease.

4.3.2 Cytokines and soluble mediators

The infection of human monocytes and mature dendritic cells results in suppression of the interferon system and increases virus replication. Type I interferon-associated genes are less activated severe dengue disease. Increased number of infected cells presenting targets for CD4+ and CD8+ T cells, results in large quantities of interleukin IL-10, IL-2, interferon (IFN)-γ and TNF which lonely or synergistically, contributes to endothelial damage and altered homeostasis (Bosch et al., 2002; Talavera et al., 2004). Sub viral particles and virions released from infected cells also damages endothelial cells. Uptake of the non-structural protein NS1 by hepatocytes promotes viral infection of the liver. During DHF, the complement cascade is also activated and the levels of the complement activation products C3a and C5a correlate with the severity of illness (Malasit, 1987). Soluble and membrane-associated NS1 have been demonstrated to activate human complement. The levels of plasma NS1 correlated with disease severity, suggesting links between the virus, complement activation and the development of DHF/DSS (Navarro-Sanchez et al., 2005).

Alternative hypothesis for dengue pathogenesis points out the role of secondary T-cell responses. Researches point that the stimulation of T-cell memory results in the production of heterotypic CD4 and CD8 cells, which are less powerful in killing but release considerable amount of pro-inflammatory cytokines that contribute to disease severity. Cross-reactivity between antibodies produced against NS with human platelets, and endothelial cells, damages these cells. In patients with DF, IFN production and activated natural killer cells can limit disease severity (Mongkolsapaya et al., 2003; Zivna et al., 2002).

4.4 DENV transmission by non-vector modes

Other mosquito-borne flavivirus, such as West Nile virus, is transmitted efficiently in breast milk, blood transfusion, organ transplantation, stem cell transplantation, intra-uterine exposure and needle stick injuries (Hong et al., 2003; Iwamoto et al., 2003). The main transmission route for DENV is by vector mosquito. It is also transmitted by needle stick injuries, bone marrow transplantation and intrapartum vertical transmissions (Rodriguez Rodriguez et al., 2009). Recent reports have demonstrated dengue viremia in blood donors from Honduras, Brazil, Australia and Puerto Rico, which are endemic areas for dengue infection. Transmission of dengue infection has been reported from donor to recipient in one case of living donor renal transplant (Tan et al., 2005). The clinical presentation and course of illness was similar to that of an immuno-competent patient, except for prolonged course of illness (19 days) and duration of thrombocytopenia. Transmission during a bone marrow transplant was reported in one instance during a dengue epidemic in Puerto Rico in 1994 (Rigau-Perez et al., 2001).

4.4.1 Individual reported cases of transfusion mediated transmission

There are only two reported instances of transmission through blood transfusion. The first involved a patient in Hong Kong who developed fever 3 days after a blood transfusion, associated with moderate neutropenia, severe thrombocytopenia and hypotension responsive to fluid therapy. The donor was asymptomatic at the time of donation but developed mild symptoms of DF 1 day after blood donation. Stored sample from the donor tested positive for dengue virus by RT-PCR (Chuang et al., 2008). The second involved the transmission of dengue from an asymptomatic blood donor from Singapore who developed an acute febrile illness the day after donating blood. Investigation confirmed dengue infection in the recipients of the three blood products from his donation. Two recipients had DF with some evidence of capillary leakage, whereas the platelet recipient had asymptomatic seroconversion and all patients recovered. A stored serum sample from the donation tested positive for DEN-2 by RT-PCR (Tambyah et al., 2008).

4.4.2 Population based study on DENV transmission through transfusion

Various studies have shown the presence of asymptomatic or subclinical infection, which can range from 0.77 to 87% depending on the population studied (Ooi et al., 2006). It is estimated that for every one symptomatic case, there can be 6.7 cases that are asymptomatic (Chen and Wilson, 2005). A study found silent transmission of dengue commonly in 15 to 40 year age group. Among 329 healthy volunteers in a province in Thailand with high rate of dengue infection, 29 (8.8%) had a serum sample positive for dengue IgM, of which two samples tested positive for viral RNA (Poblap et al., 2006). Cluster sampling studies around index cases in Indonesia detected eight asymptomatic dengue infections of 785 volunteers over a 2-year period, of which two demonstrated viraemia by RT-PCR (Beckett et al., 2005). Virus was isolated in 215 of 3189 (6.7%) persons in a study evaluating the dynamics of transmission of dengue virus in a dengue epidemic area of Colombia, most of who were asymptomatic (Mendez et al., 2006). Two recent studies reported viraemia in blood donations collected from four countries experiencing high dengue transmission rates. In the first study, twelve (0.07%) of 16,521 blood donations collected in Puerto Rico tested positive using the dengue-specific nucleic acid amplification test (NAT). Testing using RT-PCR was positive in four samples and live virus was recovered from three of the PCR-positive samples (Mohammed et al., 2008). In the second study, samples from asymptomatic blood donors in Honduras, Brazil and Australia were obtained during periods of clinical dengue outbreaks and screened using the dengue-specific TMA assay. Nine (0.30%) of 2994 Honduran samples were tested positive, of which 8 were confirmed by RT-PCR and 4 samples yielded infectious viruses. Three (0.06%) of 4858 Brazilian samples tested positive, of which 2 were RTPCR positive (Linnen et al., 2008).

Technically, it is possible for DENV to be transmitted through blood transfusions because the disease courses with a transient viremia after infection and can be asymptomatic or have only mild symptoms. DENV was identified as one of three high-priority infectious agents with actual or potential risk of transfusion transmission in the United States or Canada. The rate of asymptomatic DENV infection in blood donors has been determined retrospectively in Puerto Rico and several other countries where dengue is endemic using molecular diagnostic. Infection rates have been shown to vary with disease incidence in the community, including the seasonal variation of dengue. In Puerto Rico, nearly 1 in 1000 blood donations were positive for DENV nucleic acid by during the 2005 dengue season (Mohammed et al., 2008) versus 1 in 600 positive during the 2007 outbreak (Tomashek and Margolis, 2011). The prevalence of DENV nucleic acid in blood donations in Puerto Rico in 2005 was similar to that estimated for WNV in areas experiencing outbreaks in the United States in 2002 before universal screening was implemented in 2003.

4.5 Challenges in identifying DENV as a risk in blood transfusion

Lack of knowledge in endemic areas - researchers and clinicians may not know/ consider blood transfusion as a source of infection.

Inconclusive data of dengue cases - may have been transfusion transmitted but has not been confirmed due to unavailability of complete information and serological tests.

Presence of high rate of existing antibodies - among transfusion recipients and donors especially in endemic areas will hinder to calculate the actual risk of dengue after transfusion.

4.6 Serological testing for DENV

At present, the only approach to prevent transfusion of DENV-positive blood would be screening with sensitive nucleic acid amplification tests to detect asymptomatic DENV infections in otherwise healthy donors and asymptomatic viremia in the 24 to 48 hours before donors becoming ill with dengue. Exclusion of donors in endemic areas during the high-incidence dengue season or during an outbreak is not feasible since the entire population is at risk of DENV infection, the need for blood components is typically high during outbreaks, and outbreaks can be long lasting.

The small number of reports of transfusion transmission could be because of the fact that it is difficult to differentiate between non-mosquito transmission and mosquito mediated transmission. Future studies are needed to establish rates of transfusion-transmitted DENV by viremic donations and their clinical consequences in recipients (Chen and Wilson, 2005). These evaluations should determine the most cost and prevention-effective approaches to prevent transfusion-transmitted dengue infections.

5. Conclusion

Hence, both BDV and DENV are less studied in transfusion medicine. It might be due to the incomplete evidence of transmission in BDV and, non-availability of better testing module for DV. In both the cases, the severity of causing serious damage to health is pretty high. The evidence for causing neuropsychiatric illness in BDV has not been proven or there is lack of evidence in it, but it may worsen the situation of a patient who is suffering from any prior neuropsychiatric illness. Ignoring the need for testing of the presence of these viruses in blood transfusion might result in serious health issues at global level. So in order to prevent potential risk of BDV and DENV infection through transfusion medicine, precautionary measures should be taken to diagnose and prevent BDV and DENV infection during blood transfusion.

6. References

Alvarez, M., Rodriguez-Roche, R., Bernardo, L., Vazquez, S., Morier, L., Gonzalez, D., Castro, O., Kouri, G., Halstead, S.B., Guzman, M.G., 2006. Dengue hemorrhagic Fever caused by sequential dengue 1-3 virus infections over a long time interval: Havana epidemic, 2001-2002. Am J Trop Med Hyg 75, 1113-1117.

Alwin Prem Anand, A., 2010. Is blood transfusion safe? BDV and neuropsychiatric illness. Acta Neuropsychiatrica 22, 208-208.

Asai, Y., Hashimoto, S., Kujime, K., Gon, Y., Mizumura, K., Shimizu, K., Horie, T., 2001. Amantadine inhibits RANTES production by influenzavirus-infected human bronchial epithelial cells. Br J Pharmacol 132, 918-924.

Bacher, M., Weihe, E., Dietzschold, B., Meinhardt, A., Vedder, H., Gemsa, D., Bette, M., 2002. Borna disease virus-induced accumulation of macrophage migration inhibitory factor in rat brain astrocytes is associated with inhibition of macrophage infiltration. Glia 37, 291-306.

Batra, A., Planz, O., Bilzer, T., Stitz, L., 2003. Precursors of Borna disease virus-specific T cells in secondary lymphatic tissue of experimentally infected rats. J Neurovirol 9, 325-335.

Beckett, C.G., Kosasih, H., Faisal, I., Nurhayati, Tan, R., Widjaja, S., Listiyaningsih, E., Ma'roef, C., Wuryadi, S., Bangs, M.J., Samsi, T.K., Yuwono, D., Hayes, C.G., Porter, K.R., 2005. Early detection of dengue infections using cluster sampling around index cases. Am J Trop Med Hyg 72, 777-782.

Benveniste, E.N., 1992. Cytokines: influence on glial cell gene expression and function. Chem Immunol 52, 106-153.

Benveniste, E.N., 1997. Cytokines: influence on glial cell gene expression and function. Chem Immunol 69, 31-75.

Billaud, J.N., Ly, C., Phillips, T.R., de la Torre, J.C., 2000. Borna disease virus persistence causes inhibition of glutamate uptake by feline primary cortical astrocytes. J Virol 74, 10438-10446.

Bilzer, T., Stitz, L., 1994. Immune-mediated brain atrophy. CD8+ T cells contribute to tissue destruction during borna disease. J Immunol 153, 818-823.

Bode, L., 1995. Human infections with Borna disease virus and potential pathogenic implications. Curr Top Microbiol Immunol 190, 103-130.

Bode, L., Dietrich, D.E., Stoyloff, R., Emrich, H.M., Ludwig, H., 1997. Amantadine and human Borna disease virus in vitro and in vivo in an infected patient with bipolar depression. Lancet 349, 178-179.

Bode, L., Durrwald, R., Rantam, F.A., Ferszt, R., Ludwig, H., 1996. First isolates of infectious human Borna disease virus from patients with mood disorders. Mol Psychiatry 1, 200-212.

Bode, L., Komaroff, A.L., Ludwig, H., 1992. No serologic evidence of borna disease virus in patients with chronic fatigue syndrome. Clin Infect Dis 15, 1049.

Bode, L., Ludwig, H., 2003. Borna disease virus infection, a human mental-health risk. Clin Microbiol Rev 16, 534-545.

Bode, L., Reckwald, P., Severus, W.E., Stoyloff, R., Ferszt, R., Dietrich, D.E., Ludwig, H., 2001. Borna disease virus-specific circulating immune complexes, antigenemia, and free antibodies--the key marker triplet determining infection and prevailing in severe mood disorders. Mol Psychiatry 6, 481-491.

Bode, L., Zimmermann, W., Ferszt, R., Steinbach, F., Ludwig, H., 1995. Borna disease virus genome transcribed and expressed in psychiatric patients. Nat Med 1, 232-236.

Bosch, I., Xhaja, K., Estevez, L., Raines, G., Melichar, H., Warke, R.V., Fournier, M.V., Ennis, F.A., Rothman, A.L., 2002. Increased production of interleukin-8 in primary human monocytes and in human epithelial and endothelial cell lines after dengue virus challenge. Journal of virology 76, 5588-5597.

Briese, T., Schneemann, A., Lewis, A.J., Park, Y.S., Kim, S., Ludwig, H., Lipkin, W.I., 1994. Genomic organization of Borna disease virus. Proc Natl Acad Sci U S A 91, 4362-4366.

Campbell, I.L., Abraham, C.R., Masliah, E., Kemper, P., Inglis, J.D., Oldstone, M.B., Mucke, L., 1993. Neurologic disease induced in transgenic mice by cerebral overexpression of interleukin 6. Proc Natl Acad Sci U S A 90, 10061-10065.

Carbone, K.M., Moench, T.R., Lipkin, W.I., 1991a. Borna disease virus replicates in astrocytes, Schwann cells and ependymal cells in persistently infected rats: location of viral genomic and messenger RNAs by in situ hybridization. J Neuropathol Exp Neurol 50, 205-214.

Carbone, K.M., Park, S.W., Rubin, S.A., Waltrip, R.W., 2nd, Vogelsang, G.B., 1991b. Borna disease: association with a maturation defect in the cellular immune response. J Virol 65, 6154-6164.

Carbone, K.M., Rubin, S.A., Sierra-Honigmann, A.M., Lederman, H.M., 1993. Characterization of a glial cell line persistently infected with borna disease virus (BDV): influence of neurotrophic factors on BDV protein and RNA expression. J Virol 67, 1453-1460.

Carbone, K.M., Trapp, B.D., Griffin, J.W., Duchala, C.S., Narayan, O., 1989. Astrocytes and Schwann cells are virus-host cells in the nervous system of rats with Borna disease. J Neuropathol Exp Neurol 48, 631-644.

Chambers, T.J., Hahn, C.S., Galler, R., Rice, C.M., 1990. Flavivirus genome organization, expression, and replication. Annu Rev Microbiol 44, 649-688.

Chareonsirisuthigul, T., Kalayanarooj, S., Ubol, S., 2007. Dengue virus (DENV) antibody-dependent enhancement of infection upregulates the production of anti-inflammatory cytokines, but suppresses anti-DENV free radical and pro-inflammatory cytokine production, in THP-1 cells. The Journal of general virology 88, 365-375.

Chase, G., Mayer, D., Hildebrand, A., Frank, R., Hayashi, Y., Tomonaga, K., Schwemmle, M., 2007. Borna disease virus matrix protein is an integral component of the viral ribonucleoprotein complex that does not interfere with polymerase activity. J Virol 81, 743-749.

Chen, C.H., Chiu, Y.L., Shaw, C.K., Tsai, M.T., Hwang, A.L., Hsiao, K.J., 1999. Detection of Borna disease virus RNA from peripheral blood cells in schizophrenic patients and mental health workers. Mol Psychiatry 4, 566-571.

Chen, L.H., Wilson, M.E., 2005. Nosocomial dengue by mucocutaneous transmission. Emerging infectious diseases 11, 775.

Chuang, V.W., Wong, T.Y., Leung, Y.H., Ma, E.S., Law, Y.L., Tsang, O.T., Chan, K.M., Tsang, I.H., Que, T.L., Yung, R.W., Liu, S.H., 2008. Review of dengue fever cases in Hong Kong during 1998 to 2005. Hong Kong Med J 14, 170-177.

Clements, G.B., Kennedy, P.G., 1989. Modulation of herpes simplex virus (HSV) infection of cultured neuronal cells by nerve growth factor and antibody to HSV. Brain 112 (Pt 5), 1277-1294.

Cubitt, B., de la Torre, J.C., 1994. Borna disease virus (BDV), a nonsegmented RNA virus, replicates in the nuclei of infected cells where infectious BDV ribonucleoproteins are present. J Virol 68, 1371-1381.

Cubitt, B., de la Torre, J.C., 1997. Amantadine does not have antiviral activity against Borna disease virus. Arch Virol 142, 2035-2042.

de la Torre, J.C., 1994. Molecular biology of borna disease virus: prototype of a new group of animal viruses. J Virol 68, 7669-7675.

de la Torre, J.C., 2002. Molecular biology of Borna disease virus and persistence. Front Biosci 7, d569-579.

De La Torre, J.C., Gonzalez-Dunia, D., Cubitt, B., Mallory, M., Mueller-Lantzsch, N., Grasser, F.A., Hansen, L.A., Masliah, E., 1996. Detection of borna disease virus antigen and RNA in human autopsy brain samples from neuropsychiatric patients. Virology 223, 272-282.

Di Santo, E., Alonzi, T., Fattori, E., Poli, V., Ciliberto, G., Sironi, M., Gnocchi, P., Ricciardi-Castagnoli, P., Ghezzi, P., 1996. Overexpression of interleukin-6 in the central nervous system of transgenic mice increases central but not systemic proinflammatory cytokine production. Brain Res 740, 239-244.

Dietrich, D.E., Bode, L., Spannhuth, C.W., Lau, T., Huber, T.J., Brodhun, B., Ludwig, H., Emrich, H.M., 2000. Amantadine in depressive patients with Borna disease virus (BDV) infection: an open trial. Bipolar Disord 2, 65-70.

Dietrich, D.E., Zhang, Y., Bode, L., Munte, T.F., Hauser, U., Schmorl, P., Richter-Witte, C., Godecke-Koch, T., Feutl, S., Schramm, J., Ludwig, H., Johannes, S., Emrich, H.M., 2005. Brain potential amplitude varies as a function of Borna disease virus-specific immune complexes in obsessive-compulsive disorder. Mol Psychiatry 10, 515, 519-520.

Dunn, A.J., 2000. Cytokine activation of the HPA axis. Ann N Y Acad Sci 917, 608-617.

Dussart, P., Labeau, B., Lagathu, G., Louis, P., Nunes, M.R., Rodrigues, S.G., Storck-Herrmann, C., Cesaire, R., Morvan, J., Flamand, M., Baril, L., 2006. Evaluation of an enzyme immunoassay for detection of dengue virus NS1 antigen in human serum. Clin Vaccine Immunol 13, 1185-1189.

Ferszt, R., Kuhl, K.P., Bode, L., Severus, E.W., Winzer, B., Berghofer, A., Beelitz, G., Brodhun, B., Muller-Oerlinghausen, B., Ludwig, H., 1999. Amantadine revisited: an open trial of amantadinesulfate treatment in chronically depressed patients with Borna disease virus infection. Pharmacopsychiatry 32, 142-147.

Gamble, J., Bethell, D., Day, N.P., Loc, P.P., Phu, N.H., Gartside, I.B., Farrar, J.F., White, N.J., 2000. Age-related changes in microvascular permeability: a significant factor in the susceptibility of children to shock? Clin Sci (Lond) 98, 211-216.

Gonzalez-Dunia, D., Cubitt, B., de la Torre, J.C., 1998. Mechanism of Borna disease virus entry into cells. J Virol 72, 783-788.

Gonzalez-Dunia, D., Eddleston, M., Mackman, N., Carbone, K., de la Torre, J.C., 1996. Expression of tissue factor is increased in astrocytes within the central nervous system during persistent infection with borna disease virus. J Virol 70, 5812-5820.

Green, S., Vaughn, D.W., Kalayanarooj, S., Nimmannitya, S., Suntayakorn, S., Nisalak, A., Lew, R., Innis, B.L., Kurane, I., Rothman, A.L., Ennis, F.A., 1999. Early immune activation in acute dengue illness is related to development of plasma leakage and disease severity. The Journal of infectious diseases 179, 755-762.

Griffin, D.E., Hardwick, J.M., 1999. Perspective: virus infections and the death of neurons. Trends Microbiol 7, 155-160.

Gubler, D.J., 2002. The global emergence/resurgence of arboviral diseases as public health problems. Arch Med Res 33, 330-342.

Gubler, D.J., Meltzer, M., 1999. Impact of dengue/dengue hemorrhagic fever on the developing world. Adv Virus Res 53, 35-70.

Hallensleben, W., Zocher, M., Staeheli, P., 1997. Borna disease virus is not sensitive to amantadine. Arch Virol 142, 2043-2048.

Hans, A., Bajramovic, J.J., Syan, S., Perret, E., Dunia, I., Brahic, M., Gonzalez-Dunia, D., 2004. Persistent, noncytolytic infection of neurons by Borna disease virus interferes with ERK 1/2 signaling and abrogates BDNF-induced synaptogenesis. FASEB J 18, 863-865.

Heinrich, A., Adamaszek, M., 2010. Anti-Borna disease virus antibody responses in psychiatric patients: long-term follow up. Psychiatry Clin Neurosci 64, 255-261.

Herden, C., Herzog, S., Richt, J.A., Nesseler, A., Christ, M., Failing, K., Frese, K., 2000. Distribution of Borna disease virus in the brain of rats infected with an obesity-inducing virus strain. Brain Pathol 10, 39-48.

Honda, T., Fujino, K., Okuzaki, D., Ohtaki, N., Matsumoto, Y., Horie, M., Daito, T., Itoh, M., Tomonaga, K., 2011. Upregulation of insulin-like growth factor binding protein 3 in astrocytes of transgenic mice that express borna disease virus phosphoprotein. J Virol 85, 4567-4571.

Hong, D.S., Jacobson, K.L., Raad, II, de Lima, M., Anderlini, P., Fuller, G.N., Ippoliti, C., Cool, R.M., Leeds, N.E., Narvios, A., Han, X.Y., Padula, A., Champlin, R.E., Hosing, C., 2003. West Nile encephalitis in 2 hematopoietic stem cell transplant recipients: case series and literature review. Clinical infectious diseases : an official publication of the Infectious Diseases Society of America 37, 1044-1049.

Hornig, M., Briese, T., Lipkin, W.I., 2003. Borna disease virus. J Neurovirol 9, 259-273.

Hornig, M., Solbrig, M., Horscroft, N., Weissenbock, H., Lipkin, W.I., 2001. Borna disease virus infection of adult and neonatal rats: models for neuropsychiatric disease. Curr Top Microbiol Immunol 253, 157-177.

Iwamoto, M., Jernigan, D.B., Guasch, A., Trepka, M.J., Blackmore, C.G., Hellinger, W.C., Pham, S.M., Zaki, S., Lanciotti, R.S., Lance-Parker, S.E., DiazGranados, C.A., Winquist, A.G., Perlino, C.A., Wiersma, S., Hillyer, K.L., Goodman, J.L., Marfin, A.A., Chamberland, M.E., Petersen, L.R., 2003. Transmission of West Nile virus from an organ donor to four transplant recipients. The New England journal of medicine 348, 2196-2203.

Kamitani, W., Ono, E., Yoshino, S., Kobayashi, T., Taharaguchi, S., Lee, B.J., Yamashita, M., Okamoto, M., Taniyama, H., Tomonaga, K., Ikuta, K., 2003. Glial expression of Borna disease virus phosphoprotein induces behavioral and neurological abnormalities in transgenic mice. Proc Natl Acad Sci U S A 100, 8969-8974.

Kelley, K.W., Bluthe, R.M., Dantzer, R., Zhou, J.H., Shen, W.H., Johnson, R.W., Broussard, S.R., 2003. Cytokine-induced sickness behavior. Brain Behav Immun 17 Suppl 1, S112-118.

Kitani, T., Kuratsune, H., Fuke, I., Nakamura, Y., Nakaya, T., Asahi, S., Tobiume, M., Yamaguti, K., Machii, T., Inagi, R., Yamanishi, K., Ikuta, K., 1996. Possible correlation between Borna disease virus infection and Japanese patients with chronic fatigue syndrome. Microbiol Immunol 40, 459-462.

Kobayashi, T., Zhang, G., Lee, B.J., Baba, S., Yamashita, M., Kamitani, W., Yanai, H., Tomonaga, K., Ikuta, K., 2003. Modulation of Borna disease virus phosphoprotein nuclear localization by the viral protein X encoded in the overlapping open reading frame. J Virol 77, 8099-8107.

Konsman, J.P., Parnet, P., Dantzer, R., 2002. Cytokine-induced sickness behaviour: mechanisms and implications. Trends Neurosci 25, 154-159.

Kraus, I., Bogner, E., Lilie, H., Eickmann, M., Garten, W., 2005. Oligomerization and assembly of the matrix protein of Borna disease virus. FEBS Lett 579, 2686-2692.

Kristensson, K., 2011. Microbes' roadmap to neurons. Nat Rev Neurosci 12, 345-357.

Lee, M.S., Hwang, K.P., Chen, T.C., Lu, P.L., Chen, T.P., 2006. Clinical characteristics of dengue and dengue hemorrhagic fever in a medical center of southern Taiwan during the 2002 epidemic. J Microbiol Immunol Infect 39, 121-129.

Licinio, J., Wong, M.L., 1999. The role of inflammatory mediators in the biology of major depression: central nervous system cytokines modulate the biological substrate of depressive symptoms, regulate stress-responsive systems, and contribute to neurotoxicity and neuroprotection. Mol Psychiatry 4, 317-327.

Linnen, J.M., Vinelli, E., Sabino, E.C., Tobler, L.H., Hyland, C., Lee, T.H., Kolk, D.P., Broulik, A.S., Collins, C.S., Lanciotti, R.S., Busch, M.P., 2008. Dengue viremia in blood donors from Honduras, Brazil, and Australia. Transfusion 48, 1355-1362.

Ludwig, H., Bode, L., Gosztonyi, G., 1988. Borna disease: a persistent virus infection of the central nervous system. Prog Med Virol 35, 107-151.

Ludwig, H., Furuya, K., Bode, L., Klein, N., Durrwald, R., Lee, D.S., 1993. Biology and neurobiology of Borna disease viruses (BDV), defined by antibodies, neutralizability and their pathogenic potential. Arch Virol Suppl 7, 111-133.

Malasit, P., 1987. Complement and dengue haemorrhagic fever/shock syndrome. Southeast Asian J Trop Med Public Health 18, 316-320.

Manji, H.K., Drevets, W.C., Charney, D.S., 2001. The cellular neurobiology of depression. Nat Med 7, 541-547.

Martina, B.E., Koraka, P., Osterhaus, A.D., 2009. Dengue virus pathogenesis: an integrated view. Clinical microbiology reviews 22, 564-581.

Miranda, H.C., Nunes, S.O., Calvo, E.S., Suzart, S., Itano, E.N., Watanabe, M.A., 2006. Detection of Borna disease virus p24 RNA in peripheral blood cells from Brazilian mood and psychotic disorder patients. J Affect Disord 90, 43-47.

Mohammed, H., Linnen, J.M., Munoz-Jordan, J.L., Tomashek, K., Foster, G., Broulik, A.S., Petersen, L., Stramer, S.L., 2008. Dengue virus in blood donations, Puerto Rico, 2005. Transfusion 48, 1348-1354.

Mongkolsapaya, J., Dejnirattisai, W., Xu, X.N., Vasanawathana, S., Tangthawornchaikul, N., Chairunsri, A., Sawasdivorn, S., Duangchinda, T., Dong, T., Rowland-Jones, S., Yenchitsomanus, P.T., McMichael, A., Malasit, P., Screaton, G., 2003. Original antigenic sin and apoptosis in the pathogenesis of dengue hemorrhagic fever. Nature medicine 9, 921-927.

Montkowski, A., Landgraf, R., Yassouridis, A., Holsboer, F., Schobitz, B., 1997. Central administration of IL-1 reduces anxiety and induces sickness behaviour in rats. Pharmacol Biochem Behav 58, 329-336.

Moryl, E., Danysz, W., Quack, G., 1993. Potential antidepressive properties of amantadine, memantine and bifemelane. Pharmacol Toxicol 72, 394-397.

Navarro-Sanchez, E., Despres, P., Cedillo-Barron, L., 2005. Innate immune responses to dengue virus. Arch Med Res 36, 425-435.

Nelson, R.J., Chiavegatto, S., 2001. Molecular basis of aggression. Trends Neurosci 24, 713-719.

Neumann, P., Lieber, D., Meyer, S., Dautel, P., Kerth, A., Kraus, I., Garten, W., Stubbs, M.T., 2009. Crystal structure of the Borna disease virus matrix protein (BDV-M) reveals ssRNA binding properties. Proc Natl Acad Sci U S A 106, 3710-3715.

Nieto-Sampedro, M., Bovolenta, P., 1990. Growth factors and growth factor receptors in the hippocampus. Role in plasticity and response to injury. Prog Brain Res 83, 341-355.

Norris, J.G., Tang, L.P., Sparacio, S.M., Benveniste, E.N., 1994. Signal transduction pathways mediating astrocyte IL-6 induction by IL-1 beta and tumor necrosis factor-alpha. J Immunol 152, 841-850.

Ohlmeier, M.D., Sieg, S., Emrich, H.M., Dietrich, D.E., 2007. Amantadine in acute bipolar mania. Aust N Z J Psychiatry 41, 194.

Ohlmeier, M.D., Zhang, Y., Bode, L., Sieg, S., Feutl, S., Ludwig, H., Emrich, H.M., Dietrich, D.E., 2008. Amantadine reduces mania in borna disease virus-infected non-psychotic bipolar patients. Pharmacopsychiatry 41, 202-203.

Ojika, K., Appel, S.H., 1984. Neurotrophic effects of hippocampal extracts on medial septal nucleus in vitro. Proc Natl Acad Sci U S A 81, 2567-2571.

Olive, M.F., Hodge, C.W., 2000. Co-localization of PKCepsilon with various GABA(A) receptor subunits in the mouse limbic system. Neuroreport 11, 683-687.

Ooi, E.E., Goh, K.T., Gubler, D.J., 2006. Dengue prevention and 35 years of vector control in Singapore. Emerging infectious diseases 12, 887-893.

Planz, O., Pleschka, S., Ludwig, S., 2001. MEK-specific inhibitor U0126 blocks spread of Borna disease virus in cultured cells. J Virol 75, 4871-4877.

Pletnikov, M.V., Moran, T.H., Carbone, K.M., 2002a. Borna disease virus infection of the neonatal rat: developmental brain injury model of autism spectrum disorders. Front Biosci 7, d593-607.

Pletnikov, M.V., Rubin, S.A., Vogel, M.W., Moran, T.H., Carbone, K.M., 2002b. Effects of genetic background on neonatal Borna disease virus infection-induced neurodevelopmental damage. I. Brain pathology and behavioral deficits. Brain Res 944, 97-107.

Pletnikov, M.V., Rubin, S.A., Vogel, M.W., Moran, T.H., Carbone, K.M., 2002c. Effects of genetic background on neonatal Borna disease virus infection-induced neurodevelopmental damage. II. Neurochemical alterations and responses to pharmacological treatments. Brain Res 944, 108-123.

Poblap, T., Nitatpattana, N., Chaimarin, A., Barbazan, P., Chauvancy, G., Yoksan, S., Gonzalez, J.P., 2006. Silent transmission of virus during a Dengue epidemic, Nakhon Pathom Province, Thailand 2001. Southeast Asian J Trop Med Public Health 37, 899-903.

Poenisch, M., Unterstab, G., Wolff, T., Staeheli, P., Schneider, U., 2004. The X protein of Borna disease virus regulates viral polymerase activity through interaction with the P protein. J Gen Virol 85, 1895-1898.

Poenisch, M., Wille, S., Ackermann, A., Staeheli, P., Schneider, U., 2007. The X protein of borna disease virus serves essential functions in the viral multiplication cycle. J Virol 81, 7297-7299.

Prat, C.M., Schmid, S., Farrugia, F., Cenac, N., Le Masson, G., Schwemmle, M., Gonzalez-Dunia, D., 2009. Mutation of the protein kinase C site in borna disease virus phosphoprotein abrogates viral interference with neuronal signaling and restores normal synaptic activity. PLoS Pathog 5, e1000425.

Richt, J.A., Stitz, L., 1992. Borna disease virus-infected astrocytes function in vitro as antigen-presenting and target cells for virus-specific CD4-bearing lymphocytes. Arch Virol 124, 95-109.

Rigau-Perez, J.G., Vorndam, A.V., Clark, G.G., 2001. The dengue and dengue hemorrhagic fever epidemic in Puerto Rico, 1994-1995. Am J Trop Med Hyg 64, 67-74.

Rodriguez Rodriguez, D., Garza Rodriguez, M., Chavarria, A.M., Ramos-Jimenez, J., Rivera, M.A., Tamez, R.C., Farfan-Ale, J., Rivas-Estilla, A.M., 2009. Dengue virus antibodies in blood donors from an endemic area. Transfus Med 19, 125-131.

Rosenberger, U., Shakibaei, M., Buchner, K., 1995. Localization of non-conventional protein kinase C isoforms in bovine brain cell nuclei. Biochem J 305 (Pt 1), 269-275.

Rott, R., Becht, H., 1995. Natural and experimental Borna disease in animals. Curr Top Microbiol Immunol 190, 17-30.

Sauder, C., de la Torre, J.C., 1999. Cytokine expression in the rat central nervous system following perinatal Borna disease virus infection. J Neuroimmunol 96, 29-45.

Sauder, C., Muller, A., Cubitt, B., Mayer, J., Steinmetz, J., Trabert, W., Ziegler, B., Wanke, K., Mueller-Lantzsch, N., de la Torre, J.C., Grasser, F.A., 1996. Detection of Borna disease virus (BDV) antibodies and BDV RNA in psychiatric patients: evidence for high sequence conservation of human blood-derived BDV RNA. J Virol 70, 7713-7724.

Schmid, S., Metz, P., Prat, C.M., Gonzalez-Dunia, D., Schwemmle, M., 2010. Protein kinase C-dependent phosphorylation of Borna disease virus P protein is required for efficient viral spread. Arch Virol 155, 789-793.

Schneider, U., 2005. Novel insights into the regulation of the viral polymerase complex of neurotropic Borna disease virus. Virus Res 111, 148-160.

Schneider, U., Schwemmle, M., Staeheli, P., 2005. Genome trimming: a unique strategy for replication control employed by Borna disease virus. Proc Natl Acad Sci U S A 102, 3441-3446.

Schwardt, M., Mayer, D., Frank, R., Schneider, U., Eickmann, M., Planz, O., Wolff, T., Schwemmle, M., 2005. The negative regulator of Borna disease virus polymerase is a non-structural protein. J Gen Virol 86, 3163-3169.

Schwemmle, M., De, B., Shi, L., Banerjee, A., Lipkin, W.I., 1997. Borna disease virus P-protein is phosphorylated by protein kinase Cepsilon and casein kinase II. J Biol Chem 272, 21818-21823.

Schwemmle, M., Salvatore, M., Shi, L., Richt, J., Lee, C.H., Lipkin, W.I., 1998. Interactions of the borna disease virus P, N, and X proteins and their functional implications. J Biol Chem 273, 9007-9012.

Shankar, V., Kao, M., Hamir, A.N., Sheng, H., Koprowski, H., Dietzschold, B., 1992. Kinetics of virus spread and changes in levels of several cytokine mRNAs in the brain after intranasal infection of rats with Borna disease virus. J Virol 66, 992-998.

Shoya, Y., Kobayashi, T., Koda, T., Ikuta, K., Kakinuma, M., Kishi, M., 1998. Two proline-rich nuclear localization signals in the amino- and carboxyl-terminal regions of the Borna disease virus phosphoprotein. J Virol 72, 9755-9762.

Stitz, L., Bilzer, T., Planz, O., 2002. The immunopathogenesis of Borna disease virus infection. Front Biosci 7, d541-555.

Stitz, L., Planz, O., Bilzer, T., 1998. Lack of antiviral effect of amantadine in Borna disease virus infection. Med Microbiol Immunol 186, 195-200.

Stoyloff, R., Strecker, A., Bode, L., Franke, P., Ludwig, H., Hucho, F., 1997. The glycosylated matrix protein of Borna disease virus is a tetrameric membrane-bound viral component essential for infection. Eur J Biochem 246, 252-257.

Talavera, D., Castillo, A.M., Dominguez, M.C., Gutierrez, A.E., Meza, I., 2004. IL8 release, tight junction and cytoskeleton dynamic reorganization conducive to permeability increase are induced by dengue virus infection of microvascular endothelial monolayers. The Journal of general virology 85, 1801-1813.

Tambyah, P.A., Koay, E.S., Poon, M.L., Lin, R.V., Ong, B.K., 2008. Dengue hemorrhagic fever transmitted by blood transfusion. The New England journal of medicine 359, 1526-1527.

Tan, F.L., Loh, D.L., Prabhakaran, K., Tambyah, P.A., Yap, H.K., 2005. Dengue haemorrhagic fever after living donor renal transplantation. Nephrol Dial Transplant 20, 447-448.

Terayama, H., Nishino, Y., Kishi, M., Ikuta, K., Itoh, M., Iwahashi, K., 2003. Detection of anti-Borna Disease Virus (BDV) antibodies from patients with schizophrenia and mood disorders in Japan. Psychiatry Res 120, 201-206.

Tomashek, K.M., Margolis, H.S., 2011. Dengue: a potential transfusion-transmitted disease. Transfusion 51, 1654-1660.

Tomonaga, K., 2004. Virus-induced neurobehavioral disorders: mechanisms and implications. Trends Mol Med 10, 71-77.

Tomonaga, K., Kobayashi, T., Ikuta, K., 2002. Molecular and cellular biology of Borna disease virus infection. Microbes Infect 4, 491-500.

Volmer, R., Monnet, C., Gonzalez-Dunia, D., 2006. Borna disease virus blocks potentiation of presynaptic activity through inhibition of protein kinase C signaling. PLoS Pathog 2, e19.

Walker, M.P., Jordan, I., Briese, T., Fischer, N., Lipkin, W.I., 2000. Expression and characterization of the Borna disease virus polymerase. J Virol 74, 4425-4428.

Walker, M.P., Lipkin, W.I., 2002. Characterization of the nuclear localization signal of the borna disease virus polymerase. J Virol 76, 8460-8467.

Wilcox, C.L., Johnson, E.M., Jr., 1988. Characterization of nerve growth factor-dependent herpes simplex virus latency in neurons in vitro. J Virol 62, 393-399.

Wilcox, C.L., Smith, R.L., Freed, C.R., Johnson, E.M., Jr., 1990. Nerve growth factor-dependence of herpes simplex virus latency in peripheral sympathetic and sensory neurons in vitro. J Neurosci 10, 1268-1275.

Wilder-Smith, A., Chen, L.H., Massad, E., Wilson, M.E., 2009. Threat of dengue to blood safety in dengue-endemic countries. Emerging infectious diseases 15, 8-11.

Wu, S.J., Grouard-Vogel, G., Sun, W., Mascola, J.R., Brachtel, E., Putvatana, R., Louder, M.K., Filgueira, L., Marovich, M.A., Wong, H.K., Blauvelt, A., Murphy, G.S., Robb, M.L., Innes, B.L., Birx, D.L., Hayes, C.G., Frankel, S.S., 2000. Human skin Langerhans cells are targets of dengue virus infection. Nature medicine 6, 816-820.

Zivna, I., Green, S., Vaughn, D.W., Kalayanarooj, S., Stephens, H.A., Chandanayingyong, D., Nisalak, A., Ennis, F.A., Rothman, A.L., 2002. T cell responses to an HLA-B*07-restricted epitope on the dengue NS3 protein correlate with disease severity. Journal of immunology 168, 5959-5965.

9

Transfusion-Transmitted Bacterial, Viral and Protozoal Infections

Pankaj Abrol[1] and Harbans Lal[2]
[1]Post Graduate Institute of Medical Sciences,
University of Health Sciences,Rohtak (Haryana)
[2]Maharaja Agrasen Medical College, Agroha, Hissar (Haryana)
India

1. Introduction

Blood transmitted infection is the commonest cause of death after blood transfusion. All patients on regular packed cell volume (PCV) or any blood component are at increased risk of transfusion transmitted infections. The etiological agents can be virus, bacteria or protozoa. These organisms can cause clinical sickness in recipient, can persist in him as carrier state or can cause asymptomatic infection in him. Every blood bank follows screening procedures to prevent such infections but the infective agents escape detection due to window period – a period where in the infective agent's presence cannot be detected, though it is present in donor's blood. Blood banks in developed countries are doing Nucleic Acid Amplification Testing (NAT) since 1999 to screen donated blood. The window period for testing for HIV, Hepatitis B and Hepatitis C has been significantly reduced with NAT. NAT can detect low levels of viral genetic material in blood.

Patients having thalassemia major or any other chronic hemolytic anemia are on regular PCV infusion essential for their survival. Patients having hemophilia; on cryoprecipitate, fresh frozen plasma or on plasma based factors are also at increased risk. Hemophilia patients on recombinant factors VIII or IX, from the start of therapy are safe.

2. Nuclear acid amplification testing (NAT)

Despite improvement in HIV, HCV and HBV serological tests, we still have viral transmission of these diseases because of donations that take place while donor is:

1. In pre-seroconversion window period
2. Infected with immunovariant viruses
3. A non-sero-converting chronic carrier

In most countries, the safety of blood is ensured by donor selection, testing of donations for viral markers and in the case of blood products, the inclusion of viral inactivation steps during the manufacture of the blood products. However, transmission of HIV, HBV and HCV, continues to be a threat to safe blood transfusion, especially in developing countries. It is due to low numbers of voluntary donations, use of low sensitivity tests for viral screening and the high prevalence of these viruses. This has contributed to the high rate of transfusion transmitted infections compared with developed countries. In developing countries, where the majority of donors are still replacement donors, the risk of transfusion transmitted viral infections is much higher than in countries with a 100% voluntary donor base. The prevalence of post transfusion HBV and HCV in India is between 1 to 5% [Singh, 1999]. The prevalence of HIV varies from region to region in a country.

The implementation of nucleic acid testing (NAT) over the last decade into the blood screening process has added an extra layer of safety against transmission of transfused viral infections. NAT was first introduced by the European plasma industry in 1995 and consequently for whole blood donation screening in some parts of Europe and then Asia. HCV NAT was first introduced between 1999 and 2001 in blood banks across France, Germany, Italy, Spain, Switzerland and the United Kingdom presumably as it was already mandatory for plasma screening in these countries [Pathak & Chandrashekhar, 2010].

Serological screening of blood donor have greatly reduced, but not eliminated the risk of transmission of viral infections by transfusion of blood and blood products. Production of antibodies takes several weeks after the infection. During this **serological window period**, infective antigen is present in blood of the patient, but there are no detectable antibodies. The primary benefit of NAT is the ability to reduce residual risk of infectious window period (WP) donations [Wiedemann et al., 2007].

NAT screening reduces window period as follows:

1.   HIV - 11 Days
2.   HBV - 20 Days
3.   HCV - 15 Days

The introduction of Nucleic Acid Technology testing has reduced the risk of transfusion transmitted HCV and HIV infections to approximately 1 in 1 million and 1 in 3 million respectively in Western Europe and the USA. NAT testing can detect even low level of viral genetic material.

3. Etiology of blood transmitted infections

1.   Viruses – HIV 1 & 2 virus, Hepatitis C, Hepatitis B, Other Hepatitis Viruses, Cytomegalovirus, Human T-Cell Leukemia Virus, Cytomegalovirus, Parvovirus, Epstein Barr virus, Human herpes virus, West Nile virus.
2.   Bacterial contamination – Staphylococcus, streptococcus, Yersinia, Serratia, Acinetobacter, Pseudomonas, Escherichia etc.
3.   Protozoa – Malaria, Chagas, Toxoplasmosis, Leishmaniasis, Babesiosis
4.   Nematodes – Microfilariasis

4. Transfusion transmited viral infections

In last 2 decades, much attention has been given to prevention of viral infections like HIV-1 and 2, human T-cell lymphotropic virus (HTLV) I and II, hepatitis C virus, hepatitis B virus

(HBV) and west Nile virus (WNV). Because of potential transmission of virus during 'immunological window period', NAT is being performed. However, it has some limitations in blood components with very low levels of viremia, which can even escape detection by NAT. Despite this limitation, the combination of both serological testing and NAT has considerably reduced the risk of viral transmission by blood transfusion.

4.1 HIV

Human immune deficiency virus (HIV) is an important global public health problem. HIV infection causes a broad spectrum disease and has a varied clinical course, from mild, flu-like symptoms to AIDS; which is life threatening and the end stage of HIV infection. HIV is transmitted through sexual contact, sharing of HIV contaminated needles and/or syringes, transfusion of blood components, and nosocomial exposure to HIV contaminated blood or bodily fluids, and can be passed vertically from a mother to her infant.

Factors that can contribute to HIV transmission through blood transfusion include the window period (i.e. a short viraemic period in which the donor is infected with HIV at a very early stage and often tested negative in a donor screening test), HIV-antibody negative chronic carriers and HIV mutant infection. The primary source of transfusion transmitted HIV infection, however, is donations collected during the window period. Donated blood is tested for antibodies to HIV-1, HIV-1 p24 antigen test and HIV RNA test using NAT. Window period has been reduced from 42 days by HIV antibody assays in the 1980s to 16 days by HIV-1 p24 antigen test and 11 days by HIV NAT [Canadian Blood Services, 2001; Public Health Agency of Canada, 2003]. The risk of HIV transmission through blood transfusion was estimated to be 1 in 752,000 donations between 1987 and 1996. This risk has been estimated to be 1 in 1.3 million donations following the implementation of HIV-1 p24 testing, and 1 in 1.6 million donations following the implementation of HIV NAT on a pool of 24 samples.

4.2 HCV

Hepatitis C virus currently affects over four million people in USA. There it is the commonest transfusion transmitted infection and main indication for liver transplantation. High risk group is constituted by those who received transfusion prior to 1991 or the ones who were IV drug abusers using shared needles. Incubation period can be as long as decades and this contributes to high rate of infection. Route of infection is by and large intravenous/injection pricks. Sexual transmission is also possible. Other routes are nosocomial exposure to contaminated blood and body fluids and mother to child transmission. Hepatitis C virus subtype varies worldwide. Approximately 90% of individuals infected with HCV are either asymptomatic or have only mild symptoms. However, about 80% of acute infections progress to chronic infection, and almost half of those chronically infected individuals eventually develop cirrhosis or hepatocellular carcinoma after a few decades [Public Health Agency of Canada 2003].

In Europe, predominant genotypes are 1, 2 and 3. Types 1a and 3a are seen in north-western countries, whereas 1b is in Hungary, Germany, Russia and Turkey. Types 1a and 1b are common in North America. Types 1b, 2a and 2b predominate in Japan [Blood Book, 2011]. After infection, antibodies against Hepatitis C virus take 54-192 days to appear. The window period yielded with HCV nucleic acid amplification testing (HCV NAT) is shorter than that from the HCV antibody test. There is high risk of transfusion transmitted infection in this window. In United States there is 1 in 121,000 risk of HCV infection.

4.3 HBV

Hepatitis B surface antigen testing was introduced in 1970's and its transmission was consistently reduced since then. Still 300 million individuals are infected worldwide. HBV surface antigen is routinely included in donor screening but it fails to detect presence of HBV during window period. Chronic carriers of HBV may have low level viremia and may not have detectable HBsAg level, so some centres have started testing antibodies against HBV core protein (anti HBc). Today, the residual risk of transfusion transmitted HBV infection varies between 0.75 per million blood donations in Australia, 3.6 – 8.5 in the USA and Canada, 0.91 – 8.7 in Northern Europe, 7.5 – 13.9 in Southern Europe up to 200 per million donations in Hong Kong, largely reflecting the global epidemiology of HBV. Some countries with low level prevalence of HBV have implemented HBV NAT testing in plasma pools. The kinetics of viral antigen and antibody appearance during HBV infection create two different window periods in which one or the other test may fail: the "early acute phase", when serological markers are still negative and the "late chronic phase" when HBsAg may become gradually undetectable, although infectivity remains. NAT can potentially identify and can be of particular benefit in detecting HBV DNA in latent HBV infection in early acute phase/occult HBV infection, when HBV DNA is present in plasma and presence of anti-HBC and HBsAg is variable [Biswas et al., 2003].

4.4 Hepatitis A virus

Hepatitis A is an important vaccine preventable infectious disease. The most common mode of transmission is feco-oral. It occurs through personal contact or ingestion of contaminated food/water.

Transmission of HAV through blood transmission is not yet established. However, transmission of HAV has been reported through infusion of blood products in hemophilia patients. Since pooled plasma from multiple donors is used for preparing blood products, and the solvent-detergent method for viral inactivation is ineffective against HAV, the risk of transmission of HAV through the use of blood products, though extremely small, may still exist. Currently, blood units are not routinely tested for antibodies to HAV. It has been suggested that recipients of clotting factors receive vaccine against HAV to prevent Transfusion Transmitted hepatitis A [Moor et al., 1999].

4.5 Hepatitis E virus (HEV)

It's an acute infection caused by hepatitis E virus and is endemic in Asia and Africa. Mode of transmission as well as clinical presentation is same as in hepatitis A. Like hepatitis A, there are no carriers in hepatitis E. Periods of viremia are also short.

Although transmission of HEV through blood transfusion has not been established, possibility of its transmission through transfusion cannot be excluded in endemic areas.

5. Other hepatitis viruses

Other transfusion transmitted viruses – TTV, SEN-V and GBV-C do not cause hepatitis or other diseased states. Routine screening before blood transfusion is not recommended [Dzieczkowski & Anderson, 2008].

5.1 Human T Lymphotropic virus (HTLV)

HTLV 1 is associated with adult T cell leukemia/lymphoma and severe tropical spastic paraparesis. HTLV 2 is associated with milder forms of myelopathy / spastic paraparesis and pulmonary disorders. Both retroviruses have also been attributed a role in risk for developing severe asthma, respiratory and urinary tract infections, uveitis and dermatitis [Murphy et al., 1994, 2004]. Enzyme immunosorbent assays and particle agglutination tests are used for screening, followed by confirmatory tests of positive tests. No vaccine is available for prophylaxis and no effective antiviral drug is available for treatment.

5.2 Cytomegalovirus (CMV)

This omnipresent virus infects more than half of general population. Prevalence of CMV antibodies increases with age. Acute infection is usually asymptomatic. This is transmitted by infected WBC's found in packed red cells or platelet components. Leukoreduction reduces the risk of CMV transmission, regardless of serological status of donor. Immunocompromised patients, CMV seronegative transplant recipients, pregnant women and neonates form the high risk group. Pre-storage leukodepletion of blood components may be as effective as the use of CMV seronegative blood components [Vamvakas, 2005; Blajachman et al., 2001; Blajachman, 2006]. Donor blood is not routinely tested for CMV.

5.3 Parvovirus B-19

Blood components as well as pooled plasma products can transmit parvovirus B-19. Patients having thalassemia or hemophilia are at risk. Infection can also be transmitted through respiratory secretions as well vertically from mother to child. This is etiological agent of erythema infectiosum, or 5th disease in children. Patient may remain asymptomatic or present with mild symptoms like fever. Parvovirus B-19 has affinity for erythroid precursors and in some patients, inhibits both production and maturation of erythrocytes [Dzieczkowski & Anderson, 2008]. Patient can develop pure red cell aplasia or develop acute aplastic crisis in patients having hemolytic anemia like sickle cell disease or thalassemia. Infection of a seronegative pregnant mother may result in fetal anemia and/or fetal death.

The prevalence of antibodies to HPV-B19 among blood donors seems to be very low. Currently, blood units are not routinely screened for serologic markers of HPV-B19 infection, and the viral inactivation methods are ineffective against HPV-B19 [Koenigbauer et al., 2000]. Therefore, a very low risk of HPV-B19 transmission through blood transfusion, in particular through the infusion of blood products, may exist. It has also been suggested that high-risk individuals receive anti-HPV-B19 negative blood components in order to prevent/reduce severe complications associated with HPV-B19 infection [Wu et al., 2005; Plentz et al., 2005].

5.4 Epstein-Barr virus (EBV)

Epstein-Barr virus is common in general population. In children, infection is usually asymptomatic, whereas in adults, it often results in mild symptoms like fever and sore throat. EBV is generally associated with Burkitt's lymphoma, nasopharyngeal carcinoma and B-cell lymphoma in immune-compromised patients.

It is transmitted primarily through person to person contact via saliva. It is also transmitted through blood transfusion. Since antibodies to EBV are present in up to 90% of population, it would be impractical to eliminate sero-positive donors by serological screening tests. Leukodepletion remains best option to reduce EBV transmission through blood transfusion [Public Health Agency of Canada, 2003; Sher, 1999].

5.5 Human herpes virus 6 (HHV-6)

HHV-6 is causative agent of 6th disease. It presents in children as persistent fever. It is generally asymptomatic in adults. Significant symptoms appear in immunocompromised individuals. HHV-6 causes persistent infection and there is high prevalence of antibodies among blood donors. Currently donor blood is not routinely screened for HHV-6 serological markers [Sayers, 1994].

5.6 Human herpesvirus 8 (HHV-8)

HHV-8 is now associated with Kaposi's sarcoma in immunocompromised individuals. Though it is transmitted through organ/bone marrow transplantation, there is lack of evidence of its transfusion through blood. Serological screening of blood donors is not recommended [Engels et al., 1999].

5.7 West Nile virus

West Nile Virus (WNV) is a mosquito borne RNA virus of Flavivirus family. It is an important and emerging transfusion transmitted agent in North America. It was first isolated in 1937 from samples obtained in Uganda. It appeared in New York in 1999. This RNA virus can be detected by NAT. In 2002, 4200 cases of WNV were reported to centre for Disease Control and Prevention (CDC) and by 2003, number had risen to 9858. Most of WNV (80%) cases either remain asymptomatic or have only minor flu-like symptoms. In minority of cases (0.6%) patient can have fatal meningitis or encephalitis, especially in immune-compromised/elderly patients. In 2002, 23 cases of transfusion- and four cases of organ-transmitted WNV infection were reported and WNV-specific NAT testing was implemented as routine screening in the USA in 2003. No transfusion transmitted WNV case has been described in Europe [Bihl et al., 2007]. `

5.8 Creutzfeldt-Jakob disease and variant Creutzfeldt-Jakob disease (CJD and VCJD)

Creutzfeldt-Jakob is a form of human transmissible spongiform encephalopathy. It is characterised by mental deterioration, cerebellar dysfunction, involuntary movements and psychiatric disturbances. It occurs at a rate of 1 per million population annually. Transmission of CJD through blood is not established or ruled out.

Variant CJD is human form of bovine spongiform encephalopathy. It is spread through consumption of contaminated meat of infected cattle.

At present screening of blood donors for CJD as well as VCJD is not recommended.

6. Bacterial contamination

With improvement in screening methods for transfusion transmitted viral infections, relative risk for blood transmitted bacterial infections has increased. Approximately 57% of all Transfusion Transmitted infections and 16% of transfusion related deaths have been associated with bacterial contamination. Blood components may be contaminated with bacteria at many stages of preparation, including blood collection, processing, pooling, and transfusion. Bacteria may enter into blood components from many sources: donors' bacteremia, exposure to donor skin bacteria by venipuncture, contaminated bags and infected environment of blood banks or hospitals. The load of bacteria is determined by the storage time. Platelet units that are stored over 3 days and red cell units that are stored over 21 days are strongly associated with an increased risk of bacterial reactions.

Packed RBC's and FFP are stored at cold temperatures, so they are not common sources of bacterial contamination. Some gram negative bacterias like Yersinia, Serratia, Acinetobacter, Pseudomonas, and Escherichia species can grow at temperatures as low as 1- 6° C and can therefore be transmitted through packed red cells [Dzieczkowski et al, 2008].

Platelet concentrates are stored at room temperature and are more likely to contain the skin contaminants including coagulase-negative staphylococci. Both staphylococcus and streptococcus infections can be transmitted through stored platelets. It is estimated that 1 in 1,000-2,000 platelet component is contaminated with bacteria. Risk of death is 1 in 17,000 cases of sepsis associated transfusion with RDP's (random donor platelets) and 1 in 61,000 when transfused platelets by apheresis.

Recipients of blood contaminated with bacteria may develop fever with chills, followed by development of septic shock, DIC and death. Symptoms may develop within minutes of initiation of transfusion or may take several hours. The course may be abrupt, fast and fulminant. When reaction is suspected, transfusion should be immediately stopped. Broad spectrum antibiotics should be stopped. Shock should be treated. Blood bank should be notified. Blood component bag should be sent for Gram staining and culture.

6.1 Syphilis

Syphilis is caused by infection with Treponema pallidum. It is spread primarily through sexual contact. T. Pallidum can also be transmitted by vertical transmission from mother to fetus or through blood if donor is already infected. Its transmission through transmission has become extremely rare after implementation of the serological tests for antibodies to T. Pallidum.

6.2 Rocky mountain spotted fever (RSMF)

It is a severe tick borne disease caused by Rickettsia rickettsii – a bacterium. The disease is endemic in most part of the United States. RMSF is characterized by the sudden onset of moderate to high fever, which normally persists for 2-3 weeks, if untreated. Other typical symptoms include headache, myalgia, and petechial rash, and early RMSF may be confused with meningitis. RMSF is transmitted mainly through the bites of infected ticks. Currently, no specific questions or assays are used for screening and testing of serologic markers of *R. rickettsii* in blood donors.

6.3 Malaria

Malaria is an important parasitic infectious disease worldwide. Malaria is endemic in tropical and sub-tropical regions in Asia and Africa, with up to 300 million infections and one million deaths annually. It is caused by four species of Plasmodium, namely vivax, ovale, malariae and falciparum. P. Falciparum may result in severe complications and/or death. It is spread primarily by bite of the infected female Anopheles mosquito. It can also be transmitted from infected mother to her fetus or from an infected blood donor to the recipient. Patients of chronic hemolytic anemia, as of thalassemia are on regular packed RBC's infusion and are at risk for malaria.

6.4 Chagas disease

The etiological agent is a protozoan parasite – Trypanosoma cruzi. It is endemic in Central and South America and parts of Mexico. Acute infection presents as fever, lymphadenopathy, hepatosplenomegaly, cardiomegaly and mega-esophagus. *T. cruzi* is transmitted from an infected vector to a person through feces deposited on the skin at the time of bite. The agent can also be transmitted vertically from mother to infant and through blood transfusion and organ transplantation.

Donors who were born or have lived in endemic areas for more than 1 year are more likely to be positive for *T. cruzi* antibodies. The majority of patients diagnosed with Transfusion Transmitted Chagas disease in North America have been found to be immunosuppressed.

Screening methods, such as inquiry about travel history and testing for serologic markers, are neither sensitive nor specific enough to effectively identify asymptomatic blood donors. Leukodepletion may reduce the risk of transfusion transmitted Chagas' disease [Leiby, 2000].

7. Toxoplasmosis

Toxoplasmosis is a zoonosis caused by *Toxoplasma gondii*, a parasite that is hosted in cats and dogs and has three forms - trophozoites, cysts and oocysts. About 5 million people are affected worldwide. The infection is usually asymptomatic or causes minor symptoms like fever, malaise and cutaneous rash. It can cause myocarditis and meningo-encephalitis in immunocompromised individuals; and fetal death in a pregnant female. The seroprevalence of antibodies to *T. gondii* increases with age and varies from 8% to 60%.

It has been suggested that people who are at increased risk of toxoplasmosis, such as immunosuppressed individuals and pregnant women, receive *T. gondii* antibody-negative blood components for transfusion. The universal program of leukodepletion that is currently carried out in Canada may reduce the risk of transfusion transmitted toxoplasmosis.

7.1 Leishmaniasis

Leishmaniasis is caused by Leishmania donovani and affects nearly 12 million people in tropical and subtropical areas. Acute infection is often subclinical and chronic infection usually leads to anemia, lymphadenopathy and hepatosplenomegaly. Transmitted usually by infected vector – the sandfly, it can also be transmitted by blood transfusion. Due to global travel of diverse population and costly testing, leishmaniasis is now prevalent in 90 countries. Individuals returning to the US from combat zones in Iraq are currently deferred for blood donation for one year [Bihl et al., 2007].

7.2 Babesiosis

It is a zoonotic disease caused by Babesia microti. Babesia is a genus of protozoal piroplasm. Usually patient is asymptomatic or has mild symptoms like fever and headache. Patient may have severe anemia and hemolytic anemia. The disease is severe in infants, older patients, splenectomized and immunocompromised individuals. Usual transmission is by bite of deer ticks. There is low risk of transmission through blood. Effective screening methods for blood donors are not available.

8. Nematodes – Microfilariasis

Filaria is a disease seen in tropical countries like India in Asia. Microfilariae present in a donor's blood having filaria can be transmitted by blood transfusion. These may circulate in the recipient's blood but do not develop into adult worms. Mortality is not documented after such incidence but it may give rise to morbidity in transfusion recipients in terms of allergic reaction [Choudhary et al., 2003]. Transfusion associated filarial infection can increase morbidity in endemic areas. Blood donors with active history of filarial infection should be deferred from donating blood. Filarial antigen detection test may be employed as a screening test for blood donors.

9. Prevention of transfusion transmitted infections

1. **Transfusion of non-infected blood/blood products**: Etiological agent present in donor's blood can escape detection. Development of antibodies against the etiological organism takes time. So screening tests dependent on antibody detection fail to detect infection in early period. After use of NAT testing, this window period for HIV, Hepatitis B and Hepatitis C is reduced.
2. **Encouraging voluntary blood donation**: In developed countries, the majority of blood donors are voluntary, whereas in developing countries, majority of blood donors are replacement donors. The incidence of blood transmitted infections is much lower in the countries having majority of transfusions from voluntary donation.
3. **Donor deferral**: Current strategies to prevent transfusion transmitted malaria are based on risk group assessment and donor deferral for 4-12 months for visitors from low

endemic areas to high endemic countries and 3-5 years (or permanently) for donors with a history of residence in an endemic area. However, this policy may lead to unaffordable loss of blood donation. That is why the policy of travel based risk assessment is combined with serological screening tests in some countries.

4. **Immunization**: Hepatitis B should be prevented by vaccination. HIV vaccine is being developed. Hepatitis C vaccine is not available at present. More vaccines should be developed to prevent transfusion of transmitted infections.

5. **Prevention of infection of stored blood/blood products**: Storage system in blood bank has to provide infection free environment.

6. **Use of infection free equipment for transfusion**: Use of disposable syringes/needles etc will decrease the risk of transmission of infections.

7. **Education**: HIV transmission can be prevented by increasing awareness, and first AID education of health workers. Unnecessary blood donations should be avoided to decrease the risk factor.

10. References

[1] Bihl F., Castelli D., Marincola F., Dodd R. Y. & Brandes C. Transfusion transmitted infections. *J Transl Med* 2007; 5: 25 Available: http://www.ncbi.nlm.gov/pmc/articles/PMC1904179/ Accessed on 06/07/2011

[2] Biswas R., Tabor E., Hsia C. C., Wright D. J., Laycock M. E., Feibig E. W., Peddada L., Smith R., Schreiber G. B., Epstein J. S., Nemo G. J. & Busch M. P. Comparative sensitivity of HBV NAT and HBsAg assays for detection of acute HBV infection. *Transfusion* 2003; 43: 788-798.

[3] Blajchman M. A., Goldman M., Freedman J.J. & Sher G. D. Proceedings of a consensus conference: prevention of post-transfusion CMV in the era of universal leukoreduction. *Transfus Med Rev* 2001; 15: 1-20.

[4] Blajchman M. A. The clinical benefits of the leukoreduction of blood products. *J Trauma* 2006; 60: S83-90.

[5] Canadian Blood Services (CBS). Nucleic acid testing for HIV May 2001. Available: http://www.bloodservices.Ca/cent Apps. Accessed on 26/08/2011

[6] Choudhary N., Murthy P. K., Chatterjee R. K., Khan M. A. & Ayyagri A. Transmission of filarial infection through blood transfusion. *Ind J Pathol Microbiol* 2003; 46: 367-370.

[7] Dzieczkowski J. S. & Anderson K. C. Transfusion Biology and Therapy In: McGraw Hill: *Harrison's Principles of Internal Medicine* 2008, pp 707-713.

[8] Engels E. A., Eastman H., Ablashi D. V., Wilks R. J., Braham J. & Manns A. Risk of transfusion associated transmission of human herpes virus 8. *J Natl Can Inst* 1999; 20: 1773-1775.

[9] Koenigbauer U. F., Eastlund T. & Day J. W. Clinical illness due to parvovirus B19 infection after infusion of solvent/detergent-treated pooled plasma. *Transfusion* 2000; 40: 1203-1206.

[10] Leiby D. A. Epidemiological aspect of transfusion transmitted babesiosis and chagas' disease. The compendium. 53rd AABB annual meeting. 2000; Washington DC: 209-213.

[11] Moor A. C. E., Dubbelman T. M. A. R., VanStieveninck J. & Brank A. Transfusion transmitted diseases: risks, prevention and perspectives. *Eu J Haematol* 1999; 62: 1-18.

[12] Murphy E. L., Glynn S. A., Fridey J., Smith J. W., Wright D. J., Newman B., Gibble J. W., Ameti D. I., Nass C. C., Schreiber G. B. & Nemo G. J. Increased prevalence of infectious diseases and other adverse outcomes in human T-lymphotropic viruses types I and II- infected blood donors. Retrovirus Epidemiology Donor Study (REDS) Study Group. *J Infect Dis* 1997; 176: 1468-1475.

[13] Murphy E. L., Wang B., Sacher R. A., Fridey J., Smith J. W., Nass C. C., Newman B., Ownby H. E., Garratty G., Hutching S. T. & Schreiber G. B. Respiratory and urinary tract infections, arthritis and asthma associated with HTLV-I and HTLV-II infection. *Emerg Infect Dis* 2004; 10: 109-116.

[14] Pathak S. & Chandrashekhar M. (2010). Nucleic acid testing: Redefining security in blood screening. Available: http://www.maxhealthcare.in/max-medical-journal/september2010/nuclearacid_testing.html Accessed on 20/08/2011

[15] Plentz A., Hahn J., Knoll A., Holler E., Jilg W. & Modrow S. Exposure of hematologic patients to Parvovirus B19 as a contaminant of blood cell preparations and blood products. *Transfusion* 2005; 45: 1811–1815.

[16] Public Health Agency of Canada. Transfusion transmitted diseases/infections. Modified on 2003-05-12. Available: www.phac-aspc.gc.ca/hcai-iamss Accessed on 15/06/2011

[17] Sayers M. H. Transfusion transmitted viral infections other than hepatitis and human deficiency virus infection. Cytomegalovirus, Epstein-Barr virus, human herpes virus 6 and human parvovirus B 19. *Arch Pathol Lab Med* 1994; 118: 346-349.

[18] Sher G. D. Leukoreduction of the blood supply. May 1999 Available: http://www.bloodservices.ca/CentreApps/Internet/UW_V502_MainEngine.nsf/r esources/Leukoreduciton/$file/leuko_position_paper.pdf Accessed on 26/08/2011

[19] Singh B. Nucleic acid testing (NAT) screening of blood donors in India: a project report, *International Hospital Federation reference book* 2008/2009, pp 66-67.

[20] Transfusion transmitted diseases. – *Blood Book, Blood information for life.* Available: www.bloodbook.com/trans-tran.html Accessed on 20/08/2011

[21] Vamvakas E. C. Is white blood cell reduction equivalent to antibody screening in preventing transmission of cytomegalovirus by transfusion? A review of literature and meta-analysis. *Transfus Med Rev* 2005; 19: 181-199.

[22] Wiedemann M., Kluwick S., Walter M., Fauchald G., Howe J., Bronold M. & Zauke M. HIV-I, HCV and HBV window reduction by the new Roche Cobos (R) Taqscreen MPX test in (sero-converting donors). *J Clin Vir* 2007; 39: 282–287.

[23] Wu C. G., Mason B., Jong J., Erdman D., McKernan L., Oakley M., Soucie M., Evatt B. & Yu M. Y. Parvovirus B19 transmission by a high-purity factor VIII concentrate. *Transfusion* 2005; 45: 1003–1010.

10

Human T-Lymphotropic Viruses (HTLV)

Marina Lobato Martins[1,3], Rafaela Gomes Andrade[2,3],
Bernardo Hinkelmann Nédir[2,3] and Edel Figueiredo Barbosa-Stancioli[2,3]
[1]Gerência de Desenvolvimento Técnico Científico,
Centro de Hematologia e Hemoterapia de Minas Gerais (Fundação HEMOMINAS),
[2]Laboratório de Virologia Básica e Aplicada,
Departamento de Microbiologia,
Universidade Federal de Minas Gerais,
[3]Interdisciplinary HTLV Research Group (GIPH)
Brazil

1. Introduction

1.1 HTLV epidemiology

The Human T-lymphotropic viruses (HTLV) belong to *Retroviridae* family, genus *Deltaretrovirus*. Currently they are classified into four types: 1, 2, 3 and 4. The HTLV-1 was described in 1980 (Poiez et al., 1980) and since then has been identified on all five continents, with an estimated of 15 to 20 million infected people (Gessain, 1996). The areas are characterized as endemic, where the prevalence ranging from 0.5 to 20% in the population, depending on age and gender, or not endemic, where the prevalence is less than 0.1%. The seroprevalence rates increase with age and are higher in females than males.

Areas of great prevalence for HTLV-1 include Japan, Sub-Saharan Africa, Caribbean basin, South America, Melanesia and the Middle East. The HTLV-2 was described in 1982 (Kalyanaraman et al., 1982) and it is endemic in African and Ameridian populations, but its worldwide distribution has been ascribed to transmission among intravenous drug users. HTLV-3 and 4 were discovered in a rural area of southern Cameroon (Mahieux & Gessain, 2011; Wolfe et al., 2005) and, at present, they are restricted to that region.

HTLV-1 and 2 are transmitted sexually and vertically, firstly by breastfeeding, as well as parenterally, by contaminated blood transfusion, sharing of contaminated needles and syringes, or transplantation of infected organs and tissues. The level of HTLV-1 proviral load and anti-HTLV-1/2 antibodies are important to sexual or vertical virus transmission, besides the period of exposure to risk factors (sexual intercourse or breastfeeding). In endemic areas for HTLV-1, approximately 25% of infants breastfed by HTLV-1 seropositive mothers acquire the infection. Because of HTLV-1/2 transmission by blood transfusion, different countries have introduced at different times screening for the viruses in blood banks, some of them across the country and others only in endemic areas. The efficiency of HTLV-1 transmission by blood transfusion may depends of type and time stock of the blood component, besides the proviral load of the blood donor, since the transmission is dependent of the presence of infected cells. Lookback studies have shown different rates of seroconversion in patients who have received HTLV-1 infected blood, which is higher in areas with high prevalence than those with low prevalence (Namen-Lopes et al., 2009; Sullivan et al., 1991). Thus, HTLV-1/2 screening of blood units is important to prevents the most cases of transfusion transmitted infection, but the relatively long HTLV immunological window period (51 days) may lead to its transmission (Manns et al., 1992), been necessary stablish haemovigilance actions in blood banks.

2. HTLV-1 genome

HTLV has a particle of 110 to 140nm in diameter with a lipoprotein envelope presenting surface and transmembrane proteins, important in the diagnosis of infection. Inside the capsid is found the viral genome, constituted by two copies of single-stranded RNA, besides viral proteins, such as reverse transcriptase and integrase, essential in the process of transcription of viral RNA into complementary DNA and integration of proviral DNA in the host cell genome (Cann & Chen, 1996).

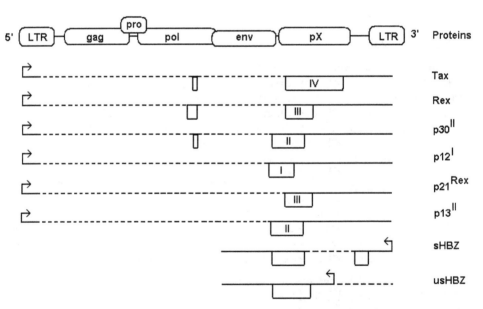

Fig. 1. HTLV-1 genomic regions, virus mRNAs and proteins. HTLV-1 encodes three classes of mRNAs from 5'-LTR: unspliced mRNA coding for gag proteins (p24, p15 and p19) and polymerases proteins (reverse transcriptase, integrase and protease); single-spliced mRNAs coding for envelope proteins (gp46 and p21), $p12^I$, $p21^{Rex}$, $p13^{II}$; and doble-spliced mRNAs coding for Tax, Rex and $p30^{II}$. In addition, two isoforms of HBZ, spliced and unspliced, are encoded from the 3'-LTR on the complementary strand of the genome.

The HTLV genome is characterized by regions called gag, pol and env, flanked by two long repeated terminations (LTRs) located at the end 5' and 3' containing viral promoters and other regulatory elements. The gag region is initially translated as a polyprotein precursor, and subsequent cleavage gives rise to mature gag proteins: the matrix protein of 19 kDa (p19), capsid protein of 24 kDa (p24) and nucleocapsid protein of 15 kDa (p15). The protease is encoded by the nucleotide sequence comprising part of the 3' gag region and part of the 5' region of pol. Thus, the synthesis of the protease is done as part of the gag polyprotein precursor accompanied by frameshift reading. The protease is responsible for processing the gag mature products and its own cleavage to generate the mature protease molecule. The pol region encodes for two proteins, the reverse transcriptase and the integrase. The env region encodes for the viral envelope proteins. The envelope precursor protein is cleaved to give mature products, the surface glycoprotein of 46 kDa (gp46) and transmembrane protein of 21 kDa (p21) (Cann & Chen, 1996). Other region, called pX, is responsible for encoding viral regulatory and acessory proteins, related to the persistence of virus infection and pathogenesis. Four ORFs (open reading frames) had been described in pX, whose alternative splices results in sequences encoding for different proteins: p40tax, p27rex and p21rex, p12, p13 and p30 (Franchini G & Streicher, 1995). HTLV-1 also shows transcriptional activity from the negative strand, through the 3' LTR, encoding a protein known as HTLV-1 basic leucine zipper factor (HBZ) (Gaudray et al, 2002). The regulatory and acessory HTLV-1 proteins have different roles in establish a persistent virus infection and to induce HTLV-1 associated diseases.

3. HTLV-1 life cycle

HTLV-1 establishes a chronic infection, usually with a long period between infection and first symptoms of the diseases associated with the virus. The principal tropism is for CD4+ T cells, but also can infect other cell types such as CD8+ T cells, dendritic cells, macrophages, nerve cells, and hematologic stem cells. The life cycle (Figure 2) is characterized by the following phases (Cann & Chen, 1996):

1. Binding of gp21/gp46 virus proteins to surface receptor on the cell membrane;
2. Fusion with membrane and penetration of viral capsid into the cell;
3. Reverse transcription of viral RNA genome into DNA by reverse transcriptase, inside the capsid;
4. Entry of viral DNA in the nucleus and its integration into the host genome, forming the provirus;
5. Synthesis of viral RNA by cellular machinery, having as template the proviral DNA, and splicing of transcripts for the formation of viral mRNAs;
6. Synthesis of viral proteins;
7. Assembly and budding of virions;
8. Proteolytic processing of capsid proteins, finally obtaining mature viral particle that is ready to infect new cells.

It is considered that during primary infection, the virus has a period of active replication by reverse transcriptase, but that the subsequent proliferation occurs mainly via clonal expansion of infected cells, or by viral sinapse, which transmit viral genome through infected cell-to-uninfected cell contact (Igakura et al., 2003). Therefore, HTLV displays low levels of intra-individual genetic variation, unlike other retroviruses.

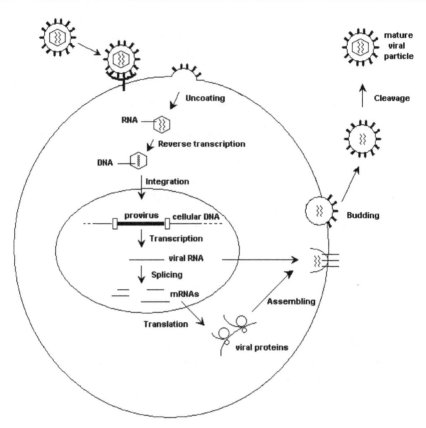

Fig. 2. HTLV life cycle. The HTLV life cycle has the following events: (1) interaction of viral envelope proteins with HTLV receptors; (2) viral particle fusion with cell membrane and uncoating of viral core; (3) reverse transcription of viral positive strand RNA into DNA; (4) integration of proviral DNA into host cellular DNA; (5) provirus transcription and splicing for formation of mRNAs; (6) translation of viral proteins; (7) virion assembly and budding of immature virions from the cellular membrane and (8) maturation of viral particle.

4. Pathological aspects of HTLV-1 infection

Human T-cell lymphotropic virus 1 is associated with distinct clinical entities including adult T-cell leukemia (ATL) and HTLV-1 associated myelopathy/tropical spastic paraparesis (HAM/TSP). Other inflammatory diseases such as uveitis, polymyositis, arthritis and alveolitis, as well as infective dermatitis and some types of skin lesions, are also associated with HTLV-1. HTLV-2 is not clearly associated with disease, but it has been associated with increased susceptibility to bacterial infections, with significant impact on the morbidity of carriers. Approximately 95% of HTLV-1 carriers remain asymptomatic throughout life, whereas about 5% develop diseases associated with the virus. The pathogenic potential of HTLV-1 requires that the virus diagnosis be accurate to define the virus type and to allow counsel of HTLV-1/2 carriers.

4.1 ATL

HTLV-1 is able to transform cells due to ability of the viral regulatory proteins to down or up-regulate the expression of cellular genes involved in cellular proliferation and DNA repair. Tax is the major viral protein that is able to interfere in different levels, acting in the up-regulation and down-regulation of transcription factors and inhibiting the activity of cell cycle regulators and tumor suppressor proteins.

According ATL pathogenesis model, only a certain level of Tax is transiently expressed in a limited population of infected cells at a time, and in other cell populations at different times, in order to maintain a low level of this protein during viral infection. During transient expression of Tax in a given population, regardless of the immune response and destruction of some of these cells, a cell expansion can be efficiently enhanced by the multiple mechanisms of action of the Tax protein: stimulation of several genes involved in cell proliferation, induction of cell cycle phases G1 to S and S2 to M, inducing accumulation of mutations and genetic abnormalities, by attenuation of the control points of the cell cycle, DNA repair system and apoptosis. This situation would happen repeatedly over a long period in the carrier, with expansion of clones of infected cells. Finally, the clonal expansion of cell population with damaged DNA, and accumulation of new mutations by Tax activity, could lead to a process of malignant transformation of a cell clone with monoclonal expansion of the malignant clone and the onset of ATL (Yoshida, 2001 and 2010). Thus, the pleiotropic effects of Tax lead to the promotion of cell proliferation, accumulation of damaged DNA and inhibition of apoptosis of abnormal cells, thus contributing to the transformation of infected cells. Despite of all the effects of Tax protein in expanding the population of infected cells, Tax expression is detected at low levels in the carriers. This seems to be due to its immunogenicity, so that if Tax expression was continuous, the infected cell would become an easy target for the host immune response. The low expression of Tax in infected cells must be controlled by viral proteins that function as negative regulators of Tax expression, being important to evasion of immune surveillance.

Recently, HBZ has taken prominence in the pathogenesis of ATL because its negative effect on the Tax expression. It was found that HBZ is constitutively expressed in ATL cells and asymptomatic carriers, and acts as a transcriptional factor that represses the expression of viral proteins encoded by the positive strand, including Tax protein. Transcripts of tax are detected in approximately 30 to 40% of ATL patients, whereas HBZ mRNA has been detected in all studied cases of ATL. HBZ antagonizes the activation of viral transcription induced by Tax, but also promotes cell proliferation, and HBZ expression has been correlated with levels of proviral load (Satou et al., 2006). It has been suggested that HBZ, along with Rex and p30, suppresses the function of Tax, protecting infected cells from attack by cytotoxic T lymphocytes, thus contributing to the persistence of mutated cells clones that can continuously advance toward the phenotype of tumor cells. In this model, Tax would be important in the early stages of infection, promoting cell growth, infection from cell to cell and genetic instability of infected cells. Later, the expression of Tax cease to escape from immune surveillance. Thus, HBZ appears to has a critical role in oncogenesis triggered by HTLV-1 (Matsuoka & Green, 2009; Yoshida, 2010).

In addition to viral proteins, host factors also play a role in determining the outcome of HTLV, such has been demonstrated by the identification of gene polymorphisms that confer susceptibility or protection to ATL, or other diseases associated with HTLV-1.

4.2 HAM/TSP

HAM/TSP (HTLV-1 associated myelopathy/tropical spastic paraparesis) is an inflammatory neurodegenerative disease of a progressive feature, leading to the motor and sensory disturbance. It is characterized by atrophy of the thoracic spinal cord involving perivascular demyelination and axonal degeneration, inflammatory response in the affected region and an infiltrate of mononuclear cells, with destruction of nerve fibers in inflammatory foci leading to loss of sensory-motor ability (Izumo et al., 2000).

The main neurological features of HAM/TSP according to the WHO (World Health Organization, 1989) are: chronic spastic paraparesis that usually progresses slowly, or sometimes remains unchanged after initial progression; weakness in the lower limbs; bladder disorder that occurs earlier and constipation observed later; sexual impotence and decreased of libido; paresthesia, backache, hyperreflexia of lower limbs, often with clonus and Babinski signal; hyperreflexia of upper limbs and signals of Hoffmann and Trömner. HAM/TSP affects, in the most cases, individuals between 35-50 years old, with a predominance of females over males (2-3 times).

The low incidence of HAM/TSP (2-3%) in HTLV-1 carriers suggests that virus-host interactions have a role in the pathogenesis of inflammatory disease. High proviral load (number of infected lymphocytes), high titers of anti-HTLV-1 antibodies in serum and cerebrospinal fluid and high levels of proinflammatory cytokines and chemokines are characteristic of patients with HAM/TSP, compared with that observed in asymptomatic carriers, suggesting that an enhanced immune response to HTLV-1 is developed in the patients (Jacobson et al., 1988; Parker et al., 1992; Yamano et al., 2002). HTLV-1 is able to cross the blood-brain barrier by migration of infected lymphocytes and, as in peripheral blood, the proliferation of infected cells within the CSF is confronted by an intense anti-HTLV-1 cellular immune response in HAM/TSP patients (Cavrois et al., 2000).

Tax appears to be the main viral antigen, triggering a cytotoxic T lymphocytes (CTL) response. It has been suggested that the efficiency of the anti-HTLV-1 CTL response is an important determinant of HAM/TSP pathogenesis, and could explain why some HTLV-1 carriers develop a high proviral load and diseases such as HAM/TSP, whereas others remain asymptomatic. It was reported that the frequency of lysis of infected cells by CTL response were significantly associated with HAM/TSP, as well as the level os Tax expression, and both are predictors of proviral load (Asquith et al., 2005). The pathogenesis of neurological disease may be related to the ability of the infected cells in cross the blood brain barrier and to invade the central nervous system (CNS), inducing a local chronic inflammatory response promoted by anti-Tax CD8+ CTL activity, leading to high levels of proinflammatory cytokines. Thus, when the CTL response is ineffective in controlling proviral load in the CNS, an exaggerated proinflammatory state may be continuously maintained, causing the kill of the glial cells and myelopathy – the bystander damage. On the other hand, individuals presenting efficient HTLV-1-specific CD8+ cells to lyse infected cells, would eliminate high rate of infected cells, mantaining the proviral load in low level. This lytic efficiency may be related to HLA class I binding affinity to viral peptides, avidity to antigens and expression of cytolytic genes (Jeffery et al., 1999; Kattan et al., 2009; MacNamara et al., 2010; Vine et al., 2004).

Other two hypothesis for HAM/TSP pathogenesis has been described: (1) the direct damage mechanism, which assumes that HTLV-1 infects cells residing in the central nervous system, such as astrocytes, neurons and oligodendrocytes. Infection of resident brain cells may suffer direct immune attack and excitotoxicity of neurons leading to their death; (2) the molecular mimicry, that considers that Tax cross-react with autoantigens in neurons leading to a state of autoimmunity. Neuronal proteins, such as nuclear riboproteins hnRNPA1 and hnRNP-A1B, show cross-reactivity with anti-Tax. In this mechanism, infiltrating CD8+ cytotoxic T cells or antibody-producing B cells specific for Tax may recognize self antigens, causing an autoimmune response and the incidental destruction of neurons.

Recently, it has been suggested that HBZ protein also has an important role in HAM/TSP development. At the same way as for Tax, HBZ-specific CD8+ T cell response appears to be important to maintain low proviral load and asymptomatic status of carriers (Hilburn et al., 2011).

5. HTLV-2: Biological characteristics, pathogenesis and epidemiology

Human T-lymphotropic virus 2 (HTLV-2) is endemic in some African populations and in Amerindians tribes from North, Central and South America, especially in Brazil, where some tribes show prevalence of 30% (Black et al., 1996; Duenas-Barajas et al., 1992; Hjelle et al., 1993; Lairmore et al., 1990; Shindo et al., 2002). HTLV-2 is also present among intravenous drug users (IDU), mainly in the United States and in Europe (De La Fuente et al., 2006; Murphy et al., 1999). HTLV-2 shares similar epidemiological determinants with HTLV-1: presence of populational clusters with high prevalence, higher prevalence in women, increase prevalence rate with age, and the same pathways of transmission.

HTLV-2 is not known to have a precise pathologic role. It is not associated with any malignancies, but only with rare cases of subacute myelopathy like HAM/TSP, that have a more slowly progression (Araujo & Hall, 2004). However, HTLV-2 appears to be associated with an increased incidence of pneumonia, asthma and bronchitis, bladder and kidney infection, inflammatory conditions, such as arthritis, and with increased mortality, being suggested that HTLV-2 may inhibit immunologic responses to respiratory infections and induce inflammatory or autoimmune reactions (Roucoux & Murphy, 2004). In addition, increased incidence of sensory neuropathy has been reported in IDU infected with HTLV-2 (Dooneief et al., 1996). This association was more pronounced in patients co-infected with HIV-1, whose risk of developing peripheral neuropathy was shown to be three times higher compared with patients infected only with HIV-1 (Zehender et al., 2002). In summary, HTLV-2 has been considered less pathogenic than HTLV-1. However, studies presented around the world have been shown occurrence of illness in individuals infected only with HTLV-2 as well as co-infected with other agents, such as HTLV-1, HIV-1, HBV, HCV, *Mycobacterium sp.* These data confirm the importance of diagnosis, monitoring and counseling for HTLV-2.

6. HTLV-1/2 diagnosis

Laboratory testing for HTLV-1 and HTLV-2 infections has become routine for blood transfusion and organ transplantation in many countries worldwide. The serological tests for anti-HTLV-1/2 antibodies are divided in two major groups: the screening serological assays and the confirmatory tests. Some antibodies that recognize HTLV-1 antigens can either recognize those from HTLV-2, and the serological screening tests are not accurate to distinguish the both viruses' infections. Thus, confirmatory tests must diferentiate between HTLV-1 and HTLV-2.

The most used tests for the diagnosis of HTLV-1/2 are enzyme immunoassays (ELISA), indirect Immunofluorescence (IFA), Western blot (WB) and polymerase chain reaction (PCR) assays. The first one is a screening assay and the others are considered confirmatory tests. However, commercial HTLV-1/2 IFA or PCR assays are not available. "In-house" tests have been developed and used elsewhere, but this requires carefully optimization with several clinical samples to establish good patterns of sensitivity and specificity.

The HTLV serological window period is not clearly known. The period of seroconvertion is related to the route of transmission and with the level of infected cells received in this event. The virus transmission through blood transfusion is considered the most efficient route and the seroconvertion of the recipients is around two months (Manns et al., 1992), while for the other routes of transmission the seroconvertion can reach six months or more. There are no reports of infected individuals who had viral clearance.

For serological diagnosis of HTLV-1/2 is recommended one or two concomitant enzyme immunoassays with different formats and antigen composition followed by a confirmatory test in case of sample be reactive. The results of ELISA test can be: reactive, non-reactive or indeterminate (absorbance value around to cut-off). The sample is usually tested in triplicate, and if two or three replicates are reactive, a new blood collection shoul be realize and the new sample tested by ELISA. The reactivity in two or three replicates implicates in the use of a confirmatory test, such as Western Blot.

Western blot is a confirmatory assay used to test samples that were repeatedly reactives in screening tests. Commercial tests normally use as antigens viral lysate of HTLV-1, besides HTLV-1 and HTLV-2 recombinant envelope proteins. The sample will be considered seronegative if no reactivity to viral antigens is observed; indeterminate if are specific reactivity for HTLV antigens but do not fulfill the criterion of seropositivity; and seropositive if presents reactivity to all antigens defined by the manufacturer as positive pattern. Depending on the reactivity profile, WB may be not able to define the diagnosis for HTLV-1 or HTLV-2.

The high proportion of indeterminate results in the screening tests for HTLV infection has been a challenge worldwide and has been an important problem faced by blood banks. The improvement in the diagnosis for HTLV has been necessary to reduce inconclusive results and to avoid unnecessary follow-up to define the status of infection (Martins et al., 2010; Costa et al., 2011). In endemic areas, indeterminate WB results can range from 0.02% to 50%. The causes of indeterminate WB tests and what is the medical importance of this status is still not clear. Molecular tests can be useful to solve the majority of these inconclusive cases, as well as to discriminate between HTLV-1 or HTLV-2 infection (Waters et al., 2011).

The techniques of molecular biology for confirmatory diagnosis of HTLV-1/2 are based primarily on the detection of viral nucleic acid in the form of proviral DNA by PCR (polymerase chain reaction). Many protocols for HTLV diagnosis by PCR has been developed in-house, with no commercial tests yet licensed. PCR for HTLV-1 and 2 has been particularly useful for: investigation of neonatal transmission, since the serological tests in infants can detect maternal antibodies (Ribeiro et al., 2010); discrimination between infection by type 1 or type 2 virus; definition of dual infection (HTLV-1 and HTLV-2); definition of virus subtypes; diagnostic in subjects with suspected of seroconversion; and resolution of cases with seroindeterminate results (Andrade et al., 2010, Costa et al., 2011; Waters et al., 2011). Since HTLV not presents large quantities of viral RNA circulating, the use of plasma or serum is not suitable for HTLV molecular diagnosis. Considering the HTLV tropism for lymphocytes, the biological sample of choice for the molecular diagnosis of infection is the blood. However, different biological samples containing potentially infected cells may be used for virus identification, in case of specific research studies. Currently, real-time PCR has been preferentially employed over conventional PCR because of its very higher sensitivity and specificity, low contamination risk, easeness of performance and rapidity in obtaining results, showing be viable to substitute confirmatory serological test for HTLV-1/2 diagnosis (Andrade et al., 2010, Costa et al., 2011; Waters et al., 2011).

In addition of molecular tests for detection of the viral genome, molecular tests are also used to quantify the level of HTLV infectivity, or proviral load. HTLV-1 proviral load is an important risk marker for the development of diseases associated with HTLV-1. Unlike HIV, where the quantification of the burden of infection is given by the number of viral particles (quantification of viral RNA copies per mL of plasma), the load for HTLV is quantified by the number of copies of proviral DNA present in a cellular population, that mean, the measure of the number of infected cells, because there is little free HTLV-1 particle in plasma. The proviral load of HTLV-1 in peripheral blood is typically high compared with infection by other retroviruses, and although the numbers vary widely among infected individuals, the mean of proviral load in healthy carriers is significantly lower than that observed in symptomatic patients (Kamihira et al., 2003; Nagai et al., 1998; Ono et al, 1995; Yakova et al., 2005).

7. Counseling HTLV-1/2 seropositive carriers

The counseling to HTLV-1/2 seropositive carriers aims to clarify aspects of infection and diseases associated with the virus, to provide guidance about virus transmission pathways and treatment, besides assess the need for emotional support. It is also necessary to clarify the significance of the serological results, mainly if the individual has not been tested by a confirmatory assay or if the result has been seroindeterminate. HTLV-1/2 seroindeterminate individuals are difficult to counseling because their status as infected or not is not defined. These individuals should be informed that the result is not defined, since false-reactive results may occur, requiring additional tests (such as molecular tests) or serological monitoring to define possible seroconvertion.

Upon diagnosis of HTLV infection, it is initially recommended that the carrier be informed about the differences between HTLV and HIV, emphasizing the fact that most individuals infected with HTLV will not develop diseases, remaining asymptomatic lifelong. However, the carrier must be advised that he/she is able of transmitting the virus, and what the ways to prevent the viral transmission: to not donate blood, organs, breast milk or sperm; to not make use of shared needles, syringes or other cutting objects; to discuss with his/her partner(s) sexual about risk of virus transmission by sexual intercourse and measures to prevent it, such as condom use; to prefer cesarean delivery; and to avoid breastfeeding by

HTLV positive mother, ensuring the nutrition of infants through natural milk from breast milk banks or artificial feeding.

It is also recommended for HTLV carriers testing for other pathogens that share the same transmission pathways, such as hepatitis B, hepatitis C and HIV. Sexual partners should be tested for HTLV, as well as all children of HTLV seropositive mothers.

In summary, counseling of infected individual is an arduous task that should involves a mutidisciplinar team, able to properly inform the carrier, take your questions and avoid hopeless attitude.

8. Acknowledgment

ML Martins and BH Nédir received fellowships from FAPEMIG, RG Andrade from CAPES, and EF Barbosa-Stancioli from CNPq. The studies developed by GIPH have received financial support from FAPEMIG, CNPq and Pro-Reitoria de Pesquisa da UFMG (PRPq).

9. References

Andrade, RG, Ribeiro, MA, Namen-Lopes, MS, Silva, SM, Basques, FV, Ribas, JG, Carneiro-Proietti, AB, Martins, ML. (2010) Evaluation of the use of real-time PCR for human T cell lymphotropic virus 1 and 2 as a confirmatory test in screening for blood donors. *Revista da Sociedade Brasileira de Medicina Tropical*, 43, pp. 111-115.

Araujo, A, Hall, WW. (2004) Human T-lymphotropic virus type II and neurological disease. *Annals of Neurology*, 56, pp. 10–19.

Asquith, B, Mosley, AJ, Heaps, A, Tanaka, Y, Taylor, GP, McLean, AR, Bangham, CR. (2005) Quantification of the virus-host interaction in human T lymphotropic virus I infection. *Retrovirology*, 2, pp. 75.

Black, FL, Biggar, RJ, Lal, RB, Gabbai, AA, Filho, JP. (1996) Twenty-five years of HTLV type II follow-up with a possible case of tropical spastic paraparesis in the Kayapo, a Brazilian Indian tribe. *AIDS Research and Human Retroviruses*, 12, pp. 1623-1627.

Cann, AJ, Chen, ISY. (1996) Human T-cell leukemia virus types I and II, In: *Fields Virology 3rd edition*, Fields, BN, Knipe, DM, Howley PM et al., pp. 1849-1879. Raven Publishers, Philadelphia.

Cavrois, M, Gessain, A, Gout, O, Wain-Hobson, S, Wattel, E. (2000) Common human T cell leukemia virus type 1 (HTLV-1) integration sites in cerebrospinal fluid and blood lymphocytes of patients with HTLV-1-associated myelopathy/tropical spastic paraparesis indicate that HTLV-1 crosses the blood-brain barrier via clonal HTLV-1-infected cells. *The Journal of Infectious Diseases*, 182, pp. 1044-1050.

Costa, EA, Magri, MC, Caterino-de-Araujo, A. (2011) The best algorithm to confirm the diagnosis of HTLV-1 and HTLV-2 in at-risk individuals from São Paulo, Brazil. *Journal of Virology Methods*, 173, pp. 280-286.

Couroucé, AM, Pillonel, J, Lemarie, JM, Saura, C. (1998) HTLV testing in blood transfusion. *Vox Sanguinis*, 74, Suppl 2, pp. 165-169.

De la Fuente, L, Toro, C, Soriano, V, Brugal, MT, Vallejo, F, Barrio, G, Jiménez, V, Silva, T, Project Itínere Working Group. (2006) HTLV infection among young injection and non-injection heroin users in Spain: prevalence and correlates. *Journal of Clinical Virology*, 35, pp. 244-249.

Dooneief, G, Marlink, R, Bell, K, Marder, K, Renjifo, B, Stern, Y, Mayeux, R. (1996) Neurologic consequences of HTLV-II infection in injection-drug users. *Neurology*, 46, pp. 1556-1560.

Dueñas-Barajas, E, Bernal, JE, Vaught, DR, Briceño, I, Durán, C, Yanagihara, R, Gajdusek, DC. (1992) Coexistence of human T-lymphotropic virus types I and II among the Wayuu Indians from the Guajira Region of Colombia. *AIDS Research and Human Retroviruses*, 8, pp. 1851-1855.

Franchini, G, Streicher, H. (1995) Human T-cell leukemia virus. *Baillières Clinical Haematology*, 8, pp. 131-148.

Gaudray, G, Gachon, F, Basbous, J, Biard-Piechaczyk, M, Devaux, C, Mesnard, JM. (2002) The complementary strand of the human T-cell leukemia virus type 1 RNA genome encodes a bZIP transcription factor that down-regulates viral transcription. *Journal of Virology*, 76, pp. 12813-12822.

Gessain, A. (1996) Epidemiology of HTLV-I and associated diseases, In: *Human T-cell lymphotropic virus I*, Hollsberg P. & Hafler DA, pp. 34-64. John Wiley and Sons, New York.

Hilburn, S, Rowan, A, Demontis, MA, Macnamara, A, Asquith, B, Bangham, CR, Taylor, GP. (2011) In vivo expression of human T-lymphotropic virus type 1 Basic Leucine-Zipper protein generates specific CD8+ and CD4+ T-lymphocyte responses that correlate with clinical outcome. *Journal of Infection Disease*, 203, pp. 529-236.

Hjelle, B, Zhu, SW, Takahashi, H, Ijichi, S, Hall, WW. (1993) Endemic human T cell leukemia virus type II infection in southwestern US Indians involves two prototype variants of virus. *Journal of Infectious Diseases*, 168, pp. 737-740.

Igakura, T, Stinchcombe, JC, Goon, PK, Taylor, GP, Weber, JN, Griffiths, GM, Tanaka, Y, Osame, M, Bangham, CR. (2003) Spread of HTLV-I between lymphocytes by virus-induced polarization of the cytoskeleton. *Science*, 299, pp. 1713-1716.

Izumo, S, Umehara, F, Osame, M. (2000) HTLV-I-associated myelopathy. *Neuropathology*, 20, Suppl. S65-68.

Jacobson, S, Zaninovic, V, Mora, C, Rodgers-Johnson, P, Sheremata, WA, Gibbs, CJJr, Gajdusek, C, McFarlin, DE. (1988) Immunological findings in neurological diseases associated with antibodies to HTLV-I: activated lymphocytes in tropical spastic paraparesis. *Annals of Neurology*, 23, Suppl. S196-200.

Jeffery, KJ, Usuku, K, Hall, SE, Matsumoto, W, Taylor, GP, Procter, J, Bunce, M, Ogg, GS, Welsh, KI, Weber, JN, Lloyd, AL,

Kalyanaraman, VS, Sarngadharan, MG, Robert-Guroff, M. (1982) A new subtype of human T-cell leukemia virus (HTLV-II) associated with a T-cell variant of hairy cell leukemia. *Science*, 218, pp. 571-573.

Kamihira, S, Dateki, N, Sugahara, K, Hayashi, T, Harasawa, H, Minami, S, Hirakata, Y, Yamada, Y. (2003) Significance of HTLV-1 proviral load quantification by real time PCR as a surrogate marker for HTLV-1-infected cell count. *Clinical and Laboratory Haematology*, 25, pp. 111-117.

Kattan, T, MacNamara, A, Rowan, AG, Nose, H, Mosley, AJ, Tanaka, Y, Taylor, GP, Asquith, B, Bangham, CR. (2009) The avidity and lytic efficiency of the CTL response to HTLV-1. *Journal of Immunology*, 182, pp. 5723-5729.

Lairmore, MD, Jacobson, S, Gracia, F, De, BK, Castillo, L, Larreategui, M, Roberts, BD, Levine, PH, Blattner, WA, Kaplan, JE. (1990) Isolation of human T-cell lymphotropic virus type 2 from Guaymi Indians in Panama. *Proceedings of National Academy of Sciences U S A*, 87, pp. 8840-844.

MacNamara, A, Rowan, A, Hilburn, S, Kadolsky, U, Fujiwara, H, Suemori, K, Yasukawa, M, Taylor, G, Bangham, CR, Asquith, B. (2010) HLA class I binding of HBZ determines outcome in HTLV-1 infection. *PLoS Pathogens*, 6, pp. e1001117.

Mahieux, R, Gessain, A. (2011) HTLV-3/STLV-3 and HTLV-4 Viruses: Discovery, Epidemiology, Serology and Molecular Aspects. *Viruses*, 3, pp. 1074-1090.

Manns, A, Wilks, R, Murphy, EL, Haynes, G, Figueroa, P, Barnett, M, Hanchard, B, Blattner, WA. (1992). A prospective study of transmission by transfusion of HTLV-I and risk factors associated with seroconversion. *International Journal of Cancer*, 51, pp. 886–891.

Martins, ML, Santos, AC, Namen-Lopes, MS, Barbosa-Stancioli, EF, Utsch, DG, Carneiro-Proietti, AB. (2010) Long-term serological follow-up of blood donors with an HTLV-indeterminate western blot: antibody profile of seroconverters and individuals with false reactions. *Journal of Medicine Virology*, 82, pp. 1746-1753.

Matsuoka, M, Green, PL. (2009) The HBZ gene, a key player in HTLV-I pathogenesis. *Retrovirology*, 6, pp. 7.

Murphy, EL, Glynn, SA, Fridey, J, Smith, JW, Sacher, RA, Nass, CC, Ownby, HE, Wright, DJ, Nemo GJ. (1999) Increased incidence of infectious diseases during prospective follow-up of Human T-Lymphotropic Virus Type II– and I– infected blood donors. *Archives of International Medicine*, 159, pp. 1485-1491.

Nagai M, Usuku K, Matsumoto W, Kodama D, Takenouchi N, Moritoyo T, Hashiguchi S, Ichinose M, Bangham CR, Izumo S, Osame M. (1998) Analysis of HTLV-I proviral load in 202 HAM/TSP patients and 243 asymptomatic HTLV-I carriers: high proviral load strongly predisposes to HAM/TSP. *Journal of Neurovirology*, 4, pp. 586-593.

Namen-Lopes, MSS, Martins, M L, Drummond, PC, Lobato, RR, Interdisciplinary HTLV Research Group (GIPH), Carneiro-Proietti, ABF. (2009) Lookback study of HTLV-1 and 2 seropositive donors and their recipients in Belo Horizonte, Brazil. *Transfusion Medicine*, 19, pp. 180-188.

Ono, A, Mochizuki, M, Yamaguchi, K, Miyata, N, Watanabe, T. (1995) Increased number of circulating HTLV-1 infected cells in peripheral blood mononuclear cells of HTLV-1 uveitis patients: a quantitative polymerase chain reaction study. *British Journal of Ophthalmology*, 79, pp. 270-276.

Parker, CE, Daenke, S, Nightingale, S, Bangham, CR. (1992) Activated, HTLV-1-specific cytotoxic T-lymphocytes are found in healthy seropositives as well as in patients with tropical spastic paraparesis. *Virology*, 188, pp. 628-636.

Poiez, BJ, Ruscetti, FW, Gazdar, AF, Bunn, PA, Minna, JD, Gallo, RC. (1980) Detection and isolation of type C retrovirus particles from fresh and cultured lymphocytes of a patient with cutaneous T-cell lymphoma. *Proceedings of National Academy of Sciences U S A*, 77, pp. 7415-7419.

Ribeiro, MA, Proietti, FA, Martins, ML, Januário, JN, Ladeira, RVP, Oliveira, MF, Carneiro-Proietti, ABF. (2010) Geographic distribution of human T-lymphotropic virus types 1 and 2 among mothers of newborns tested during neonatal screening, Minas Gerais, Brazil. *Revista Panamerica de Salud Publica*, 27, pp. 330-337.

Roucoux, DF, Murphy, EL. (2004) The epidemiology and disease outcomes of Human T-Lymphotropic Virus type II. *AIDS Reviews*, 6, pp. 144-154.

Satou, Y, Yasunaga, J, Yoshida, M, Matsuoka, M. (2006) HTLV-I basic leucine zipper factor gene mRNA supports proliferation of adult T cell leukemia cells. *Proceedings of National Academy of Sciences U S A*, 103, pp. 720-725.

Shindo, N, Alcantara, LC, Van Dooren, S, Salemi, M, Costa, MC, Kashima, S, Covas, DT, Teva, A, Pellegrini, M, Brito, I, Vandamme, AM, Galvão-Castro, B. (2002) Human retroviruses (HIV and HTLV) in Brazilian Indians: seroepidemiological study and molecular epidemiology of HTLV type 2 isolates. *AIDS Research and Human Retroviruses*, 18, pp. 71-77.

Silva, EA, Otsuki, K, Leite, AC, Alamy, AH, Sá-Carvalho, D, Vicente, AC. (2002) HTLV-II infection associated with a chronic neurodegenerative disease: clinical and molecular analysis. *Journal of Medicine Virology*, 66, pp. 253-257.

Sullivan, MT, Williams, AE, Fang, CT, Gradinetti, T, Poiez, BJ, Enrich, GD. (1991). Transmission of human T-lymphotropic virus types I and II by blood transfusion: a retrospective study of blood components (1983 through 1988): the American Red Cross HTLV-I/II Collaborative Study Group. *Archives of Internal Medicine*, 151, pp. 2043–2048.

Vine, AM, Heaps, AG, Kaftantzi, L, Mosley, A, Asquith, B, Witkover, A, Thompson, G, Saito, M, Goon, PKC, Carr, L, Martinez-Murillo, F, Taylor, GP, Bangham, CRM. (2004) The Role of CTLs in Persistent Viral Infection: Cytolytic Gene Expression in CD8- Lymphocytes distinguishes between Individuals with a High or Low Proviral Load of Human T Cell Lymphotropic Virus Type 1. *Journal of Immunology*, 173, pp. 5121–5129.

Waters, A, Oliveira, AL, Coughlan, S, de Venecia, C, Schor, D, Leite, AC, Araújo, AQ, Hall, WW. (2011) Multiplex real-time PCR for the detection and quantitation of HTLV-1 and HTLV-2 proviral load: addressing the issue of indeterminate HTLV results. *Journal of Clinical Virology*, 52, pp. 38-44.

Wolfe, ND, Heneine, W, Carr, JK, Garcia, AD, Shanmugam, V, Tamoufe, U, Torimiro, JN, Prosser, AT, Lebreton, M, Mpoudi-Ngole, E, McCutchan, FE, Birx, DL, Folks, TM, Burke, DS, Switzer, WM. (2005) Emergence of unique primate T-lymphotropic viruses among central African bushmeat hunters. *Proceedings of National Academy of Sciences U S A*, 102, pp. 7994-7999.

World Health Organization. Report of the Scientific Group on HTLV-I and Associated Diseases, Kagoshima, Japan, December 1988: Virus diseases. Human T Lymphotropic Virus Type I, HTLV-I. (1989) *Wkly Epidem. Rec.*, 49, pp. 382-383.

Yakova, M, Lézin, A, Dantin, F, Lagathu, G, Olindo, S, Jean-Baptiste, G, Arfi, S, Césaire, R. (2005) Increased proviral load in HTLV-1-infected patients with rheumatoid arthritis or connective tissue disease. *Retrovirology*, 2, pp. 4.

Yamano, Y, Nagai, M, Brennan, M, Mora, CA, Soldan, SS, Tomaru, U, Takenouchi, N, Izumo, S, Osame, M, Jacobson, S. (2002) Correlation of human T-cell lymphotropic virus type 1 (HTLV-1) mRNA with proviral DNA load, virus-specific CD8(+) T cells, and disease severity in HTLV-1-associated myelopathy (HAM/TSP). *Blood*, 99, pp. 88-94.

Yoshida, M. (2001) Multiple viral strategies of HTLV-1 for dysregulation of cell growth control. *Annual Review of Immunology*, 19, pp. 475-495.

Yoshida, M. (2010) Molecular approach to human leukemia: Isolation and characterization of the first human retrovirus HTLV-1 and its impact on tumorigenesis in Adult T-cell Leukemia. Proceedings of the Japan Academy. Series B, Physical and Biological Sciences, 86, pp. 117-129.

Zehender, G, Colasante, C, Santambrogio, S, De Maddalena, C, Massetto, B, Cavalli, B, Jacchetti, G, Fasan, M, Adorni, F, Osio, M, Moroni, M, Galli, M. (2002) Increased risk of developing peripheral neuropathy in patients coinfected with HIV-1 and HTLV-2. *Journal of Acquired Immune Deficiency Syndrome*, 31, pp. 440-447.

Part 4

Alternative Strategies to Allogenic Blood Transfusion

11

Autotransfusion: Therapeutic Principles, Efficacy and Risks

A.W.M.M. Koopman-van Gemert

Department of Anaesthesiology, Albert Schweitzer Hospital, 3300AK Dordrecht
The Netherlands

1. Introduction

The safety of allogenic blood products has been increased in the following ways: strict rules for donor selection following new insights in infectious; testing of donor blood with techniques to minimise window-period; reduction of leukocyte-count of blood products (in some countries); introduction of disinfectant techniques of plasma; introduction of quarantined plasma; culture of thrombocyte products. Other adverse effects, such as transfusion reactions, human errors, graft versus host disease, alloimmunisation, signs of an increase in nosocomial infections, as well as a possible immunosuppressive effect have contributed to the demand for alternative blood products or techniques decreasing the transfusion of allogeneic blood products, the so-called "blood-saving techniques". To reach this goal, these techniques can be used separately. However, in most cases a combination of several methods will be employed, often referred to generally as "blood management".

Momentarily, both pharmacological and non-pharmacological methods are available. Each technique has its' own efficacy. Each technique however, may also carry its' own adverse effects or complications. Most adverse effects are published in case reports or retrospective studies. Literature published studying aprotinin shows the importance of controlled randomised trials or cohort studies large enough to detect the incidence of adverse effects and to measure any differences in side effects. At the moment, haemovigilance for blood transfusion saving techniques is not regulated. However, the Dutch experiences highlight the importance of awareness of adverse effects.

Autotransfusion (red cell salvage) is one of these techniques and involves the infusion of blood collected intra-operatively from the operative field, or postoperatively from the drains, and will be discussed in this chapter. This method is one of the most commonly used techniques of autologous blood transfusion. The collected blood can be re-infused either directly or after filtration of cellular and other debris via a blood cell separator, referred to as the "washed method". In this chapter, efficacy, quality and safety of both methods will be described.

2. Definitions of the different techniques

2.1 Unprocessed or unwashed method of autotransfusion

This is the oldest technique, first suggested in 1818 by James Blundell and first performed by Brainard in 1860 (Blundell 1818, Brainard 1860, Koopman 1993). Blood is collected under low vacuum pressure (< 100 mm Hg) in a container and in most cases only filtered through a 170 micron filter. Several pore-sized filters are now available on the market. Originally this technique was also used intra-operatively, but because of serious adverse effects during reinfusion it was, until recently, only used for reinfusion of wound blood lost in the postoperative phase (drain blood) (Stachura et al. 2010). The blood is predominately collected without addition of anticoagulants, because the added anticoagulant is not removed by washing, and anticoagulant other than citrate may cause coagulopathy. Due to the risk of bacterial growth in the collected blood maintained at room temperature, collection and reinfusion is advised to be completed within a time span of a maximum of six hours. In cardiac surgery, longer periods of holding at lower temperature have been applied without complications (Schmidt et al.1998). Unwashed techniques are not advised for children.

2.2 Processed or washed methods of autotransfusion

With this approach, anticoagulant (heparin or citrate) is added to the tip of the vacuum by means of a double-lumen suction catheter. The aspirated blood is filtered through a 170 micron filter. Thereafter, the blood is centrifuged in a blood cell separator, removing the plasma which contains cell remnants. The remaining erythrocytes are washed with a saline solution and infused through a 40 micron blood filter. Postoperatively, the drain-blood, with or without anticoagulant, can be collected and processed in a time span of 6 hours. There is no limit to the amount of reinfusion of washed salvaged blood. One has to realise that only erythrocytes are recovered and consequently, massive blood loss replacement of plasma and platelets must be done by means of allogeneic blood products. For children devices available to process smaller volumes of blood are available.

3. Quality of the recovered blood

When blood comes into contact with non-endothelial tissue, due to the activation of the coagulation and complement cascade, platelets and leukocytes are activated and erythrocytes are destroyed (Krohn et al. 2001, Sinardi et al. 2005 , Stachura et al. 2010). Aspiration of blood increases this damage by air contact and turbulence. The amount of haemolysis depends on the type of surgery. Suction of a small amount of blood increases the risk of haemolysis and reduces the efficacy of erythrocyte recovery. The infusion of activated proteins and damaged cells may cause serious organ damage (Faught et al.1998). Moreover, aspirated blood must be anti-coagulated with a high-dose heparin or citrate to prevent clotting which, without removal. may cause coagulopathy.

Complications described include Acute Respiratory Distress Syndrome (ARDS), Disseminated Intravascular Coagulopathy (DIC), renal failure, Multi Organ Failure (MOF) (so-called "blood-salvage" syndrome), air embolism and coagulopathy (Bull & Bull 1990, Tawes & Duvall 1996). Washing of the blood product prevents these complications.

Blood collected postoperatively from wound-drains is less activated. The recovered blood contains free haemoglobin (Dalén 1995, 1997), activated cells, and mediators of the activated coagulation pathway. These factors can be measured in recipient's plasma. Dalén showed that approximately 0.5% of the recovered erythrocytes in drain-blood are haemolysed (Dalén & Enström 1998, 1999). The haematocrit level is lower in drain-blood due to dilution with chyle. Filtration of drain blood through a leukocyte-reducing filter previous to collection in the container, and avoiding filtration after collection, may reduce erythrocyte damage (Dalén & Enström 1998, 1999).

Unwashed drain-blood contains no fibrinogen and therefore addition of anticoagulant should not be necessary. However, clot-formation in the recovered blood has been described in 0,3 % of cases (Horstmann et al. 2010). Generally, no obvious clinical side-effects have been shown, but confusion may arise with diagnostic tests e.g. biochemical confirmation of myocardial infarction (Pleym et al. 2005).

The suction tip and the collection bag may be a cause of bacterial contamination (Wollinsky 1997), but antibiotic prophylaxis is generally effective. If autotransfusion is applied following advised methods, bacterial contamination is not a major risk (Wollinsky et al. 2007, Bowley et al. 2006).

3.1 Quality of the recovered erythrocytes

The efficacy of erythrocyte recovery is determined by the type of surgery, suction-technique, the pressure of the vacuum, and the prevention foaming and turbulence of the aspirated blood. Aspiration of small volumes destroys more erythrocytes than aspiration of larger volumes. Depending on these factors, recovery of erythrocytes is between 65% (e.g. orthopaedic) and 95% (e.g. vascular surgery) (Koopman 1993). Filtration of the collected drain-blood through a leukocyte-filter before collection in the container also reduces erythrocyte damage (Jensen et al. 1999), in contrast to filtration after collection of the blood. The haematocrit of a bag of washed red cells is approximately 0.50 l/l, slightly less than that of stored allogenic erythrocytes (Ht 60 l/l). Due to haemolysis during the suction process, regular measurement of the patient's haemoglobin level is advised.

The survival of recovered erythrocytes is normal and seems uninfluenced by the different types of autotransfusion or the type of surgery (Thorley et al. 1990, Kent et al. 1991, Wixson et al.1994). Room temperature incubation of drain-blood causes lactate formation and swelling of the erythrocytes. Some older studies show that the osmotic resistance and 24-hour survival of stored erythrocytes after processing in a cell saver is slightly decreased (Marcus et al. 1987, Schmidt et al.1996) compared to fresh recovered wound-blood, but more recent studies found no difference (Alleva 1995, Schmidt et al.1996). Oxygen delivery and 2,3-DPG levels are not influenced by cell salvage or processing (McShane et al. 1987, Schmidt et al.1996). The function of recovered leukocytes and platelets is marginally investigated, but may be depressed (McShane et al.1987).

3.2 Washing efficacy

Processing of salvaged blood by means of centrifugation and washing removes most free haemoglobin and anticoagulant, 95 and 98%, respectively (Koopman 1993). Even in massive transfusions of more than 100 units of salvaged red cells, just 5000 IU of heparin are re-infused. Most modern devices have a haemolysis sensor controlling the wash procedure. This is of great import, reducing the amount of free haemoglobin infused, thereby reducing excretion in the renal tubules and the risk of acute renal failure.

Fat embolism is a complication due to aspiration of fat particles, orthopaedic surgery displaying the highest risk. Fat globules may adhere to the tubing and/or filters and are of no risk for patients (figure 1). However, fat particles < 40 micron will be infused to the patient, unfiltered. A surface- or fat-filter is more effective than a screen-filter. A leukocyte filter is the most favourable (Ramirez et al. 2002, de Vries et al. 2003, 2006), but decreases reinfusion flow greatly.

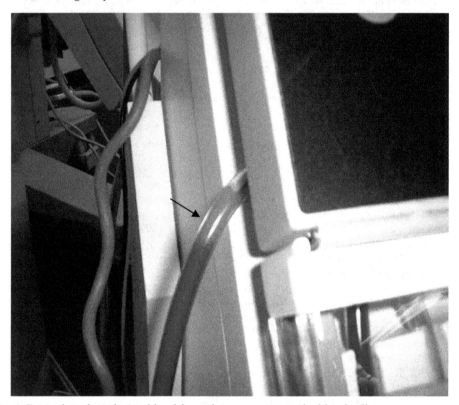

Fig. 1. Fat in the tube infusing blood from the reservoir into the blood cell separator processing bowl (arrow)

Salvaged blood of patients recovered from the area on and around a disfunctioning hip prosthesis may contain Cobalt or Chromium - washing of the salvaged blood removes, respectively, 76.3 and 78.6% of the content (Reijngoud et al. 2009).

In cardiac surgery, heart enzymes are recovered in the salvaged blood. Diagnosing perioperative complications such as myocardial infarction will be subject to error. The troponin level remains, however, uninfluenced and is therefore the most reliable indicator (Pleym et al. 2005).

4. Adverse reactions

As mentioned, reinfusion of aspirated unprocessed salvaged blood can induce serious organ damage such as ARDS, DIC, renal failure, MOF or coagulopathy. Filtration and washing largely removes toxic factors and reduces complications. Due to operating errors, however, serious complications are reported (Faugt et al. 1998, Zijlker et al. 2011). Most research has been published investigating the safety of reinfusion of unwashed drain-blood. A Dutch study of 1819 patients undergoing orthopaedic surgery showed adverse reactions in 3.6% of cases (Horstmann et al. 2009). Most reactions were mild, such as fever (> 38,5⁰C) and shivering. Two patients experienced a severe adverse reaction: cardiac arrest and atrial fibrillation due to a pulmonary embolism subsequent to reinfusion of 30 and 50 ml of autologous drain-blood, respectively. Both patients survived. Other authors describe mild adverse reactions (So-Osman et al. 2006, Kirkos et al. 2006, Hendrych 2006). Some found no relationship (Faught 1998, Moonen et al. 2008). Reinfusion of IL-6 may be a contributing factor. A 7-fold increase in normal baseline levels has been found (Handel et al. 2006). Filtration by means of a leukocyte-filter has been shown to reduce the level of interleukins but may actually instigate complement activation during the filtration process itself (Dalén & Engström 1998).

Reinfusion of unwashed blood had no effect on lung perfusion (Attinel et al, 2007). However, there was a slight decrease in thrombocyte levels found (de Jong et al, 2007).

A study of 120 patients investigating the immunological response to several methods of blood transfusion showed a decrease in Natural Killer (NK-) cells and interferon gamma levels by all methods except reinfusion of unwashed drain-blood, which saw an increase (Gharehbaghian et al. 2004). The IL-10 levels did not change. Gharehbaghian argues that higher concentrations of interferon gamma or NK-cells indicate a more favourable immunological response.

Reinfusion of unwashed drain-blood is often used in the context of cardiac surgery. However, recent studies showed greater haemodynamic instability, probably caused by infusion of the abovementioned cytokines and activated complement (Marcheix et al. 2008, Boodwhani et al. 2008). Moreover, increases in cognitive dysfunction (15 vs. 6%) after unwashed autotransfusion have been witnessed (Djaiani et al. 2007). Laboratory values showed increased indicators of fibrinolysis or DIC (Krohn et al. 2001, Sinardi et al. 2005). These changes seemed to be clinically irrelevant in general, but some authors showed an increase in postoperative blood loss in cases of reinfusion of >750ml (Schönbergen et al. 1992, Wiefferink et al. 2007). Not all authors confirmed these results (Schroeder et al. 2007, Sirvinskas et al. 2007). Washing of the salvaged blood prevents these adverse events and is obligatory for processing intra-operative aspirated blood. Furthermore, in cardiac surgery this can be extended to drain-blood collected postoperatively.

There is no literature referring to the maximum amount of drain-blood that can be re-infused unwashed. In most studies, a mean of 500 ml is re-infused. Greater than 1500 ml is re-infused in just a handful of cases, 0.5% (Huët 1999, Horstman 2010). Some authors advise a maximum of 15% of circulating volume (Krohn et al. 2001, Sinardi et al. 2005). Therefore, a guideline could be a maximum 15% of the circulating blood volume, with a cut-off value of 1500 ml. In addition, reinfusion of collected drain should be performed following filtration of the blood through a 40 micron filter. For children, there are no data available. However, re-infusion of unwashed blood is not advisable.

A preventable complication is air embolism, particularly when blood is infused under pressure (Faugt et al. 1998). As reinfusion bags and tubing from all systems contain air, an air detector placed in the infusion system is then mandatory.

5. Indications

Perioperative autotransfusion may be indicated for all operations with great blood loss. Most experiences are in the context of vascular surgery. In a retrospective study of 9918 patients, Giordano (Giordano et al.1993) concluded that cell salvage an efficient method of reducing use of allogenic blood transfusions. Most randomised studies, however, are conducted in cardiac, vascular or orthopaedic surgery (Carless et al. 2010; table 1). For all other types of surgery, data regarding efficacy is sparse.

Author and study protocol	Study groups	Results	Adverse events	Level of evidence
Carless 2010 Cochrane CD 001888	1966-2009 75 RCT: - ortho: n = 36 - Cardio: n = 33 - Vasc: n = 6 Washed: n = 27 Unwashed: n = 40 Other: n = 8 BT-protocol: n = 60 - 75 55 x postop. - 76 21 x intra- and postoperative No BT-protocol: n = 15 Patients: n = 3857	Overall: RR = 0.62 Ortho: RR = 0.46 - 77 washed: RR = 0.48 - 78 unwashed: RR = 0.47 Cardio: RR = 77 - 79 washed: RR = 0.66 - 80 unwashed: RR = 0.85 Vasc: RR = 0.63 n.s. BT-protocol: RR = 0.61 No BT-protocol: RR = 0.56 Mean 0.68 EC less	Mortality, re-operations, (wound) infections, thrombosis, stroke, myocardial infarction, hospital stay: n.s.	A1

Abbreviations: Ortho = orthopedic; Cardio = cardiology; Vasc = vascular surgery; B.T. = Blood Transfusion; N.S. = Not significant; RCT = Randomised Controlled Trial; RR = Relative Risk for allogeneic blood transfusion

Table 1. Meta-analysis 75 RCT.

5.1 Autotransfusion during cardiac surgery

Reinfusion of intra- and postoperative collected blood reduces the need for allogenic blood transfusions (Ferrari et al. 2007, Klein et al. 008). Washed techniques are more efficacious (RR washed 0.61 vs. unwashed 0.87) (Huët et al.1999, Carless et al. 2010). Most complications, such as increase in bleeding and cognitive dysfunction, are described under unwashed methods (see 4.0). In conclusion, washed techniques reduce adverse events, especially the frequency of cognitive dysfunction up to > 50% (Carrier et al. 2006, Westerberg 2005, Djaiani et al. 2007, Svenmarker et al. 2004). In cardiac surgery this should be state-of-the-art.

5.2 Autotransfusion in orthopaedic surgery

Reinfusion of intra- and postoperative collected blood is in most studies an efficacious method of reducing the need for allogenic blood transfusions. (Huët et al. 1999, Tylman et al. 2001, Jones et al. 2004, Carless et al. 2010, Tsumara et al. 2006, Smith et al. 2007, Zacharopoulos et al 2007, Amin et al. 2008, Tripkovic et al. 2008, Munoz et al. 2011). The haematocrit of drain-blood is approximately 0.25-0.30 l/l due to mixture with chyle. The Cochrane analysis shows an RR of 0.48 for washed techniques vs. 0.47 for unwashed techniques (Carless et al. 2010). A disadvantage is the lack of inclusion of transfusion protocol in all trials. Moreover, surgical techniques have changed in the last few years, questioning the validity of older studies, as shown in our recent multicenter, randomied study of 2579 patients (So-Osman et al. 2011).

Approximately 75% of postoperative blood loss occurs in the ensuing 6 hours, falling within the 6-hour window recommended for re-infusion (Wood et al. 2008). Wood also showed that increase in the collection time leads to augmented wound healing.

5.3 Autotransfusion in vascular surgery

Although intra-operative autotransfusion is most widely used in vascular surgery, and yet few randomised studies (Wong et al. 2002, Takagi et al. 2007, Carless et al. 2010, Huët et al. 1999) have been published. Adverse events are never published.

5.4 Autotransfusion in obstetrics

Autotransfusion of washed shed blood may be used for Extra Uterine Pregnancies (EUP) or caesareans. Use of a cell saver for EUP improved the haematocrit level at discharge significantly (Thomas D. 2005, Selo-Ojeme & Feyi-Waboso2007, Allam et al. 2008). In the past, intra-operative autotransfusion during obstetric haemorrhage has been discouraged because of the risk of amniotic fluid embolism. Reinfusion of amniotic fluid may cause amniotic fluid syndrome with DIC, ARDS and sometimes death. Recent literature, however, shows that harmful substances are removed during the washing process (Thomas D. 2005). A consequence of leukocyte filtration is improved removal of all foetal substances in all cases. Foetal erythrocytes are present in amniotic fluid with subsequent induction of irregular antibody formation in the mother after reinfusion. However, the quantity of foetal erythrocytes seems comparable with that circulating normally amount normally circulating in the mother's blood during delivery. Use of unwashed techniques is inadvisable.

5.5 Autotransfusion in urology

Autotransfusion of washed unradiated shed blood is often employed during cystectomies and prostatectomies (Nieder et al. 2004, 2007, Davis et al. 2003, Ford et al. 2007, Gallina et al. 2007, Stoffel et al. 2005, Waters et al. 2004). In these studies, blood was collected from the surgical field subsequent to prostatic manipulation. Stoffel performed measurements of the Prostate Specific Antigen (PSA) in subjects' blood: 1 hour prior to surgery; immediately subsequent to reinfusion of the shed blood; and 3-5 weeks following surgery (Stoffel et al. 2005). He also measured the PSA level in the processed salvaged blood. He found PSA expressing cells in 88% of the samples of the salvaged blood and in 13% of the preoperative samples. Furthermore, PSA-expressing cells were found in 16% of the autotransfused patients and in 4% of the non-autotransfused patients, immediately following transfusion. No PSA-expressing cells were detected in the peripheral blood samples taken 3-5 weeks postoperatively. Authors suggest PSA expressing cells are damaged by processing of the blood and the damaged cells are removed by the immune system of the subject.

5.6 Autotransfusion in traumatology

Autotransfusion is often applied during trauma surgery, especially in cases of liver or splenic ruptures. In this field, just one randomised study has been published, subjects experiencing abdominal trauma in combination with bowel perforations (n = 44; Bowley et al. 2006). Bowel perforation is generally considered a contraindication to autotransfusion. Somewhat unexpectedly, this study displayed no difference in survival or complications. However, necessity for erythrocyte transfusions was significantly less (6.47 vs. 11.17U). All operations were performed with antibiotic prophylaxis. Grossly contaminated blood with faeces or other debris was collected in a separate reservoir and not used for autotransfusion. In conclusion, this study shows that in emergency situations with abdominal trauma, washed autotransfusion may be used, provided that is under antibiotic prophylaxis.

5.7 Jehovah's Witnesses

Many Jehovah's Witnesses accept the use of perioperative autotransfusion provided that the machine is transformed to a closed system such as a heart-lung machine, and is completely filled with a saline solution prior to commencement of the procedure, and connected to the patient by means of an intravenous line. Some contraindications may be relative in this situation when autotransfusion may increase survival (McInroy 2005, Van Wolfswinkel 2009, Wooley 2005,). In the context of operative treatment of neoplasms, when irradiation of the washed blood product is not possible, the use of a leukocyte filter will provide a 1 log reduction of the tumour load.

5.8 Other indications

Autotransfusion may be contraindicated in subjects with haemoglobinopathies. In a case of a patient with Beta-thalassaemia requiring caesarean section which involved 9L of blood loss, increased haemolysis was noticed in the aspirated blood. This was counteracted by increasing the wash-volume. A sensor measuring the level of haemolysis in the effluent wash fluid was, in this case, a useful instrument (Waters et al. 2003).

Sickle cell disease (SCD) is an absolute contraindication due to erythrocyte haemolysis during hypoxic stress. Reinfusion of this blood caused serious coagulopathies (Fox et al. 1994).

Less absolute is autotransfusion in patients with the milder sickle cell trait. Storage of autologous blood has been described, without sickling (Romanoff 1988). Recently, in two case reports, sickling was displayed in 15-20% of the washed salvaged product, with subjects experiencing uneventful recovery (Okunuga & Skelton 2009). However, the proportion of HbS differs among the various carrier states (Hulatt & Fisher 2010). When applied, measurement of sickling in the collected blood prior to reinfusion is advisable.

6. Contraindications

6.1 Bacterial contamination

Not all authors consider bacterial contamination an absolute contraindication. It has been demonstrated that bacteria are not completely removed by centrifugation and washing (5-21% subsequently present) (Boudraux et al. 1983, Faugth et al. 1998). As described in the trauma study (Bowley et al. 2006), in emergency cases, autotransfusion can be life-saving without causing harm to the patient. A few other case-reports confirm that prophylactic intravenous antibiotic therapy or addition of antibiotics to the anticoagulant solution could prevent bacteraemia or sepsis (Faught et al. 1998, Wollinsky et al. 1997).

6.2 Tumour surgery

Tumour surgery is considered an absolute contraindication to the use of autotransfusion due to fear of inducing metastases. Centrifugation and washing during processing of the aspirated blood does not remove all tumour cells and resulted in <1 log reduction in tumour load (Hanssen et al. 2002, 2004 (2x), 2006, Thomas MJG1999, Stoffel et al. 2005). Tumour load in aspirated blood may be as high as 10^7 cells/litre (Hanssen 2002, 2006). The tumour cells remain viable and proliferate, as shown in in-vitro and animal models. Furthermore, leukocyte filtration can achieve just less than one more log reduction (Hanssen et al. 2004 (2x), 2006, Thomas MJG 1999). Radiation of the aspirated blood with 50 Gy resulted in a 10 log reduction in tumour load, after which no DNA-metabolism could be found (Thomas MJG 1999, Hanssen et al. 2002). There are special bags on the market for irradiation. The duration of the procedure is 6-15 minutes and is a complicated logistic process. However, combination of leukocyte filtration with irradiation has been found to remove all active tumour cells (Poli et al. 2008). Detailed studies showed that irradiation does not damage the red cells and that recovery in the first the 24 hours is improved, presumed due to selective loss of senescent erythrocytes (Hanssen et al. 2002). Experience with transfusion of irradiated salvaged blood has been described in more than 700 patients without adverse effects (Valbonesi et al. 1999). Comparison of subject outcome with regard to differences between filtration or the irradiation techniques have not been published. Therefore, based on non-clinical studies, the irradiation technique is the only method that can be safely used.

A personal opinion is that in life-threatening bleeding during tumour surgery in the case of a Jehovah's Witness, reinfusion of autotransfused blood through a leukocyte filter may be considered.

6.3 Other contraindications

The following are described in guidelines, but not investigated in randomised studies: cleansing of the wound with toxic fluids; usage of haemostatic medicines on collagen or thrombin base; or aspiration of fat.

7. Haemovigilance

Risks of allogenic blood transfusions have been one of the motives for introduction of blood-saving techniques and employment of alternative methods. Years ago, haemovigilance was introduced to monitor the safety of allogenic blood transfusions. Currently, haemovigilance for blood transfusion-saving techniques is not regulated. The Dutch foundation for haemovigilance (Transfusion Reactions In Patients: TRIP) has formulated a guideline comparable with that for allogenic blood transfusions, and begun with registration on a voluntary basis.

In 2004, a number of hospitals spontaneously reported incidents with autologous blood transfusion techniques (Zijlker et al. 2011). An annual increase in participation of other hospitals has been witnessed. The biggest hurdle is that registration of the total number of autotransfusions performed in Dutch hospitals (cell savers, drain blood reinfusion) in the Netherlands is not known, and a more complicated registration compared with allogenic blood transfusions which involve compulsory registration. In 2009, 2384 events were reported (2.9/1000 units of blood products), 98 of them were serious events (0.19%) including 3 involving autotransfusion techniques. In total, 35 incidents with cell savers or drain blood were reported (www.tripnet.nl). Momentarily, 18 hospitals not only report their adverse events, but also the total amount of procedures performed. Participation of other hospitals is encouraged by TRIP. More insight in risks may result in greater prevention in the future. In addition, long term outcome may be important as the study involving Aprotinin showed us (Mangano 2006, 2007, Karkouti 200). In summary, registration of long-term outcome should be encouraged for allogenic blood transfusions as well as for alternative techniques.

8. Conclusion

Perioperative autotransfusion started with reinfusion of unwashed shed blood intra- and postoperatively and soon appeared to be potentially dangerous (Koopman 1993). Results showed that blood collected intra-operatively was more dangerous than that collected postoperatively. This is explained by the damage caused by suction, high negative pressure, and contact with the air. Removal of the supernatant plasma and cell fragments by centrifugation and washing reduces side effects and the recovered product appeared safe for intra-operative use. Initially, infusion of unwashed drain blood was considered quite dangerous, but experience in recent years shows that despite the presence of potentially harmful substances, transfusion may be safe when used within certain limits. Such limits are: negative pressure not exceeding 100 mm Hg; reinfusion via a 40 micron filter; and a volume restriction of 15% of circulating volume with a maximum of 1500 ml for adults (this volume restriction is based on lack of randomised studies using larger volumes).

Provided all safety precautions are adhered to with regard to collection and apparatus used, there seems to be no volume restriction for the use of washed shed blood. Equipment with reliable optic sensors and a haemolysis controlling sensor are of import.

Several clinical and laboratory studies show that the quality of the saved erythrocytes (reflected in oxygen transport, osmotic fragility and survival) is equal to the circulating erythrocytes of the subjects, and better than stored autologous or allogeneic erythrocytes.

Massive blood loss can be managed by autotransfusion of recovered erythrocytes. Plasma and platelet concentrates, however, must be supplemented according to guidelines for massive blood loss.

With regard to all risks involved, and in comparison with allogeneic transfusion, a 50-60% decrease is witnessed with autotransfusion.

In the case of children, only specialised apparatus may be employed in washing techniques.

Disadvantages of autotransfusion in the case of tumour surgery or bacterially-contaminated surgical fields may be less than originally feared. In the context of a low degree of contamination, antibiotic prophylaxis may be adequate. Aspirated tumour cells are not sufficiently removed by filtration and washing. Currently, only irradiation of the recovered washed blood with 50 Gy has shown to give an adequate (10 log) reduction of tumour load. This requires, however, additional time, transport, validation of the irradiation process, labelling, and identification. This all adds to the costs of an irradiated unit. Filtration of the blood by means of a leukocyte depletion filter, taking 15 to 40 minutes, gives only a 2-3 log reduction of tumour load, and is therefore considered unsafe for employment in cancer surgery. However, in emergency cases or for Jehovah's Witnesses, it may be in certain circumstances an option to discuss with the patient. With an eye on the future, it is worthwhile to investigate if more simplistic methods of tumour cell reduction can be developed.

Blood saving techniques also have there side effects and incidents. At the moment haemovigilance of these incidents is not regulated. The Dutch experiences however highlight the importance of registration of these incidents comparable with those of allogeneic blood products.

9. References

Allam, J., Cox, M., jentis, S.M.. (2008) Cell slvage in obstetrics. *Internal Journal Obstetrics* Vol. 17: 37-45.

Amin,A., Watson, A., Mangwani, J., Nawabi, D., Ahluwalia, R. & Loeffler, M. (2008) A prospective randomised controlled trial of autologous retransfusion in total knee replacement. *Journal of Bone Joint Surgery.* Vol. 90(4):451-454. ISSN: 0021-9355

Blundell, J. (1818) Experiences on the transfusion of blood by syringe. *Medical Chirgical Transfusion* Vol. 9: 56-92.

Boodhwani, M., Nathan, H.J., Mesana, T.G. & Rubens, F.D. (2008) Cardiotomy Investigators. Effects of shed mediastinal blood on cardiovascular and pulmonary function: a randomized, doubleblind study. *Annals Thoracic Surery.* Vol. 86(4):1167-1173. ISSN 0003-4975

Boudreaux, J.P., Bornside, G.H. & Cohn, I. jr. (1983) Emergency autotranfusion: partial cleansing of bacteria-laden blood by cell washing. *J Trauma* Vol.23: 31-35. ISSN: 0022-5282

Bowley, D.M., Barker, P. & Boffard, K.D. (2006) Intraoperative blood salvage in penetrating abdominal trauma: a randomised, controlled trial. World Journal Surgery. Vol. 30(6):1074-1080. ISSN: 0364-2313

Brainard, D.M.D.. (1860) Amputation of the thigh for diseases of the knee joint. Transfusion of blood. *Chirurgical Medical Journal.* Vol. 18: 116-117.

Bull, B.S. & Bull, M.H. (1990) The salvaged blood syndrome: a sequel to mechanochemical activation of platelets and leukocytes? *Blood Cells.* Vol. 16(1):5-20; discussion 20-23. ISSN 0340-4684

Carless, P.A., Henry, D.A., Moxey, A.J., O'Connell, D.L. & Fergusson, D.A. Cell salvage for minimising perioperative allogenic blood transfusion. *The Cochrane Database of Systematic Reviews* 2010, Issue 4. Art. No.: CD001888. DOI: 10.1002/14651858.CD001888.pub4

Carrier, M., Denault, A., Lavoie, J. & Perrault, L.P. (2006) Randomized controlled trial of pericardial blood processing with a cell-saving device on neurologic markers in elderly patients undergoing coronary artery bypass graft surgery. *Annals Thoracic Surgery.* Vol. 82(1):51-55. ISSN 003-4975

Dalén, T., Broström, L., & Gunnar-Enström, K. (1995) Cell Quality of salvaged blood after total knee arthroplasty. Acta Orthopedica Scandinavica.Vol. 66 (3): 329-333. ISSN 0001-6470

Dalén, T., Broström, L., & Gunnar-Enström, K. (1997) Autotransfusion after total knee arthroplasty. Effects on blood cells, plasma chemistry, and whole blood rheology. *Journal of Arthroplasty.* Vol. 12 (5): 517-525. ISSN 083-5403

Dalén, T. & Engström, K.G. (1998) Filterability of autotransfusion Blood Cells and plasma after total knee arthroplasty. *Clinical Hemorheology Microcirculation* Vol. 19:181-195. ISSN 1386-0291

Dalén, T. & Engström, K.G. (1999) Microrheology of filtered autotransfusion drain blood with and without leukocyte reduction. *Clinical Hemorheology Microcirculation.* Vol. 21:113-123. ISSN 1386-0291

Davis, M., Sofer, M., Gomez-Marin, O., Bruck, D. & Soloway, M.S.(2003) The use of cell salvage during radical retropubic prostatectomy: does it influence cancer recurrence? *Britsh Journal Urology International .* Vol. 91(6):474-476. ISSN: 1464-4096

Djaiani, G., Fedorko, L., Borger, M.A., Green, R., Carroll, J., Marcon, M. & Karski, J. (2007) Continuous-flow cell saver reduces cognitive decline in elderly patients after coronary bypass surgery. *Circulation.* Vol. 23;116(17):1888-1895. ISSN: 0009-7322

Faught, C., Wells, P., Fergussion, D. & Laupacis, A. (1998) Adverse effects of methods for minimizing perioperative allogenic transfusion: a critical review of the literature. *Transfusion Medicine Review.* Vol. 12:206-225. ISSN 0887-7963

Ferraris, V.A. et al. (2007) for the working force of the society of thoracic surgeons and the society of cardiovascular anesthesiologists clinical practice guideline: Perioperative blood transfusion and blood conservation in cardiac surgery: *Annals Thoracic Surgery.* Vol. 83: S27-86. ISSN 003-4975

Ford, B.S., Sharma, S., Rezaishiraz, H., Huben, R.S. & Mohler, J.L. (2008). Effect of perioperative blood transfusion on prostate cancer recurrence. *Urology Oncology.* Vol. 26(4):364-367. ISSN 1078-1439

Fox, J.S., Amalanath, L., Hoeltge, G.A., Andrish, J.T.. (1994) Autolgous blood transfusion and intraoperative salvaged in a patient with homozygous sickle cell disease. *Cleve Clinical Journal Medicine* vol 61: 137-40.

Gallina, A., Briganti, A., Chun, F.K., Walz, J., Hutterer, G.C., Erbersdobler, A., Eichelberg, C., Schlomm,

T., Ahyai, S.A., Perrotte, P., Saad, F., Montorsi, F., Huland, H., Graefen, M. & Karakiewicz, P.I. (2007) Effect of autologous blood transfusion on the rate of biochemical recurrence after radical prostatectomy. *Britsh Journal Urology International.* Vol. 100(6):1249-1253. ISSN: 1464-4096

Gharehbaghian, A., Haque, K.M., Truman, C., Evans, R., Morse, R., Newman, J., Bannister, G., Rogers ,C. & Bradley, B.A. (2004) Effect of autologous salvaged blood on postoperative natural killer cell precursor frequency. *Lancet*. Vol. 363(9414):1025-1030. ISSN: 0140-6736

Giordano, G.F., Giordano, D.M., Wallace, B.A., Giordano, K.M., Prust, R.S. & Sandler, S.G. (1993) An analysis of 9,918 consecutive perioperative autotransfusion. *Surgical Gynecology Obstetrics* Vol. 176(2):103-110. ISSN 0039-6087

Handel, M., Boluki, D., Loibl, O., Schaumburger, J., Kalteis,T., Matussek, J. & Grifka, J. (2006) Postoperative autologous retransfusion of collected shed blood after total knee arthroplasty with the cell saver. *Zeitschrift Orthopädie und Ihre Grenzgebiet.* Vol. 144(1):97-101. ISSN 0044-3220

Hansen, E., Bechmann, V. & Altmeppen, J. (2002) Intraoperative blood salvage in cancer surgery: safe and effective? *Transfusion Apheresis Science.* Vol. 27(2):153-157. ISSN 1473-0502

Hansen, E., Bechmann, V., Altmeppen, J., Wille, J. & Roth, G. (2004). Quality assurance in blood salvage and variables affecting quality. Anasthesiol Intensivmed Notfallmed Schmerzther. Vol. 39(9):569-575. ISSN 0939-2661

Hansen, E., Pawlik, M., Altmeppen, J., Bechmann, V. (2004). Autologous transfusion -- from euphoria to reason: clinical practice based on scientific knowledge (Part II). Intraoperative blood salvage with blood irradiation -- from an anaesthesiological point of view. *Anasthesiol Intensivmed Notfallmed Schmerzther.* Vol. 39(11):676-682. ISSN 0939-2661

Hansen, E. (2006). Failed evidence of tumour cell removal from salvaged blood after leucocyte depletion. *Transfusion Medicine.* Vol. 16(3):213-4; author reply 215-216. ISSN 0958-7578

Hendrych, J. (2006). Use of post-operative drainage and auto-transfusion sets in total knee arthroplasty. *Acta Chir Orthop Traumatol Cech.* Vol. 73(1):34-38. ISSN 0001-5415

Horstmann, W.G., Slappendel, R., Hellemondt van, G.G., Castelein, R.M. & Verheyne, C.C.P.M. (2009). Safety of retransfusion of filtered shed to minimize blood in 1819 patients after total hip or knee arthroplasty. *Transfusion Alternatives in Transfusion Medicine.* Vol. 10: 174-181. ISSN 1295-9022

Hüet, C., Salmi, L.R., Fergusson, D., Koopman-van Gemert, A.W.M.M., Rubens, F. & Laupacis, A., ISPOT investigators. (1999). A meta-analysis of the effectiveness of cell salvage perioperative allogenic blood transfusion in cardiac and orthopedic surgery. *Anesthesia Analgesia.* Vol. 89:861-869. ISSN 0003-2999

Hulatt, L.J. & Fisher. (2010) H. Intra-operative cell salvage and sickle ceel carrier state. *Anaesthesia.* Vol. 65: 649. ISSN: 0003-2409

Jensen, C.M., Pilegaard, R., Hviid, K., Nielsen, J.D. & Nielsen, H.J. (1999). Quality of reinfused drainage blood after total knee arthroplasty. *Journal of Arthroplasty.* Vol. 14(3):312-318. ISSN 0883-5403

Jones,H.W., Savage, L., White, C., Goddard, R., Lumley, H., Kashif, F. & Gurusany, K. (2004). Postoperative autologous blood salvage drains--are they useful in primary uncemented hip and knee arthroplasty? A prospective study of 186 cases. *Acta Orthopedica Belgica.* Vol. 70(5):466-473. ISSN 0001-6462

Jong de, M., Ray, M., Crawford, S., Whitehouse, S.L. & Crawford, R.W. (2007). Platelet and leukocyte activation in salvaged blood and the effect of its reinfusion on the circulating blood. *Clinical Orthopaedics and Related Research.* Vol. 456:238-242. ISSN 0009-921X

Karkouti, K., Beattie, W.S., Dattilo, K.M., McCluskey, S.A., Ghannam, M. & Hamdy, A. (2006). A propensity score case-control comparison of aprotinin and tranexamic acid in high transfusion-risk cardiac surgery. *Transfusion*. Vol. 46: 327-338. ISSN: 0041-1132

Kent, P., Ashley, S., Thorley, P.J., Shaw, A., Parkin, A. & Kester, R.C. (1991). 24-hour survival of autotransfused red cells in elective aortic surgery: a comparison of two intraoperative autotransfusion systems. *British Journal Surgery*. Vol. 78:1473-1475. ISSN: 0007-1323

Kirkos, J.M., Krystallis, C.T., Konstantinidis, P.A., Papavasiliou, K.A., Kyrkos, M.J. & Ikonomidis, L.G. (2006). Postoperative re-perfusion of drained blood in patients undergoing total knee arthroplasty: is it effective and cost-efficient? *Acta Orthopedica Belgica*. Vol. 72(1):18-23. ISSN 0001-6462

Klein,A.A., Nashef, S.A., Sharples, L., Bottrill, F., Dyer, M., Armstrong, J. & Vuylsteke, A. (2008). A randomized controlled trial of cell salvage in routine cardiac surgery. *Anesthesia Analgesia*. Vol. 107(5):1487-1495. ISSN 0003-2999

Koopman-van Gemert, A.W.M.M. (1993) Peri-operative autotransfusion by means of a blood cell separator [2e edition]. Publisher: J.J.H.M. van Gemert & J.J.R.M. van Gemert uitgeverij De Alk, ISBN 90-9005755-2, Alkmaar

Krohn, C.D., Reikerås, O., Bjørnsen, S. & Brosstad, F. (2001). Fibrinolytic activity and postoperative salvaged untreated blood for autologous transfusion in major orthopaedic surgery. *European Journal Surgery*. Vol. 67(3):168-172. ISSN 1753-1934

Mangano, D.T., Tudor, I.C. & Dietzel, C. (2006). Multicenter Study of Perioperative Ischemia Research Group; Ischemia Research and Education Foundation. The risk associated with aprotinin in cardiac surgery. *New England Journal of Medicine*. Vol. 26;354(4):353-365. ISSN: 0028-4793

Mangano, D.T., Miao, Y., Vuylsteke, A., Tudor, I.C., Juneja, R. & Filipescu, D. (2007). Investigators of The Multicenter Study of Perioperative Ischemia Research Group; Ischemia Research and Education Foundation. Mortality associated with aprotinin during 5 years following coronary artery bypass graft surgery. *Journal of the American Medical Association*. Vol. 7;297(5):471-479. ISSN: 0098-7484

Marcheix, B., Carrier, M., Martel, C., Cossette, M., Pellerin, M., Bouchard, D. & Perrault, L.P. (2008). Effect of pericardial blood processing on postoperative inflammation and the complement pathways. *Annals Thoracic Surgery*. Vol. 85(2):530-535. ISSN 003-4975

Marcus, C.S., Myhre, A., Angulo, M.C., Salk, R.D., Essex, C.E. & Demianew, S.H. (1987). Radiolabeled red cell viability. Comparison of 51 Cr, 99mTc and 111In for measuring the viability of autologous stored red cells. *Transfusion*. Vol. 27: 315-319. ISSN: 0041-1132

McInroy, A. (2005). Blood transfusion and Jehovah's Witnesses: the legal and ethical issues. *British Journal of Nursing*. Vol. 14(5):270-274. ISSN 0966-0461

McShane, A.J., Power, C., Jackson, J.F., Murphy, D.F., MacDonald, A., Moriarty, D.C. & Otridge, B.W. (1987). Autotransfusion: quality of blood prepared with a red cell processing device. *British Journal Anaesthesia*. Vol. 59: 1035-1039. ISSN 0007-0912

Moonen, A.F., Knoors, N.T., Os van, J.J., Verburg, A.D. & Pilot P. (2007). Retransfusion of filtered shed blood in primary total hip and knee arthroplasty: a prospective randomized clinical trial. *Transfusion*. Vol. 47(3):379-384. ISSN: 0041-1132

Muñoz,M., Slappendel, R. & Thomas, D. (2011). Laboratory characteristics and clinical utility of post-operative cell salvage: washed or unwashed Blood Transfus? *Blood Transfusion*. Vol. 9(3):248-261. ISSN: 1723-2007

Nieder, A.M., Simon, M.A., Kim, S.S., Manoharan, M. & Soloway, M.S. (2004). Intraoperative cell salvage during radical prostatectomy: a safe technique for Jehovah's Witnesses. *International Brazilian Journal Urology*. Vol. 30(5):377-379. ISSN 1677-5538

Nieder, A.M., Manoharan, M., Yang, Y. & Soloway, M.S. (2007). Intraoperative cell salvage during radical cystectomy does not affect long-term survival. Urology. Vol. 69(5):881-884. ISSN: 0090-4295

Okunuga, A. & Kleton, V.A. (2009). Use of cell salvage in patients with sickle cell trait. *International Journal Obstetric Anesthsia*.Vol. 18 (1): 90-91. ISSN 0959-289X

Pleym, H., Tjomsland, O., Asberg, A., Lydersen, S., Wahba, A., Bjella, L., Dale, O. & Stenseth, R. (2005). Effects of autotransfusion of mediastinal shed blood on biochemical markers of myocardialdamage in coronary surgery. *Acta Anaesthesiologica Scandinavica*. Vol. 49(9):1248-1254. ISSN 0001-5172

Poli, M., Camargo, A., Villa, L., Moura, R., Colella, R. & Deheinzelin, D. (2008). Intraoperative autologous blood recovery in prostate cancer surgery: in vivo validation using a tumour marker. *Vox Sanguinis*. Vol. 95(4):308-312. ISSN: 0042-9007

Ramírez, G., Romero, A., García-Vallejo, J.J. & Muñoz, M. (2002). Detection and removal of fat particles from postoperative salvaged blood in orthopedic surgery. *Transfusion*. Vol. 42(1):66-75. ISSN: 0041-1132

Reijngoud, L.W.P., Pattyn, C., De Haan, R., De Somer ,F., Campbell, P.A., Harinderjit, S., Gil, H.S. & De

Smet, K.A. (2009). Does Intraoperative Cell Salvage Remove Cobalt and Chromium from Reinfused Blood? *Journal of Arthroplasty*.Vol. 24(7):1125-1129. ISSN 0883-5403

Schmidt, H., Bendtzen, K. & Mortensen, P.E. (1998). The inflammatory cytokine response after autotransfusion of shed mediastinal blood. Acta Anaesthiololyca Scandinavica. Vol. 42:558-564. ISSN 0001-5172

Schmidt, H., Lund, J.O. & Steen, L.N. (1996). Autotransfused shed mediastinal blood has normal erythrocyte survival. *Annals Thoracic Surgery*. Vol. 62: 105-108. ISSN 003-4975

Schönberger, J.P., Everts, P.A., Bredee, J.J., Jansen, E., Goedkoop, R. & Bavinck, J.H. (1992). The effect of postoperative normovolaemic anaemia and autotransfusion on blood saving after internal mammary artery bypass surgery. *Perfusion*. Vol. 7:257-262. ISSN 0267-6591

Schroeder, S., Spiegel von, T., Stuber, F., Hoeft, A., Preusse, C.J., Welz, A., Kampe, S. & Lier, H. (2007). Interleukin-6 enhancement after direct autologous retransfusion of shed thoracic blood does Not influence haemodynamic stability following coronary artery bypass grafting. *Thoracic Cardiovascular Surgery*. Vol. 55(2):68-72. ISSN 0022-5223

Selo-Ojeme, D.O., Feyi-Waboso, P.A. (2007). Salvage autotransfusion versus homologous blood transfusion for ruptured ectopic pregnancy. *International Journal Gynaecology Obstetrics*. Vol. 96(2):108-111. ISSN 1470-0328

Sinardi, D., Marino, A., Chillemi, S., Irrera, M., Labruto, G. & Mondello, E.. (2005). Composition of the blood sampled from surgical drainage after joint arthroplasty: quality of return. *Transfusion*. Vol. 45(2):202-207. ISSN: 0041-1132

Sirvinskas, E., Veikutiene, A., Benetis, R., Grybauskas, P., Andrejaitiene, J., Veikutis, V. & Surkus, J. (2007). Influence of early re-infusion of autologous shed mediastinal blood on clinical outcome after cardiac surgery. *Perfusion*. Vol. 22(5):345-352. ISSN 0267-6591

So-Osman, C., Nelissen, R.G., Eikenboom, H.C. & Brand, A. (2006). Efficacy, safety and user-friendliness of two devices for postoperative autologous shed red blood cell re-infusion in elective orthopaedic surgery patients: A randomized pilot study. *Transfusion Medicine*. Vol. 16(5):321-328. ISSN 0958-7578

So-Osman, C., Nelissen, R.G.H.H., Koopman-van Gemert, A.W.M.M., Kluyver, E., Pöll, R., Onstenk, R.,

Van Hilten, J.A., Jansen-Werkhoven, T.M., Brand, R. & Brand A. (2011). A randomised controlled trial on erythropoietin and blood salvage as transfusion alternative in orthopedic surgery using a restrictive transfusion policy. *Transfusion Alternatives in Transfusion Medicine*. Vol. 12 (1): 25. ISSN 1295-9022

Smith, L.K., Williams, D.H. & Langkamer, V.G.(2007). Post-operative blood salvage with autologous retransfusion in primary total hip replacement. *Journal Bone Joint Surgery British*. Vol.89(8):1092-7. ISSN: 0301-620X

Stoffel, J.T., Topjian, L. & Libertino, J.A. (2005). Analysis of peripheral blood for prostate cells after autologous transfusion given during radical prostatectomy. *British Journal Urology International*. Vol. 96(3):313-315. ISSN: 1464-4096

Stachura,A., Król, R., Poplawski,T., Michalik, D., Pomianowski, S., Jacobsson,M., Åberg, M. & Bengtsson, A. (2010). Transfusion of intra-operative autologous whole blood: influence on complement activation and interleukin formation. *Vox Sanguinis*. Vol. 2; 239-246. ISSN: 0042-9007

Svenmarker,S., Engström, K.G., Karlsson, T., Jansson, E., Lindholm, R. & Aberg, T. (2004). Influence of pericardial suction blood retransfusion on memory function and release of protein S100B. *Perfusion*. Vol. 19(6):337-343. ISSN 0267-6591

Takagi, H., Sekino, S., Kato, T., Matsuno, Y. & Umemoto, T. (2007). Intraoperative autotransfusion in abdominal aortic aneurysm surgery: meta-analysis of randomized controlled trials. *Archives Surgery*. Vol. 142(11):1098-1101. ISSN 0096-6908

Tawes, R.L. Jr. & Duvall, T.B. (1996). Is the "salvaged-cell syndrome" myth or reality? *American Journal Surgery*. Vol. 172 (2):172-174. ISSN: 0002-9610

Thomas, D. (2005). Facilities for blood salvage (cell saver technique) must be available in every obstetric theatre. *International Journal Obstetric Anesthesia*. Vol. 14(1):48-50. ISSN 0959-289X

Thomas, M.J.G. (1999. Infected and malignant fields are an absolute contraindication to intraoperative cell salvage: fact or fiction? *Transfusion Medicine*. Vol. 9:269-278. ISSN 0958-7578

Thorley, P.J., Shaw, A., Kent, P., Ashley, S., Parkin, A. & Kester, R.C. (1990). Dual tracer technique to measure salvaged red cell survival following autotransfusion in aortic surgery. *Nuclear Medicine Communication*. Vol. 11:369-374. ISSN 0143-3636

Tripković, B., Buković, D., Sakić, K., Sakić, S., Buković, N. & Radaković, B. (2008). Quality of the blood sampled from surgical drainage after total hip arthroplasty. *Collegium Antropologicum*. Vol. 32(1):153-160. ISSN 0350-6134

Tsumara, N., Yoshiya, S., Chin, T., Shiba, R., Kohso, K. & Doita, M. (2006). A prospective comparison of clamping the drain or post-operative salvage of blood in reducing blood loss after total knee arthroplasty. *Journal Bone Joint Surgery British*. Vol. 88(1):49-53. ISSN: 0301-620X

Tylman,M., Bengtson, J.P., Avall, A., Hyllner, M. & Bengtsson, A. (2001). Release of interleukin-10 by reinfusion of salvaged blood after knee arthroplasty.*Intensive Care Medicine*. Vol. 27(8):1379-84. ISSN 0342-4642

Van Wolfswinkel, M.E.. (2009). Maternal mortality and serious maternal morbidity in Jehovah's Witnesses in the Netherlands. *British Journal Obstetrics Gynaecology*. Vol. 116: 1103-1110. ISSN: 1470-0328

Valbonesi, M., Bruni, R., Lercari, G., Florio, G., Carlier, P. & Morelli, F. (1999). Autoapheresis and intraoperative blood salvage in oncologic surgery. *Transfusion Science*. Vol. 21:129-139. ISSN 0955-3886

Vries de, A.J., Gu, Y.J., Post, W.J., Vos, P., Stokroos, I., Lip, H. & Oeveren van, W. (2003). Leucocyte depletionduring cardiac surgery: a comparison of different filtration strategies. *Perfusion*. Vol. 18(1):31-38. ISSN 0267-6591

Vries de, A.J., Vermeijden, W.J., Gu, Y.J., Hagenaars, J.A. & Oeveren van, W. (2006). Clinical efficacy and biocompatibility of three different leukocyte and fat removal filters during cardiac surgery. *Artificial Organs*. Vol. 30(6):452-457. ISSN 0160-564X

Waters, J.H., ShinJung Lee, J., Klein, E., O'Hara, J., Zippe, C. & Potter, P.S . (2004). Preoperative Autologous Donation Versus Cell Salvage in the Avoidance of Allogeneic Transfusion in Patients Undergoing Radical Retropubic Prostatectomy. *Anesthesia Analgesia*. Vol. 98:537–542. ISSN 0003-2999

Westerberg, M., Gäbel, J., Bengtsson, A., Sellgren, J., Eidem, O. & Jeppsson, A. (2006). Hemodynamic effects of cardiotomy suction blood. *Journal Thoracic Cardiovascular Surgery*. Vol. 131(6):1352-1357. ISSN 0022-5223

Wiefferink, A., Weerwind, P.W., Heerde van, W., Teerenstra, S., Noyez, L., Pauw de, B.E. & Brouwer, R.M. (2007). Autotransfusion management during and after cardiopulmonary bypass alters fibrin Degradation and transfusion requirements. *Journal Extra Corporeal Technology*. Vol. 39(2):66-70. ISSN 0022-1058

Wixson, R.L., Kwaan, H.C/\., Spies, S.M. & Zimmer, A.M. (1994). Reinfusion of postoperative wound drainage in total joint arthroplasty: Red blood cell survival and coagulopathy risk. *Journal Arthroplasty* Vol. 9:351-357. ISSN 0883-5403

Wollinsky, K.H., Oethinger, M., Buchele, M., Kluger, P. & Puhl, W., Hinrich-Mehrkens H. (1997). Autotransfusion bacterial contamination during hip arthroplasty and efficacy of cefurocime prophylaxis: a randomized controlled study of 40 patients. *Acta Orthopedica Scandinavica*. Vol. 68:225-230. ISSN 0001-6470

Wong, J.C.L., Torella, F., Haynes, S.L., Dalrymple, K., Mortimer, A.J. & McCollum, C.N., ATIS Investigators.(2002). Autologous versus allogenic transfusion in aortic surgery. *Annals Surgery* Vol. 235:145-151. ISSN: 0003-4932

Wood, G.C., Kapoor, A. & Javed, A. (2008). Autologous drains in arthroplasty a randomized control trial. *Journal of Arthroplasty*. Vol. 23(6):808-813. ISSN 0883-5403

Woolley, S. (2005). Jehovah's Witnesses in the emergency department: what are their rights? *Emergency Medicine Journal*. Vol. 22(12):869-71. ISSN: 1472-0205

Zacharopoulos, A., Apostolopoulos, A. & Kyriakidis, A . (2007). The effectiveness of reinfusion after total knee replacement. A prospective randomised controlled study. *International orthopaedics*. Vol. 31(3):303-308. ISSN 0341-2695.

Zijlker-Jansen, P.Y.,   Tilborgh- de Jong van. J.W., Wiersum-Osselton, J.C., Streefkerk, I.,
       Beunis, M.H., Maaren van, Y., Rohrbach, A., Koopman-van Gemert, A.W.M.M. &
       Schipperus, M.R..(2011). Transfusion reactions and blood   management
       techniques: a pilot study in the Netherlands. *Blood Transfusion* Vol. 9; suppl 1: S 34.
       ISSN:1723- 2007

12

Bloodless Medicine and Surgery

Nathaniel I. Usoro

Department of Surgery, University of Calabar Teaching Hospital, Calabar, Nigeria

1. Introduction

Bloodless Medicine and Surgery (BMS) is the provision of quality health care to patients without the use of allogeneic blood with the aim of improving outcome and protecting patients' rights.[1, 2] It involves the use of Blood Conservation techniques in combinations that are specific to the individual patient, ideally following a protocol and a multidisciplinary approach, and is synonymous with **Transfusion-free Medicine and Surgery**.[3, 4]

The term **Patient Blood Management** has crept into popular use in some circles, and has been recently defined by the Society for the Advancement of Blood Management as "the application of evidence-based medical and surgical concepts aimed at relying on a patient's own blood rather than on donor blood and achieving better patient outcomes".[5] The basic principles or 'pillars' of Patient Blood Management were ratified by the 63rd World Health Assembly, and are identical to those of BMS as discussed herein.[6]

BMS has traditionally been considered in clinical situations where patients refuse blood, and when 'safe' blood is unavailable or in short supply.[1] Many clinicians are surprised to learn that blood transfusion is based on tradition and associated with a poorer outcome (unrelated to infectious hazards) in a wide variety of patients.[7] Today, BMS has emerged as the standard of care appropriate for all patients because it is evidence-based and associated with a better outcome.[1, 2]

2. A brief history of bloodless medicine & surgery

For about 2000 years up until the 19th century bloodletting rather than blood transfusion was the standard practice in medicine.[8] Virtually all surgeries prior to the 20th century were essentially 'bloodless', and some were remarkably successful. Theodore Kocher, for instance, did his first thyroidectomy in 1872, and by the end of his career he had done 5000 thyroidectomies with only 1% mortality. Kocher never transfused any patient and he won a Nobel Prize.[9]

Karl Landsteiner's discovery of the ABO blood groups in 1900 started off the modern era of transfusion medicine. In 1915 Richard Lewisohn introduced anticoagulation with sodium citrate. Blood transfusion was used for World War I and II military casualties. Bernard Fantus set up the first hospital based blood bank in Chicago, USA about 1937.[10] From then on blood transfusion became a universal practice in medicine, so that the popular dictum seemed to be "When in doubt transfuse!".[3]

BMS started as an attempt by some dedicated surgeons in the 1960s to accommodate patients who declined blood transfusion, notably Jehovah's Witnesses.[11, 12] Their religious belief is based on a distinctive interpretation of specific passages from the Bible, such as:

"You are to abstain from ... blood" – Acts Ch. 15 v. 29 (New English Bible)[13, 14]

Denton Cooley, widely regarded as the founding father of modern bloodless surgery, performed the first bloodless open-heart surgery on one of Jehovah's Witnesses on May 18th, 1962.[2, 12] In 1977 Ott and Cooley published a pioneer report of 542 open-heart surgeries without allogeneic blood transfusion in patients ranging in age from one day to 89 years,[15] demonstrating that the "impossible" was possible – and safer. Other surgeons joined, but their ingenious techniques did not gain wide acceptance then.[2]

The advent of HIV/AIDS in 1981 forced a reconsideration of blood transfusion practices and a desire for BMS on account of the epidemic proportions of HIV, and the fact that the surest (though not the commonest) route of transmission is through blood transfusion. Many other pathogens old and new that are transmitted by blood (Table 1),[16] and many non-infectious hazards (Table 2)[17] received renewed attention and prominence. The cost of making blood "safe" rose astronomically while the supply of "safe" blood shrank. This added further impetus to the search for transfusion alternatives and the promotion of blood conservation techniques.[1, 2]

Recently however, the focus has shifted from the hazards of allogeneic blood to its efficacy – or lack of it. The Canadian Critical Care Trials Group study on Transfusion Requirements in Critical Care (TRICC) by Hérbert and co-workers in 1999 was a landmark prospective randomized study of 838 ICU patients comparing a liberal transfusion versus restricted transfusion policy. It revealed better results with the restricted transfusion group: lower ICU mortality, lower hospital mortality, lower 30-day mortality, and a trend towards decreased organ failure.[18] Several other studies have confirmed adverse outcome in transfused patients not related to infectious hazards.[19-24] Allogeneic blood has been found to increase hemorrhage, impair perfusion of the microcirculation, impair oxygen release from hemoglobin, and *worsen* rather than improve tissue oxygenation.[25-29] Some of these effects are thought to be due to storage lesions. On the other hand, it has not been possible to demonstrate the benefits of RBC transfusion.[7, 19, 29, 30]

Thus, while BMS started as an advocacy and then became widespread because of the infectious hazards and high cost/scarcity of allogeneic blood, Evidence-Based Medicine has recently emerged as the driving force behind its current practice, with improvement of outcome as the major aim.

3. Blood conservation techniques

Blood conservation techniques form the basis of the practice of BMS, and may be grouped under of four basic categories or "pillars":[3]

1. Optimizing the Hematocrit
2. Minimizing blood loss
3. Optimizing tissue oxygenation
4. Lowering the 'Transfusion Trigger' (tolerance of anemia)

Viruses
    Hepatitis viruses
    Hepatitis A virus (HAV)
    Hepatitis B virus (HBV)
    Hepatitis C virus (HCV)
    Hepatitis D virus (HDV) (requires co-infection with HBV)
    Hepatitis E virus (HEV)
    Retroviruses
    Human immunodeficiency virus (HIV) 1 and +2
    (+ + other sub-types)
    Human T-cell leukemia virus (HTLV) I and II
    Herpes viruses
    Human cytomegalovirus (HCMV)
    Epstein–Barr virus (EBV)
    Human herpes virus 8 (HHV-8)
    Parvoviruses
    Parvovirus B19
    Miscellaneous viruses
    GBV-C [previously referred to as hepatitis G virus (HGV)]
    TTV
    West Nile virus

Bacteria
  Endogenous
    Treponema pallidum (syphilis)
    Borrelia burgdorferi (Lyme disease)
    Brucella melitensis (brucellosis)
    Yersinia enterocolitica
    Salmonella spp.
  Exogenous (environmental species and skin commensals)
    Staphylococcal spp.
    Pseudomonas
    Serratia spp.
    Rickettsiae
    Rickettsia rickettsii (Rocky Mountain spotted fever)
    Coxiella burnettii (Q fever)

Protozoa
    Plasmodium spp. (malaria)
    Trypanosoma cruzi (Chagas disease)
    Toxoplasma gondii (toxoplasmosis)
    Babesia microti/divergens (babesiosis)
    Leishmania spp. (leishmaniasis)

Prions
    Variant Creutzfeldt–Jakob disease (vCJD)

Table 1. Infectious agents transmissible by blood transfusion[16]

Immune mediated
Hemolytic transfusion reactions
Febrile nonhemolytic transfusion reactions
Allergic/urticarial/anaphylactic transfusion reactions
Transfusion-related acute lung injury (TRALI)
Posttransfusion purpura (PTP)
Transfusion-associated graft versus host disease (TA-GVHD)
Microchimerism
Transfusion-related immunomodulation (TRIM)
Alloimmunization
Nonimmune mediated
Septic transfusion reactions
Nonimmune hemolysis
Mistransfusion
Transfusion-associated circulatory overload (TACO)
Metabolic derangements
Coagulopathic complications from massive transfusion
Complications from red cell storage lesions
Over/undertransfusion
Iron overload

Table 2. Noninfectious Serious Hazards of Transfusion (NISHOTs)[17]

Virtually all techniques of blood conservation are meant to buttress one or other of these pillars, and when used in combination they effectively reduce or eliminate the use of allogeneic blood with its costs and hazards, and improve clinical outcome (Table 3).

3.1 Optimizing the hematocrit

Optimizing the hematocrit increases the tolerable blood loss or the margin of safety in the event of blood loss in surgery, and reduces morbidity and mortality in non-surgical patients. Iron therapy is at the center of current efforts in this regard with or without Erythropoiesis Stimulating Agents (ESAs), even in the absence of absolute iron deficiency. [1,2, 31]

a. **Oral Iron Therapy** is the modality of choice for eligible patients. Ferrous sulfate, gluconate or fumarate may be used to administer ideally 200-220mg of elemental iron per day. Adjuncts to be given daily include Vitamin C 500mg, Vitamin B_{12} 150μg, Folic Acid 5mg, Multivitamins, and nutritional support.[4, 31] The author avoids folic acid in malignant disease.[32]

b. **Parenteral Iron Therapy** corrects anemia more rapidly, and may be used alone or in conjunction with ESAs. Intravenous iron is also preferred in anemia of chronic disease Iron dextran is the classical preparation and a low molecular weight iron dextran is available. However, less allergenic preparations are currently favored, especially iron sucrose.[31] Dose in mg = *weight x [normal Hb – actual Hb (g/L)] x 0.24 + 500,*[31] or *[normal Hb – actual Hb (g/dL)] x 200 + 500.*[4]

Iron dextran is diluted in normal saline at a ratio of 5ml (250mg):100mL saline and administered intravenously initially at 20 drops/min for 5 minutes, then 60 drops/min if no side effects occur. The total dose may be given at once to a maximum of 20mg/kg body weight over 4-6 hours or in divided doses on alternate days (preferably).[4, 31] The author found that administering Hydrocortisone 100mg *i.v.* 15 minutes before iron dextran, and diluting 5ml (250mg) of iron dextran in 250-500mL of normal saline successfully averts allergic reactions, even in a patient who previously reacted when those measures were not taken.[31]

Iron sucrose is less allergenic and is also administered safely in normal saline infusion 100mg:50mL or 200mg:100mL over 30 minutes, or 500mg:250mL administered over 3 hours. The total dose may be given at once to a maximum of 7mg/kg body weight over 3-3.5 hours (some workers have given 1000mg safely) or in divided doses on alternate days.[4]

c. **Erythropoietin alfa** which was in use for blood conservation in oncology since 1989 was approved for perioperative use in the US in 1996. **Beta** preparations are also available. In general surgery 100-150U/kg *s.c.* for 6 doses (e.g. twice weekly for 3 weeks) is recommended.[4] In oncology 150U/kg *s.c.* 3 times weekly or 40,000U *s.c.* weekly is the recommended starting dose.[33] **Darbopoietin alfa** is a long-acting ESA that can be administered *s.c.* weekly (2.25µg/kg) or 3 weekly (500µg). Intravenous iron is recommended in conjunction with ESAs as it potentiates the response and averts functional iron deficiency.[4, 34]

    ESAs stimulate RBC production by up to 4 times the basal marrow rate. Reticulocyte count increases by Day 3 and hemoglobin typically increases at 1g/dL every 4-7 days.[34] Use of ESAs is not recommended when the hemoglobin is above 12g/dl in oncology.[33]

Optimizing the hemoglobin with the appropriate medication is indicated in virtually all surgical patients, in elective and emergency cases, as it is in treatment and prophylaxis of anemia in non-surgical patients.[4] Interventions in this regard do not start working slowly after 21 days as some may imagine, but start working immediately and build up over time.[31, 34] Provided the main pathology is properly and promptly treated, the patient's improvement with bloodless care is sometimes dramatic, compared with patients who are transfused.

3.2 Minimizing blood loss

Efforts towards minimizing blood loss in the surgical patient start from the first contact and span through the entire perioperative period.

a. **Good history, physical examination, and laboratory investigations** are essential even in emergencies, taking note of the following among others:
    i.   History of bleeding disorders
    ii.   Anticoagulant therapy
    iii. Site of external hemorrhage (to be promptly arrested)
    iv.   Estimate of blood loss
    v.   Full Blood Count
    vi.   Clotting profile (if indicated)
b. **Pharmacological agents** that can reduce hemorrhage include:[4]
    i.   **Vitamin K** 10mg (2.5-50mg) *p.o., i.m., s.c., i.v.*
    ii.   **Tranexamic acid** 1.5g 3x/day – 1g 6x/day for 5-7 days, first *i.v.* then *p.o.* (for prophylaxis, 1g *p.o.* preop).

    iii. **Aprotinin** 500,000KIU *i.v.* then 150,000KIU/h in infusion (low-dose regimen, for noncardiac surgery); or 2,000,000KIU *i.v.* then 2,000,000KIU in CPB prime, then 500,000KIU in infusion for duration of surgery (Hammersmith high-dose regimen for cardiac surgery).

    iv. **Epsilon Aminocaproic acid** (EACA) 0.1g/kg *i.v.* over 30-60 min then 8-24g/day or 1g every 4 hours. When bleeding stops, 1g 6 hourly. Same dosage can be given *p.o.*

    v. **Desmopressin** (1 –deamino-8-D-arginine vasopressin or DDAVP) 0.3µg/kg *i.v.* or *s.c.* x2 periop, second dose 6-8 hours after the first; or 2 intranasal "standard puffs" totaling 300µg for home use (e.g. menorrhagia), repeated as necessary after 8-12 hours.

    vi. **Recombinant Factor VIIa** 90µg/kg *i.v.*, repeat dose every 2-3 hours or as needed.

    vii. Somatostatin

    viii. Vasopressin

    ix. **Misoprostol** 600 µg *p.o.* to prevent postpartum hemorrhage

c. **Non-invasive monitoring** such as pulse oximetry, whenever possible, minimizes blood loss.

d. **Restriction of diagnostic phlebotomies** reduces blood wastage. **Microsampling** is a recent technique that drastically reduces the volume of blood needed for tests, with obvious benefits in blood conservation.

e. **Intraoperative strategies** that could be employed to reduce blood loss include:

    i. **Normothermia** averts coagulopathy due to hypothermia,[1, 4, 35] and may be achieved by

        1. Maintaining room temperature above 27⁰ C

        2. Thermal suits or blankets

        3. Warming of intravenous infusions

    ii. **Acute Normovolemic Hemodilution (ANH)** involves withdrawal of some of the patient's blood in the operating room prior to incision, and replacement with colloids and/or crystalloids, so that intraoperatively the patient loses dilute blood with less effect on the total red cell mass. The withdrawn blood is kept within view in the operating room and is re-infused at the end of surgery.

    Up to 4 units may be withdrawn safely using the formula $V = [Baseline\ HCT – Target\ HCT]/Average\ HCT \times EBV$. (V = volume, HCT = hematocrit, EBV = estimated blood volume).[36]

    iii. **Regional anesthesia** results in less intraoperative blood loss than general anesthesia through mechanisms not yet fully elucidated.[4]

    iv. **Positioning** of patients to minimise blood loss is guided by two principles:[2]

        1. Elevate the operation site above the right atrium e.g. Trendelenburg for prostatectomy, reverse Trendelenburg for thyroidectomy;

        2. Avoid compression of venous drainage e.g. tilting patient in supine position slightly to the left to avoid compression of inferior vena cava in abdominal surgery.

    v. **Meticulous hemostasis** and good operative technique can save up to 1 or more units of blood.[1] Simple techniques like Pringle's manoeuvre in liver surgery and B-lynch suture in postpartum haemorrhage can be employed to great benefit. Use of diathermy and topical adhesives like fibrin glue and Surgicel® (Johnson & Johnson, Somerville, NJ, USA) limits blood loss, as does judicious use of tourniquet. Argon

Beam Coagulator and Cavitron Ultrasonic Surgical Aspirator (CUSA) are blood conserving innovations in hemostasis and dissection respectively.[1, 4, 37]

vi. **Cell salvage and autotransfusion** can be performed effectively by techniques ranging from simple manual scooping of blood from a wound, filtration then re-infusion, to use of sophisticated computerized cell salvage machines that return washed blood into the patient.

vii. **Laparoscopic surgery** and **interventional radiology** can effectively reduce blood loss in many surgical procedures.

viii. Other techniques like **controlled hypotension** and **hypothermia** may be used cautiously in selected patients.[2, 4]

Options	Number of Units of blood conserved
Preoperative	
Tolerance of anemia (lowering the transfusion trigger)	1-2
Increasing preoperative RBC mass	2
Intraoperative	
Meticulous hemostasis and operative technique	1 or more
ANH	1-2
Blood salvage	1 or more
Postoperative	
Restricted phlebotomy	1
Blood salvage	1

Table 3. Approximate contributions of selected modalities to blood conservation in the surgical patient *(adapted from Goodnough et al, 2003[1])*

3.3 Optimizing tissue oxygenation

This principle is often omitted from the "pillars" of BMS or Patient Blood Management.[6, 7] Nevertheless, it can be deduced as a separate and indispensable element since tissue oxygenation is the major function of blood.

Many clinicians transfuse blood in the hope of improving the patient's tissue oxygenation. However, allogeneic blood transfusion has been shown not to improve but to decrease tissue oxygenation.[27-29] Rather, tissue oxygenation can be improved by other methods avoiding blood transfusion by considering the equation for oxygen delivery:[38] $DO_2 = CO$ x $CaO_2 = CO$ x $\{(Hb$ x SaO_2 x $1.39) + (PaO_2$ x $0.003)\}$. (DO_2 = oxygen delivery, CO = cardiac output, CaO_2 = arterial O_2 content, Hb = hemoglobin concentration, SaO_2 = fraction of hemoglobin saturated with O_2, PaO_2 = partial pressure of O_2 dissolved in arterial blood). Thus, even when Hb is low, DO_2 can be improved by improving the CO and CaO_2 (SaO_2 and PaO_2).

a. **Volume replacement** with crystalloids (e.g. normal saline and Ringer's lactate) or colloids (e.g. Hetastarch, Hemacel®, Dextran, and Isoplasma®) reduces blood viscosity and improves cardiac output. Crystalloid requirement is 3 times blood volume lost, while colloid requirement is equivalent to volume lost and is therefore preferable when there is danger of circulatory overload with crystalloids.

b. **Oxygen therapy** increases SaO_2 and PaO_2. Intraoperative hyperoxic ventilation not only improves tissue oxygenation but also can augment ANH and avert allogeneic blood transfusion.[2, 4] Hyperbaric oxygen is rarely needed but may be used when indicated and available.[2, 4]

c. **Minimizing oxygen consumption** may be achieved through appropriate interventions such as:
    i.   Adequate analgesia
    ii. Treatment of sepsis
    iii. Mechanical ventilation (to reduce the work of breathing)

d. **Treating causes of tissue hypoxia** promptly e.g. pneumonia, bronchial asthma.

e. **Inotropic and vasoactive agents** may be used in extreme cases to improve cardiac output. Low dose dopamine (2-5µg/kg/minute) also improves renal perfusion, but higher doses cause vasoconstriction.

f. **Artificial Oxygen carriers** are still largely experimental. They include Perflourocarbon emulsions and modified hemoglobin-based solutions. They have been used successfully in Augmented ANH (A-ANH).[2, 4]

3.4 Lowering the transfusion trigger (tolerance of anemia)

Lowering the 'transfusion trigger' means accepting lower hemoglobin/hematocrit levels for treatment without blood transfusion. The "10/30" (hemoglobin/hematocrit) transfusion trigger employed for decades to dictate blood transfusion practices was based on a study in dogs by Adams and Lundy in 1942, and has been demonstrated not to be valid in humans. Lowering the transfusion trigger from 10g/dl to 7g/dl in critically ill patients in intensive care reduced red cell unit transfusions by 54% and improved clinical outcomes.[2, 20]

The Association of Anaesthetists of Great Britain and Ireland affirms that "a haemoglobin concentration of 8-10 g.dL[-1] is a safe level even for those patients with significant cardiorespiratory disease".[39] The current guidelines of The Society of Thoracic Surgeons and the Society of Cardiovascular Anesthesiologists suggests a transfusion trigger of hemoglobin less than 7g/dL.[40] However, patients have survived with hemoglobin below 3g/dl, and so currently there is no universal transfusion trigger.[41]

4. Bloodless medicine and surgery programs

Bloodless medicine and surgery programs (BMSPs) are specialized programs offering non-blood treatment by a committed multidisciplinary staff to a wide variety of registered patients within a hospital setting. There are up to 240 of such programs worldwide.[42] Depending on the emphasis, various institutions have adopted various names for their program, such as Blood Conservation Program or Transfusion-Free Medicine Program. These programs provide the standard of care for patients without the use of allogeneic blood products. They invariably record superior results.[2]

5. Newer innovations in bloodless medicine & surgery

One of the selling points of **robotic surgery** is a drastic reduction in blood loss due to the increased precision obtainable (figure 1).

Non-invasive continuous monitoring of total hemoglobin is now possible with the Rainbow **Pulse CO-Oximeter**® by Masimo® Corporation (figure 2), licensed for use in the US in 2010. This is of great advantage during certain types of surgeries traditionally associated with much blood loss like cardiac surgery, liver surgery, and in monitoring ANH.

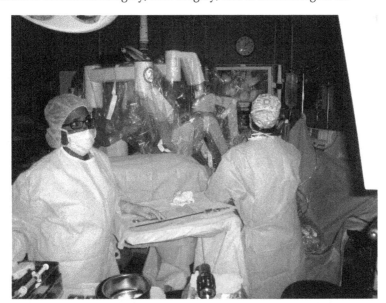

Fig. 1. Robotic surgery

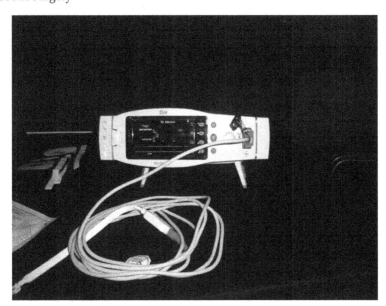

Fig. 2. Pulse CO-Oximeter®

Thromboelastometry during cardiac surgery, liver transplantation and other similar surgeries has greatly reduced transfusion rates.[43, 44] It monitors the coagulation status of the patient and greatly minimizes undue intervention with blood products.

Plasmajet® by Plasma Surgical Limited is the product of newer technology for hemostasis during surgery (figure 3). It works in a similar manner to the argon beam coagulator.

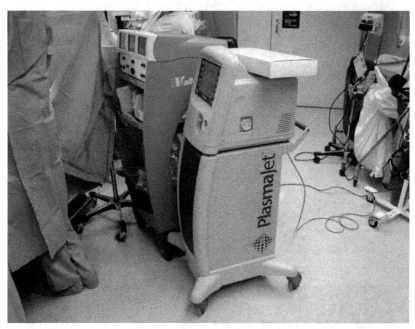

Fig. 3. Plasmajet®

6. The future of bloodless medicine and surgery

BMS is evidence-based.[7] It results in faster recovery, lower morbidity, lower mortality, shorter hospital stay, lower cost and better patient (and physician) satisfaction.[1, 2] Furthermore, patient autonomy is respected and the hazards of allogeneic blood transfusion are avoided, in accordance with the principles of nonmaleficence and beneficence in the Hippocratic Oath.[7, 41, 45] Understandably then, BMS is no longer an 'alternative' but the current standard of care.[4] BMS may also be considered a crucial step in the journey towards universal ethical, scientific, and evidence-based practice of medicine.

The Government of Western Australia is the first in the world to implement Patient Blood Management as an official policy starting from 2008.[7] In 2010 the 63rd World Health Assembly of the World Health Organization officially recognized and adopted the "pillars" of Patient Blood Management.[6] BMS is obviously therefore the universal standard of future ethical practice of medicine, having survived prejudice and being propelled by scientific evidence.

Blood conservation in BMS is not 'a technique' but a combination of techniques tailored to the needs and physiological status of the individual patient in order to avoid transfusion of allogeneic blood. It requires planning and a multidisciplinary team approach, but usually little technology, to achieve the best results. Setting up a BMSP with written protocols, standardizes the practice of bloodless medicine and surgery, thus ensuring that patients receive the best care.

7. Acknowledgments

My sincere thanks go to my dear friend, Dr Anton Camprubi, for his kind encouragement and assistance with the literature review, and for presenting me with a copy of the book *Basics of Blood Management* which makes it easy for me to write on this subject. My heartfelt appreciation also goes to Professor Nadey S. Hakim, past World President of the International College of Surgeons, for presenting me with copies of his books *Hemostasis in Surgery* and *Surgical Complications,* from which I drew some of the information herein.

I am greatly indebted to Professor Aryeh Shander, Dr David Moskowitz, Sherri Ozawa-Morriello, surgeons, anesthesiologists, and members of staff of Englewood Hospital, New Jersey, USA, where I have been repeatedly accepted as a visiting clinician/volunteer in the Bloodless Medicine and Surgery Program. Shannon Farmer, Axel Hoffman, James Reynolds and other members of the Society for the Advancement of Blood Management have also provided me much information on Bloodless Surgery, and encouragement to practice and teach it, for which I am thankful. I appreciate the invaluable institutional support of University of Calabar Teaching Hospital and University of Calabar, Calabar, Nigeria.

8. References

[1] Goodnough LT, Shander A, Spence R. Bloodless medicine: clinical care without allogeneic blood transfusion. *Transfusion* 2003; 43: 668-676.

[2] Martyn V, Farmer SL, Wren MN, Towler SCB, Betta J, Shander A, Spence RK, Leahy MF. The theory and practice of bloodless surgery. *Transfusion and Apheresis Science* 2002; 27: 29-43.

[3] Usoro NI. Blood conservation in surgery: current concepts and practice. *Int Surg* 2011; 96: 28-34.

[4] Seeber P, Shander A. *Basics of blood management.* New York, NY: Blackwell Publishing, 2007.

[5] Shander A, Waters AH. Committee on Blood Management: Developments in Patient Blood Management. *ASA Newsletter* June 2011; 75 (6): 30-32.

[6] Availability, safety, and quality of blood products. *63rd World Health Assembly (WHA 63.12)* WHO, Geneva, Switzerland, May 2010.

[7] Spahn DR, Moch H, Hofmann A, Isbister JP. Patient blood management: the pragmatic solution for the problems with blood transfusions. *Anesthesiology* 2008; 109 (6): 951-953.

[8] Curtis P. Family practice history: bloodletting. *Can Fam Physician* 1981; 27: 1030-1032.

[9] Haas LF. Emil Theodore Kocher (1841-1917). *J Neurol Neurosurg Psychiatry* 2000 ; 69 (2):171.

[10] The History of Blood Transfusion Medicine. *Bloodbook.com* 2005.
      http://www.bloodbook.com/trans-history.html

[11] Kickler TS. Blood conservation and transfusion alternatives: introduction. In: *Blood Conservation and Transfusion Alternatives: Educational Satellite Symposium Syllabus of the 28th World Congress of the International Society of Hematology,* Toronto, Ontario, Canada, 2000.

[12] Spence RK. Brief history of bloodless medicine and surgery. In: *Transfusion medicine and alternatives to blood transfusion* 2000.
      http://www.nataonline.com/index.php?NumArticle=71

[13] *How can blood save your life?* Brooklyn, NY: Watchtower Bible and Tract Society, 1990.

[14] Gohel MS,Bulbulia RA, Slim FJ, Poskitt KR, Whyman MR. How to approach major surgery where patients refuse blood transfusion (including Jehovah's Witnesses). *Ann R Coll Surg Engl* 2005; 87: 3-14.

[15] Ott DA, Cooley DA. Cardiovascular surgery in Jehovah's Witnesses: report of 542 operations without blood transfusion. *JAMA* 1977; 238 (12): 1256-8.

[16] Kitchen AD, Barbara JAJ. Current information on the infectious risks of allogeneic blood transfusion. *Transfusion Alternatives in Transfusion Medicine* 2008; 10: 102-111.

[17] Hendrickson JE, Hillyer CD. Noninfectious serious hazards of transfusion. *Anesth Analg* 2009; 108: 759-69.

[18] Hérbert PC, Wells G, Blajchman MA, et al. A multicenter, randomized, controlled clinical trial of transfusion requirements in critical care: transfusion requirements in critical care investigators, Canadian Critical Care Trials Group. *N Engl J Med.* 1999; 340: 409-417.

[19] Marik PE, Corwin HL. Efficacy of red blood cell transfusion in the critically ill: a systematic review of the literature. *Crit Care Med* 2008; 36 (9): 2667-2674.

[20] Surgenor SD, Kramer RS, Olmstead EM, et al. The Association of Perioperative Red Blood Cell Transfusions and Decreased Long-Term Survival After Cardiac Surgery. *Anesth Analg* 2009; 108: 1741-6.

[21] Bernard AC, Davenport DL, Chang PK, Vaughan TB, Zwischenberger JB. Intraoperative Transfusion of 1 U to 2 U Packed Red Blood Cells Is Associated with Increased 30-Day Mortality, Surgical-Site Infection, Pneumonia, and Sepsis in General Surgery Patients. *J Am Coll Surg* 2009; 208: 931-937.

[22] Sadjadi J, Cureton EL, Twomey P, Victorino GP. Transfusion, Not Just Injury Severity, Leads to Posttrauma Infection: A Matched Cohort Study. *The American Surgeon* 2009; 75: 307-312.

[23] Atzil S, Arad M, Glasner A, et al. Blood Transfusion Promotes Cancer Progression: A Critical Role for Aged Erythrocytes. *Anesthesiology* 2008; 109: 989–97.

[24] Stone TJ, Riesenman PJ, Charles AG. Red blood cell transfusion within the first 24 hours of admission is associated with increased mortality in the pediatric trauma population: a retrospective cohort study. *Journal of Trauma Management & Outcomes* 2008, 2:9.

[25] Reinhart WH, Zehnder L, Schulzki T. Stored erythrocytes have less capacity than normal erythrocytes to support primary haemostasis. *Thromb Haemost* 2009; 101: 720–723.

[26] Frenzela T, Westphal-Vargheseb B, Westphal M. Role of storage time of red blood cells on microcirculation and tissue oxygenation in critically ill patients. *Curr Opin Anaesthesiol* 2009; 22: 275–280.

[27] Reynolds JD, Ahearn GS, Angelo M, et al. S-nitrosohemoglobin deficiency: A mechanism for loss of physiological activity in banked blood. *Proc Natl Acad Sci* 2007; 104 (43): 17058-17062.

[28] Bennett-Guerrero E, Veldman TH, Doctor A, et al. Evolution of adverse changes in stored RBCs *Proc Natl Acad Sci* 2007; 104 (43): 17063-17068.

[29] Marik PE, Sibbald WJ. Effect of stored-blood transfusion on oxygen delivery in patients with sepsis. *JAMA* 1993; 269: 3024-3029.

[30] Rawn J. The silent risks of blood transfusion. *Curr Opin Anaesthesiol* 2008; 21: 664-668.

[31] Beris P. The use of iron to increase red cell mass. *Can J Anesth* 2003; 50 (6): S3-S9.

[32] Usoro NI, Asuquo MI, Ebughe GA, Ilori IU. Blood conservation in breast cancer care in a resource-poor setting. *POS-A357, UICC World Cancer Congress* 2008. Geneva, Switzerland.

[33] Arbuckle RB, Griffith NL, Iacovelli LM, Johnson PE, Jorgenson JA, Kloth DD, Lucarelli CD, Muller RJ. Continued Challenges with the Use of Erythropoiesis-Stimulating Agents in Patients with Cancer: Perspectives and Issues on Policy-Guided Health Care. *Pharmacotherapy* 2008; 28 (5 Pt 2): 1S-15S.

[34] Goodnough LT. The use of erythropoietin to increase red cell mass. *Can J Anesth* 2003; 50 (6): S10-S18.

[35] Ozier Y, Lentschener C. Non-pharmacological approaches to decrease surgical blood loss. *Can J Anesth* 2003; 50 (6): S19-S25.

[36] Loubser P. Acute normovolemic hemodilution. *NoBlood.org* 2009.
http://www.noblood.org/content/142-acute_normovolemic_hemodilution

[37] Pai M, Canelo R, Habib N. Haemostasis in Liver Surgery. In: Hakim NS, Canelo R (eds). *Hemostasis in Surgery*. London: Imperial College Press, 2007: 153-164.

[38] Henny CP, Trouwborst A. Physiology of acute vs chronic anemia. *Can J Anesth* 2003; 50 (6): S48-S52.

[39] *Blood Transfusion and the Anaesthetist: Red Cell Transfusion.* London, UK: The Association of Anaesthetists of Great Britain and Ireland, 2008.
http://www.aagbi.org/sites/default/files/red_cell_08.pdf

[40] The Society of Thoracic Surgeons Blood Conservation Guideline Task Force, Ferraris VA, Ferraris SP, Saha SP, Hessel EA 2nd, Haan CK, Royston BD, Bridges CR, Higgins RS, Despotis G, Brown JR; Society of Cardiovascular Anesthesiologists Special Task Force on Blood Transfusion, Spiess BD, Shore-Lesserson L, Stafford-Smith M, Mazer CD, Bennett-Guerrero E, Hill SE, Body S. Perioperative Blood Transfusion and Blood Conservation in Cardiac Surgery: The Society of Thoracic Surgeons and The Society of Cardiovascular Anesthesiologists Clinical Practice Guideline. *Ann Thorac Surg* 2007; 83: S27– 86.

[41] Spence RK. Current Concepts and Issues in Blood Management. *Orthopedics.* 2004; 27 (6 Suppl): s643-51.

[42] Bloodless Hospitals. www.mybloodsite.com 2009.

[43] Goerlinger K. Reduction of blood transfusion rate by point-of-care coagulation management in liver transplantation, visceral, and cardiac surgery. *International Forum on Quality and Safety in Healthcare.* Berlin. Mar. 2009.

[44] Anderson L, Quasim I, Soutar R, Steven M, Macfie A, Korte W. An audit of red blood cell and blood product use after the institution of thromboelastometry in a cardiac intensive care unit. *Transfusion Medicine* 2006; 16: 31-39.

[45] Mansell VJ, Mansell MA. Medico-Legal Issues. In: Hakim NS, Papalois VE (eds). *Surgical Complications.* London: Imperial College Press, 2007: 953-977.

13

Impact of Acute Normovolemic Hemodilution in Organ and Cell Structure

D.A. Otsuki, D.T. Fantoni and J.O.C. Auler Junior
LIM08-Anesthesiology, Faculdade de Medicina da Universidade de São Paulo
Brazil

1. Introduction

Rigorous control procedures adopted presently by blood banks have reduced transfusion-associated risks, such as transmission of infectious diseases. Nevertheless, other complications related with blood-transfusions remain, such as transfusion-related acute lung injury (TRALI) and other immune disorders. In critically ill patients, transfusion has been associated with increase in morbidity and mortality, so that restrictive transfusion strategies have been proposed, which have reduced incidence of organ dysfunction as well as of other complications (Hajjar et al., 2010; Hebert et al., 1999).

In order to reduce or even avoid the need for transfusions in surgeries involving massive blood-loss, alternatives such as tolerance of lower hemoglobin levels or use of acute normovolemic hemodilution (ANH) have been considered. However, both strategies involve reduction of arterial oxygen content and alteration of rheological blood properties, which can affect oxygen delivery to organs and tissues. Acute anemia elicits a number of responses, such as decrease in vascular resistance and compensatory increases in heart rate and cardiac index (Ickx et al., 2000). These compensatory mechanisms provide maintenance of oxygen transport to tissues until a critical hemoglobin limit is reached.

When performing ANH, two important aspects that must be considered are the target hemoglobin level and the type of replacement fluid to maintain volemia. During acute anemia, oxygen content decreases and myocardial oxygen consumption increases because of increases in stroke work and heart rate (Ickx et al, 2000). Regarding the hemoglobin or hematocrit level, the main organs of concern are the heart and brain because of their high oxygen demand.

The objective of this review is to discuss the impact of acute normovolemic anemia on specific organs and tissues, focusing on experimental studies.

2. Heart tolerance to acute anemia

During acute anemia, the decrease in oxygen supply is compensated with increases in stroke index and heart rate. However, if a critical limit is reached, the heart may not be able to sustain the increased pumping requirement (Crystal et al., 1988). Although in normal conditions the heart is capable of tolerating extreme hemodilution, moderate anemia can jeopardize myocardial oxygenation and contractility in specific patients, particularly in those with coronary artery disease. Therefore the detection of early signs of inadequate oxygen delivery is of paramount importance and, for this reason, cardiac tolerance to ANH has been extensively investigated. Cardiovascular function monitoring as well as systemic and regional markers of hypoxia have been used to identify critical oxygen delivery (Diebel et al., 2000; Mekontso-Dessap et al., 2002; Torres Filho et al., 2005). Conventional hemodynamic monitoring is a poor means to detect early cellular oxygen deprivation. Alterations in ECG, increases in lactate levels and hemodynamic instability occur only after tissue hypoxia has ensued. In healthy human volunteers, acute anemia (hemoglobin 5-7g/dL) promoted signs that were suggestive but not conclusive of myocardial ischemia, as evaluated by ECG ST-segment changes (Leung et al., 2000).

Few studies have addressed the effect of hemodilution in patients with cardiovascular diseases. A study demonstrated that ANH to a mean hemoglobin value of 8.6 g/dL was well tolerated in anesthetized patients with coronary artery disease who were receiving beta-blockers. These patients presented no ECG abnormalities or hemodynamic instability (Licker et al., 2004). A recent study comparing transfusion strategies in 512 patients, submitted to cardiac surgery, found that a restrictive strategy, defined as a transfusion performed when the hematocrit reached values of $\geq 24\%$, was as safe as the liberal strategy, defined as hematocrit $\geq 30\%$. The resulting mean hemoglobin values were 9.1 g/dL and 10.5 g/dL for the restrictive and liberal groups, respectively (Hajjar et al, 2010).

Except for few reports involving Jehovah's Witnesses patients (Gutierrez & Brotherton, 2011; Hashem & Dillard, 2004), data concerning use of exceedingly low hematocrit or hemoglobin thresholds derive from experimental studies. Such studies, performed with different species and various situations, demonstrated critical hematocrit levels between 10 and 15% (Fraga et al., 2005; Hiebl et al., 2010; van Bommel et al., 2002). In a study performed with dogs submitted to continuous hemodilution with lactated Ringer's solution, a decrease in heart function (ejection fraction and fractional shortening) was observed when hemoglobin levels reached 3.5 g/dL. Also, at this hemoglobin level, oxygen delivery decreased to the point of impairing oxygen consumption (Fraga et al, 2005).

In a recent study, a critical hematocrit of 10% was determined for the pig myocardium. Lower levels resulted in insufficient myocardial partial oxygen pressure and circulatory collapse (Hiebl et al , 2010). In all of these studies, the critical hematocrit was identified only after the observation of signs of global hypoxia, as represented by hemodynamic instability, cardiac arrhythmias and/or increase in lactate levels. However, in another experimental study, hemoglobin levels of 4-5 g/dL were associated with changes in heart rate variability (HRV), obtained by time- and frequency-domain analysis of ECG data, but ST-segment changes were not observed until a mean hemoglobin level of 3 g/dL, at which point oxygen consumption also decreased (Lauscher et al., 2011) . Other ECG changes not related to the ST-segment were observed in another experimental study by the same group, in which ANH induced gradual prolongation of the QT and QTc interval and reduction in the amplitude of the T wave (Scheller et al., 2011). In both studies, early ECG alterations were observed in the absence of traditional transfusion triggers, such as increase in serum lactate levels, elevation of the ST-segment or arrhythmias. The determination of early indicators of tissue hypoxia is very important to help establish safe limits for ANH.

In spite of these results, it is necessary to consider that most studies involving ANH were performed in young, healthy and anesthetized animals. Anesthesia may induce changes in tolerance to anemia by lowering oxygen comsumption and the critical hematocrit or suppressing compensatory mechanisms (Fantoni et al., 2005; Tircoveanu & Van der Linden, 2008).

The effect of anesthesia depth on hemodilution was shown in a study performed with dogs, in which increase of anesthesia depth either with halothane (from 1.0 to 1.5 MAC) or ketamine (from 0.2 to 0.4 mg/kg/min) resulted in decreased tolerance to acute anemia, with significant increase in critical hemoglobin concentration (from 2.3 to 4.1 g/dL with halothane and 2.5 to 3.7 g/dL with ketamine) (Van der Linden et al., 2003). As previously stated, decreases in arterial oxygen content caused by ANH are compensated by increases in cardiac output. This compensatory response may be blunted depending on the anesthetic protocol. High doses of negative inotropic agents may also blunt the cardiac output response by direct depression of the myocardial function. (Van der Linden et al, 2003). Cardiac output also depends on heart rate which may be affected by drugs such as opioids, which induce vagal stimulation, or β-adrenergic antagonists, which impair the expected cardiac response (Clarke et al., 1980; Ickx, 2000; Ragoonanan et al., 2009; Spahn et al., 1997). Even equipotent MACs of different inhalational anesthetics may induce different hemodynamic responses to ANH. Hemodilution performed in dogs anesthetized with 1 MAC of halothane, isoflurane or sevoflurane had the same pattern of hemodynamic response, though differences in oxygen consumption and oxygen extraction rate were observed among groups (Fantoni et al, 2005).

Ventilation and oxygenation also impact tolerance to anemia. A simple example involves hyperoxic ventilation. Ventilation with 21% oxygen induced ECG changes associated with ischemia at hemoglobin levels of 2.3 ± 0.2 g/dL. When increased to 100% oxygen, ECG readings improved until hemoglobin levels of 1.2 ± 0.4 g/dL were reached (Meier et al., 2005).

3. Impact of ANH on brain

Reduction in oxygen transport may lead to tissue hypoxia, and this may bear important consequences to the brain, including cognitive dysfunction. Available data regarding safe hematocrit levels for the nervous system derive mostly from experimental studies and a few clinical studies that associate anemia with neurological outcome after cardiopulmonary bypass (Hare et al., 2007). In healthy young human subjects, ANH to hemoglobin of 5.7 g/dL elicited subtle cognitive dysfunction and memory deficits that were reversible with erythrocyte transfusion or increase in oxygen concentration (Weiskopf et al., 2002). Such effects seem to be worse in aged patients, given the greater incidence of cognitive dysfunction in this population (Moller et al., 1998). This hypothesis was demonstrated in an experimental study by Li et al (2010), who showed the association between acute anemia (i.e. hemoglobin 5 g/dL) and age-dependent visual-spatial working memory and learning impairment in rats. They also showed an increase in hypoxia-inducible factor (HIF) and related molecular markers of cellular hypoxia, in the presence of normal systemic and local cerebral tissue oxygenation, which was more evident in older animals (Li et al., 2010).

In an ongoing experimental study with healthy pigs, cerebral cortex and hippocampus neuronal apoptosis proteins Bax and Bcl-x, as well as caspase-3 and -9 activities, presented no alterations during ANH to hematocrit 15% or 10%. However, a slight increase in cerebral nuclear and mitochondrial DNA fragmentation was observed, indicating possible cellular hypoxia (Frazilio et al., 2011).

The disagreement among results regarding different molecular markers of cellular hypoxia and global or even tissue oxygen parameters point out the difficulty in diagnosing hypoxia during hemodilution. Hemodilution may lead to decreased microvascular oxygen tension (PO2) and increased expression of hypoxic molecules (iNOS, nNOS, HIF) in the absence of lactate level increase or of hemodynamic instability. However more studies are necessary to determine whether these are sensitive and effective markers for early detection of hypoxia (Tsui et al., 2010).

For traumatic brain injury (TBI), higher hematocrit levels have been proposed. In the normal subject, ANH induces a redistribution of blood flow that favors brain oxygenation (Ragoonanan et al, 2009; van Bommel et al, 2002). However, such changes in the setting of TBI may bear deleterious effects. A reduction in hematocrit below 30% may promote an increase in intracranial pressure and a consequent decrease in cerebral perfusion. In a dog model of cryogenic brain injury, decrease in hematocrit to 27% by hemodilution with lactated Ringer's or hydroxyethyl starch was associated with additional increase in intracranial pressure and decrease in cerebral perfusion. In contrast, animals submitted to ANH with target hematocrit 35% had a response similar to the non-hemodiluted animals (Tango et al., 2009).

In an experimental study with rats, Hare et al (2007) demonstrated that hemodilution following TBI could accentuate cerebral injury. Although regional cerebral blood flow had increased similarly in healthy and TBI rats after ANH, the TBI-hemodilution group presented with decrease in brain tissue oxygenation and increase in jugular vein oxygen saturation, indicating impairment in oxygen extraction. This group also showed an increase in cerebral contusion area and greater cell death (TUNEL-positive cells) (Hare et al, 2007).

4. The impact of fluid replacement on tissues

As with other clinical situations that require fluid replacement (e.g. hemorrhagic shock, sepsis), the choice of fluids to maintain normovolemia during ANH is a subject of great controversy. Critical hemoglobin levels are expected to vary according to the type of fluid employed. In an experimental study with dogs submitted to ANH, volume replacement with 6% hydroxyethyl starch 200/0.5 maintained heart contractility at hematocrit levels as low as 10%, while replacement with lactated Ringer's to the same target yielded significant decrease in contractility, with reduction in systolic function, as defined by ejection and shortening fractions. Furthermore, analysis of the myocardial ultrastructure revealed loss in its cellular integrity in the group treated with lactated Ringer's solution (Fraga et al, 2005).

The infusion of large amounts of acellular fluids promotes important circulatory changes, such as reduction in blood viscosity and alteration in osmolality and oncotic pressure. Such properties determine the period for which the fluid remains within the intravascular space, which impacts maintenance of stroke volume and of cardiac output directly. Likewise, fluid extravasation from the intravascular space may lead to edema. Great variations in osmolality may have deleterious effects on cell homeostasis. Cardiomyocyte swelling after hypotonic stress has been demonstrated *in vitro* (Butler et al., 2009; Mizutani et al., 2005). Butler and cols. have demonstrated that ischemia may also induce cardiac myocyte swelling (Butler et al, 2009). Cardiac myocyte edema may affect ventricular compliance, thereby compromising cardiac function (Rubboli et al., 1994).

In an ANH protocol using lactated Ringer´s to a target hematocrit of 15%, cardiac function was preserved and no microscopic evidence of myocardial cell injury or edema was found, but ultrastructure analysis revealed disorganization of myofibrils and myofilaments (Otsuki et al., 2007). The observation of such structural alteration only in the crystalloid group points to the possibility that osmolarity and coloidosmotic pressure must be involved in the process. In a similar study by our group, with the same ANH protocol, a significant decrease in serum osmolarity (from 298 ± 4.0 to 279.5 ±2.1 mOsm/kgH2O) was observed with lactated Ringer's (Margarido et al., 2007).

The lung is one of the main organs affected by the administration of large quantities of fluids. Since crystalloids bear smaller permanence within the intravascular space, these solutions leaks out of the circulation into the tissues or interstitial space and may lead to lung impairment with decrease in lung compliance, atelectasis and even the development of alveolar edema. Data regarding the effects of ANH on lungs are mostly based on cardiopulmonary bypass studies. In such scenario, hemodilution and inflammatory response are associated with capillary leak and edema in different organs, including the lungs (Hirleman & Larson, 2008).

In pigs submitted to ANH with lactated Ringer´s to hematocrit 15%, lung microscopy showed areas of alveolar collapse while ventilatory mechanics and oxygenation parameters presented diminished lung compliance with decrease in PaO_2/FIO_2 ratio and increases in Qs/Qt and dead space. Ultra-structurally, there was enlargement of the alveolar basement membrane, which may explain the observed decrease in arterial oxygenation. Conversely, ANH with hydroxyethyl starch preserved pulmonary mechanics and oxygenation (Margarido et al, 2007).

Another ANH study with dogs using Lactated Ringer´s to hematocrit 10% showed an increase in lung water content as evaluated by presence of fluid in the peribronchial space and by gravimetric analysis. The restoration of oncotic pressure by albumin administration reversed these alterations (Cooper et al., 1975).

Different fluids may also affect microcirculation differently. Recent studies have demonstrated that even with maintenance of systemic perfusion variables (cardiac index, arterial blood pressure), decrease in blood viscosity may result in impairment of microcirculatory function (Cabrales & Tsai, 2006; Cabrales et al., 2004; Tsai et al., 1998).

This effect of blood viscosity on the microcirculation was demonstrated by Cabrales et al, who used a hamster window chamber model. Extreme ANH to a final hematocrit of 11% was performed with high- (dextran 500) or low-viscosity (dextran 70) plasma expanders. The maintenance of blood viscosity promoted by dextran 500 was associated with maintenance of microvascular capillary diameter, flow and functional capillary density whereas with dextran 70 it was observed an impairment of microvascular hemodynamics (Cabrales & Tsai, 2006).

An additional important aspect regarding ANH pertain the effect of fluid choice on the immune system. The effects of different fluids on immune system response have been demonstrated *in vitro* and *in vivo* studies during sepsis, hemorrhagic shock and hemodilution. The activation of the inflammatory system following massive fluid resuscitation is intimately related to negative outcomes (Cotton et al., 2006; Lee et al., 2005; Rhee et al., 1998; Welters et al., 2000). Several studies have shown divergent results because different colloids may bear pro-inflammatory (Alam et al., 2004; Lee, 2005; Rhee et al., 2000) and anti-inflammatory effects (Alam et al., 2000; Jaeger et al., 2001; Lang et al., 2003). When compared with 6% hydroxyethyl starch 200/0.5 or lactated Ringer´s, resuscitation with gelatin following hemorrhagic shock seems to exacerbate levels of interleukin-6 and TNF-α and decrease IL-10 production. Furthermore, neutrophil and mononuclear cell aggregation and important histological changes were observed in animals lungs treated with gelatin (Lee et al, 2005).

Systemic and pulmonary inflammatory effects of ANH with 6% hydroxyethyl starch 130/0.4, saline solution 0.9%, and gelatin 4% were evaluated in pigs submitted to ANH to hematocrit 15%. Gelatin was associated with increases in serum cytokines (TNF-α, Il-1, Il-6 and Il-10) and pulmonary COX-2 and E-selectin expression was higher in gelatin and hydroxyethyl starch-treated animals (Kahvegian et al., 2009; Kahvegian et al., 2010).

Endothelial activation after ANH was demonstrated by Morariu et al using real-time PCR of E- and P-selectin gene expression in different organs. Hemodilution in pigs with hydroxyethyl starch 3% (200/0.5) triggered pro-inflammatory endothelial activation as evidenced by E- and P-selectins mRNA up-regulation in the lung and other tissues (Morariu et al., 2006).

5. Conclusion

In particular settings, ANH has been proposed as an alternative to blood transfusion. However, safe limits for this procedure have not been properly established, and hypoxia remains a major concern, particularly for its effect on the heart and brain. Proper markers must be identified to monitor the effects of critical levels of hemoglobin in the various clinical settings and further studies must be conducted before ANH may be implemented in daily medical practice.

6. References

Alam, H.B., Stanton K., Koustova E., Burris D., Rich N. & Rhee P. (2004).Effect of different resuscitation strategies on neutrophil activation in a swine model of hemorrhagic shock. *Resuscitation*.V.60, No. 1, pp.91-9.

Alam, H.B., Sun L., Ruff P., Austin B., Burris D. & Rhee P. (2000).E- and P-selectin expression depends on the resuscitation fluid used in hemorrhaged rats. *The Journal of Surgical Research*.V.94, No. 2, pp.145-52.

Butler, T.L., Egan J.R., Graf F.G., Au C.G., McMahon A.C., North K.N. & Winlaw D.S. (2009).Dysfunction induced by ischemia versus edema: does edema matter? *The Journal of Thoracic and Cardiovascular Surgery*.V.138, No. 1, pp.141-7, 7 e1.

Cabrales, P. & Tsai A.G. (2006).Plasma viscosity regulates systemic and microvascular perfusion during acute extreme anemic conditions. *American Journal of Physiology*.V.291, No. 5, pp.H2445-52.

Cabrales, P., Tsai A.G. & Intaglietta M. (2004).Microvascular pressure and functional capillary density in extreme hemodilution with low- and high-viscosity dextran and a low-viscosity Hb-based O2 carrier. *American Journal of Physiology*.V.287, No. 1, pp.H363-73.

Clarke, T.N., Foex P., Roberts J.G., Saner C.A. & Bennett M.J. (1980).Circulatory responses of the dog to acute isovolumic anaemia in the presence of high-grade adrenergic beta-receptor blockade. *British Journal of Anaesthesia*.V.52, No. 3, pp.337-41.

Cooper, J.D., Maeda M. & Lowenstein E. (1975).Lung water accumulation with acute hemodilution in dogs. *The Journal of Thoracic and Cardiovascular Surgery*.V.69, No. 6, pp.957-65.

Cotton, B.A., Guy J.S., Morris J.A., Jr. & Abumrad N.N. (2006).The cellular, metabolic, and systemic consequences of aggressive fluid resuscitation strategies. *Shock*.V.26, No. 2, pp.115-21.

Crystal, G.J., Rooney M.W. & Salem M.R. (1988).Regional hemodynamics and oxygen supply during isovolemic hemodilution alone and in combination with adenosine-induced controlled hypotension. *Anesthesia and Analgesia*.V.67, No. 3, pp.211-8.

Diebel, L.N., Tyburski J.G. & Dulchavsky S.A. (2000).Effect of acute hemodilution on intestinal perfusion and intramucosal pH after shock. *The Journal of Trauma*.V.49, No. 5, pp.800-5.

Fantoni, D.T., Otsuki D.A., Ambrosio A.M., Tamura E.Y. & Auler J.O., Jr. (2005).A comparative evaluation of inhaled halothane, isoflurane, and sevoflurane during acute normovolemic hemodilution in dogs. *Anesthesia and Analgesia*.V.100, No. 4, pp.1014-9.

Fraga, A.O., Fantoni D.T., Otsuki D.A., Pasqualucci C.A., Abduch M.C. & Junior J.O. (2005).Evidence for myocardial defects under extreme acute normovolemic hemodilution with hydroxyethyl starch and lactated ringer's solution. *Shock* .V.24, No. 4, pp.388-95.

Frazilio, F.D., Otsuki D.A., Ruivo J.M., Noel-Morgan J., Chadi G., Auler Junior J.C. & Fantoni D.T. Evaluation of Neuronal Apoptosis Precursors BAX, BCL-X and Activity of Caspase 3 and 9 in an Experimental Model of Acute Normovolemic Hemodilution with Target Hematocrits 10% and 15% *Proceeding of Anesthesiology 2011*; Chicago; 2011.

Gutierrez, G. & Brotherton J. (2011).Management of severe anemia secondary to menorrhagia in a Jehovah's Witness: a case report and treatment algorithm. *American journal of obstetrics and gynecology*.[Epub ahead of print].

Hajjar, L.A., Vincent J.L., Galas F.R., Nakamura R.E., Silva C.M., Santos M.H., Fukushima J., Kalil Filho R., Sierra D.B., Lopes N.H., Mauad T., Roquim A.C., Sundin M.R., Leao W.C., Almeida J.P., Pomerantzeff P.M., Dallan L.O., Jatene F.B., Stolf N.A. & Auler J.O., Jr. (2010).Transfusion requirements after cardiac surgery: the TRACS randomized controlled trial. *JAMA*.V.304, No. 14, pp.1559-67.

Hare, G.M., Mazer C.D., Hutchison J.S., McLaren A.T., Liu E., Rassouli A., Ai J., Shaye R.E., Lockwood J.A., Hawkins C.E., Sikich N., To K. & Baker A.J. (2007).Severe hemodilutional anemia increases cerebral tissue injury following acute neurotrauma. *Journal of Applied Physiology: respiratory, environmental and exercise physiology*.V.103, No. 3, pp.1021-9.

Hashem, B. & Dillard T.A. (2004).A 44-year-old Jehovah's Witness with life-threatening anemia from uterine bleeding. *Chest*.V.125, No. 3, pp.1151-4.

Hebert, P.C., Wells G., Blajchman M.A., Marshall J., Martin C., Pagliarello G., Tweeddale M., Schweitzer I. & Yetisir E. (1999).A multicenter, randomized, controlled clinical trial of transfusion requirements in critical care. Transfusion Requirements in Critical Care Investigators, Canadian Critical Care Trials Group. *The New England journal of medicine*.V.340, No. 6, pp.409-17.

Hiebl, B., Mrowietz C., Ploetze K., Matschke K. & Jung F. (2010).Critical hematocrit and oxygen partial pressure in the beating heart of pigs. *Microvascular Research*.V.80, No. 3, pp.389-93.

Hirleman, E. & Larson D.F. (2008).Cardiopulmonary bypass and edema: physiology and pathophysiology. *Perfusion*.V.23, No. 6, pp.311-22.

Ickx, B.E., Rigolet M. & Van Der Linden P.J. (2000).Cardiovascular and metabolic response to acute normovolemic anemia. Effects of anesthesia. *Anesthesiology*.V.93, No. 4, pp.1011-6.

Jaeger, K., Heine J., Ruschulte H., Juttner B., Scheinichen D., Kuse E.R. & Piepenbrock S. (2001).Effects of colloidal resuscitation fluids on the neutrophil respiratory burst. *Transfusion*.V.41, No. 8, pp.1064-8.

Kahvegian, M., Fantoni D.T., Otsuki D.A., Holms C.A., Massoco C.O. & Auler Jr J.O. COX-2 and E-selectin expression evaluation after acute normovolemic hemodilution. In: Vincent J-L, editor. *29th International Symposium on Intensive Care and Emergency Medicine*; 2009; Brussels: BioMed Central; 2009. p. 1.

Kahvegian, M., Fantoni D.T., Otsuki D.A., Holms C.A., Massoco C.O. & Auler Jr J.O. Cytokine levels evaluation during acute isovolemic anemia. In: Vincent J-L, editor. *30th International Symposium on Intensive Care and Emergency Medicine*; 2010; Brussels: BioMed Central; 2010. p. S128.

Lang, K., Suttner S., Boldt J., Kumle B. & Nagel D. (2003).Volume replacement with HES 130/0.4 may reduce the inflammatory response in patients undergoing major abdominal surgery. *Canadian journal of anaesthesia*.V.50, No. 10, pp.1009-16.

Lauscher, P., Kertscho H., Raab L., Habler O. & Meier J. (2011).Changes in heart rate variability across different degrees of acute dilutional anemia. *Minerva anestesiologica*.[Epub ahead of print].

Lee, C.C., Chang I.J., Yen Z.S., Hsu C.Y., Chen S.Y., Su C.P., Chiang W.C., Chen S.C. & Chen W.J. (2005).Effect of different resuscitation fluids on cytokine response in a rat model of hemorrhagic shock. *Shock*.V.24, No. 2, pp.177-81.

Leung, J.M., Weiskopf R.B., Feiner J., Hopf H.W., Kelley S., Viele M., Lieberman J., Watson J., Noorani M., Pastor D., Yeap H., Ho R. & Toy P. (2000).Electrocardiographic ST-segment changes during acute, severe isovolemic hemodilution in humans. *Anesthesiology*.V.93, No. 4, pp.1004-10.

Li, M., Bertout J.A., Ratcliffe S.J., Eckenhoff M.F., Simon M.C. & Floyd T.F. (2010).Acute anemia elicits cognitive dysfunction and evidence of cerebral cellular hypoxia in older rats with systemic hypertension. *Anesthesiology*.V.113, No. 4, pp.845-58.

Licker, M., Sierra J., Tassaux D. & Diaper J. (2004).Continuous haemodynamic monitoring using transoesophageal Doppler during acute normovolaemic haemodilution in patients with coronary artery disease. *Anaesthesia*.V.59, No. 2, pp.108-15.

Margarido, C.B., Margarido N.F., Otsuki D.A., Fantoni D.T., Marumo C.K., Kitahara F.R., Magalhaes A.A., Pasqualucci C.A. & Auler J.O., Jr. (2007).Pulmonary function is better preserved in pigs when acute normovolemic hemodilution is achieved with hydroxyethyl starch versus lactated Ringer's solution. *Shock*.V.27, No. 4, pp.390-6.

Meier, J., Kemming G., Meisner F., Pape A. & Habler O. (2005).Hyperoxic ventilation enables hemodilution beyond the critical myocardial hemoglobin concentration. *European Journal of Medical Research*.V.10, No. 11, pp.462-8.

Mekontso-Dessap, A., Castelain V., Anguel N., Bahloul M., Schauvliege F., Richard C. & Teboul J.L. (2002).Combination of venoarterial PCO2 difference with arteriovenous O2 content difference to detect anaerobic metabolism in patients. *Intensive Care Medicine*.V.28, No. 3, pp.272-7.

Mizutani, S., Prasad S.M., Sellitto A.D., Schuessler R.B., Damiano R.J., Jr. & Lawton J.S. (2005).Myocyte volume and function in response to osmotic stress: observations in the presence of an adenosine triphosphate-sensitive potassium channel opener. *Circulation*.V.112, No. 9 Suppl, pp.I219-23.

Moller, J.T., Cluitmans P., Rasmussen L.S., Houx P., Rasmussen H., Canet J., Rabbitt P., Jolles J., Larsen K., Hanning C.D., Langeron O., Johnson T., Lauven P.M., Kristensen P.A., Biedler A., van Beem H., Fraidakis O., Silverstein J.H., Beneken J.E. & Gravenstein J.S. (1998).Long-term postoperative cognitive dysfunction in the elderly ISPOCD1 study. ISPOCD investigators. International Study of Post-Operative Cognitive Dysfunction. *Lancet*.V.351, No. 9106, pp.857-61.

Morariu, A.M., Maathuis M.H., Asgeirsdottir S.A., Leuvenink H.G., Boonstra P.W., van Oeveren W., Ploeg R.J., Molema I. & Rakhorst G. (2006).Acute isovolemic hemodilution triggers proinflammatory and procoagulatory endothelial activation in vital organs: role of erythrocyte aggregation. *Microcirculation*.V.13, No. 5, pp. 397-409.

Otsuki, D.A., Fantoni D.T., Margarido C.B., Marumo C.K., Intelizano T., Pasqualucci C.A. & Costa Auler J.O., Jr. (2007).Hydroxyethyl starch is superior to lactated Ringer as a replacement fluid in a pig model of acute normovolaemic haemodilution. *BritishJournal of Anaesthesia*.V.98, No. 1, pp.29-37.

Ragoonanan, T.E., Beattie W.S., Mazer C.D., Tsui A.K., Leong-Poi H., Wilson D.F., Tait G., Yu J., Liu E., Noronha M., Dattani N.D., Mitsakakis N. & Hare G.M. (2009).Metoprolol reduces cerebral tissue oxygen tension after acute hemodilution in rats. *Anesthesiology*.V.111, No. 5, pp.988-1000.

Rhee, P., Burris D., Kaufmann C., Pikoulis M., Austin B., Ling G., Harviel D. & Waxman K. (1998).Lactated Ringer's solution resuscitation causes neutrophil activation after hemorrhagic shock. *The Journal of Trauma*.V.44, No. 2, pp.313-9.

Rhee, P., Wang D., Ruff P., Austin B., DeBraux S., Wolcott K., Burris D., Ling G. & Sun L. (2000).Human neutrophil activation and increased adhesion by various resuscitation fluids. *Critical Care Medicine*.V.28, No. 1, pp.74-8.

Rubboli, A., Sobotka P.A. & Euler D.E. (1994).Effect of acute edema on left ventricular function and coronary vascular resistance in the isolated rat heart. *The American Journal of Physiology*.V.267, No. 3 Pt 2, pp.H1054-61.

Scheller, B., Pipa G., Kertscho H., Lauscher P., Ehrlich J., Habler O., Zacharowski K. & Meier J. (2011).Low hemoglobin levels during normovolemia are associated with electrocardiographic changes in pigs. *Shock*.V.35, No. 4, pp.375-81.

Spahn, D.R., Seifert B., Pasch T. & Schmid E.R. (1997).Effects of chronic beta-blockade on compensatory mechanisms during acute isovolaemic haemodilution in patients with coronary artery disease. *British Journal of Anaesthesia*.V.78, No. 4, pp.381-5.

Tango, H.K., Schmidt A.P., Mizumoto N., Lacava M., Cruz R.J., Jr. & Auler J.O., Jr. (2009).Low hematocrit levels increase intracranial pressure in an animal model of cryogenic brain injury. *The Journal of Trauma*.V.66, No. 3, pp.720-6.

Tircoveanu, R. & Van der Linden P. (2008).Hemodilution and anemia in patients with cardiac disease: what is the safe limit? *Current Opinion in Anaesthesiology*.V.21, No. 1, pp.66-70.

Torres Filho, I.P., Spiess B.D., Pittman R.N., Barbee R.W. & Ward K.R. (2005).Experimental analysis of critical oxygen delivery. *American Journal of Physiology*.V.288, No. 3, pp.H1071-9.

Tsai, A.G., Friesenecker B., McCarthy M., Sakai H. & Intaglietta M. (1998).Plasma viscosity regulates capillary perfusion during extreme hemodilution in hamster skinfold model. *The American Journal of Physiology*.V.275, No. 6 Pt 2, pp.H2170-80.

Tsui, A.K., Dattani N.D., Marsden P.A., El-Beheiry M.H., Grocott H.P., Liu E., Biro G.P., Mazer C.D. & Hare G.M. (2010).Reassessing the risk of hemodilutional anemia: Some new pieces to an old puzzle. *Canadian journal of anaesthesia*.V.57, No. 8, pp.779-91.

van Bommel, J., Trouwborst A., Schwarte L., Siegemund M., Ince C. & Henny Ch P. (2002).Intestinal and cerebral oxygenation during severe isovolemic hemodilution and subsequent hyperoxic ventilation in a pig model. *Anesthesiology*.V.97, No. 3, pp.660-70.

Van der Linden, P., De Hert S., Mathieu N., Degroote F., Schmartz D., Zhang H. & Vincent J.L. (2003).Tolerance to acute isovolemic hemodilution. Effect of anesthetic depth. *Anesthesiology*.V.99, No. 1, pp.97-104.

Weiskopf, R.B., Feiner J., Hopf H.W., Viele M.K., Watson J.J., Kramer J.H., Ho R. & Toy P. (2002).Oxygen reverses deficits of cognitive function and memory and increased heart rate induced by acute severe isovolemic anemia. *Anesthesiology*.V.96, No. 4, pp.871-7.

Welters, I.D., Spangenberg U., Menzebach A., Engel J., Menges T., Langefeld T.W. & Hempelmann G. (2000).[The effect of different volume expanders on neutrophil granulocyte function in vitro]. *Der Anaesthesist*.V.49, No. 3, pp.196-201.

14

Cryopreservation of Blood

Miloš Bohoněk
Department of Hematology,
Biochemistry and Blood Transfusion,
Central Military Hospital Prague, Praha,
Czech Republic

1. Introduction

Various methods of cryopreservation of blood, especially erythrocytes, are generally known and have been used for a long time. Storage of blood in the frozen state presented one of the alternative ways of storing blood components; this possibility was intensively explored in the 1950's and 60's, when the shelf life of non-frozen red blood cells did not exceed 21 days at those times. This time limitation significantly reduced flexibility of usage of RBC products and contributed to their dramatically high and wasteful expiration reaching up to 30%. The short shelf life of the RBCs resulted in the transfusion services not being able to meet demands of quickly evolving surgical disciplines, particularly cardiovascular surgery and radical surgical oncology. In military and emergency healthcare, utilization of these three-week products as a way of creating blood supplies was even more complicated, almost unthinkable. The storage of frozen red blood cells therefore presented a great prospect.

Following the implementation of modern resuspension solutions with addition of polysaccharides, phosphates and adenine into everyday practice in the 1970's and 80's, the general emphasis on the long-term storage of erythrocytes was withdrawn into background. In many fields, the now-normal 42-day-long life virtually eliminated the need to perform further research since no more than 5 percent of the stored RBC products had to be destroyed due to expiration.

Nevertheless, some areas with a need for long-term storage of red blood cells still remained – example being the military transfusion, emergency transfusion service, storage of rare blood cells or special autostransfusion programs. In these cases, substantially higher costs of the red blood cells production are accepted (when compared to the common storage in liquid state). Blood substitution and blood supply is a permanent strategic and logistic problem of the military medical services across the world arising from the blood, which is a biological drug, has a limited shelf life and needs the special transport and conditions of use. The same problem must solve the national health-care authorities in programs of the national blood crisis policy, where to get a huge amount of blood supply any time at any place in the case of disaster, terrorist attack and war. The therapeutic problems in immunohematolgy cases can solve by stock of rare blood, storage of autologous blood for patients with rare erythrocyte antigens and storage of autologous blood for patients with red blood cell alloantibodies with no chance to use common blood. All mentioned demands highly correspond with stock of frozen blood. New global security risks exalt this problem to all-society relevancy.

2. Methods of cryopreservation of living tissues and cells

Throughout the years, tackling the matter of cryopreservation of cells and tissues has been deriving from findings about the protection of cells against the impacts of frost, especially from the knowledge about production of ice crystals that cause the subsequent destruction of cellular structures and membranes [1916]. As early as 1866, French naturalist Félix-Archimède Pouchet first described that frozen erythrocytes are destroyed after thawing [16]. This effect had long been attributed solely to the mechanical damage that cells suffer from ice crystals generated in the course of freezing.

As we know now thanks to physical chemistry, however, during the changing process of aqueous solutions into solid state, it is water that changes its state of matter first. Water crystals are created from pure water, while the space in between them is filled with concentrated electrolyte. This leads to cellular dehydration and to the pH change. Based on this knowledge, James Lovelock came up with a hypothesis in 1953, suggesting that the damage effects of frost to cells first induce the cells dehydration and pH changes. Those mechanisms destroy cell membrane before mechanical injury caused by ice crystals. This evolved into a generally accepted theory [6,10,11,19].

Protection of cells from freezing is achieved by adding so-called cryoprotective substances. Since these cryoprotectants usually cause a significant increase in osmolality, it is nevertheless necessary to have all the procedures monitored, and to have osmotic changes under control, in order to avoid an irreversible damage to cellular structures and membranes caused by them [6,11,17] .

With regard to the types of their effects, cryoprotectants are divided into two groups:

2.1 Intracellular (penetrative) cryoprotectants

Due to their relatively simple chemical structure, these substances penetrate the cellular membrane and do not present any toxic danger for the cell when in low concentration. Glycerol, dimethyl sulfoxide (DMSO) and certain types of glycol (ethanol, propylenglycol, methanol, etc.) belong among them. In terms of utilization, they are mostly applied when the long-term preservation of frozen tissues is needed (e.g., sperm banks, erythrocyte cryobanks, banks for stem cells and umbilical cells).

There has not been fully clarified the mechanism of the effect of penetrative cryoprotectants yet. Initially, the damage of cells was associated with the effect of ice crystals only. Cryoprotective substances, nevertheless, besides limiting the creation or frozen crystals, also modify these crystals' shape and size, and by changing their ionic ratio intracellularly as well as extracellularly, they also eliminate the damage caused by osmotic shock which otherwise occurs during freezing. During the freezing process, penetrative cryoprotectants increase output of intracellular water, maintaining the osmotic balance in a partially frozen extracellular solution in this way. It results in not only reducing the cells' volume but also in the reduction of the osmotic load. With regard to subsequent survival of cells after their thawing, a significant effect is the inhibition of APT caused by some of the cryoprotectants such as glycerol and DMSO [15,23].

Glycerol: Cryoprotective effect of glycerol, that is also called low-molecular nonelectrolyte, was first described on sperms. Its cryoprotective effect lies in penetrating the cellular membrane into the cell's nucleus and creating a hyperosmotic environment. It used to be utilized for cryopreservation of large numbers of mammals' cells, as well as for embryos and unfertilized eggs. Now it is mostly used for erythrocyte cryopreservation. Glycerol is mostly used in concentration of 1.0 - 2.0 M, 20 - 40% (55% max.) respectively.

Dimethyl sulfoxide (DMSO): Just like glycerol, DMSO is a nonelectrolyte with low molecular mass. With regard to its cryoprotective quality, it has a similar effect to glycerol. As opposed to glycerol, however, it is more likely to become toxic - already at a concentration of 1.0 M.

Propylene glycol (PROH): Its cryprotective effects are caused by its entirely amorphous state that it reaches in an aqueous solution. PROH excels in stability in temperatures below the freezing point. Thereby it limits crystallization during the freezing and de-freezing process. PROH is usually used in combination with other substances, aiming to limit the possibility of a specific toxic and osmotic damage to tissues and cells.

2.2 Extracellular (non-penetrative) cryoprotectants

Due to their molecular mass, these substances do not penetrate cellular membrane and are mostly used for rapid and ultra-rapid freezing. There are many possible examples, of which several should be named: monosaccharides (glucose, hexose), disaccharides (sucrose, trehalose), trisaccharides (raffinose) and polymers (polyvinylpyrrolidone, polyethylene glycol) and other macromolecular substances such as dextran, modified gelatin, hydroxyethyl starch or albumin.

The mechanism of the non-penetrative cryoprotectants effect lies in their ability to stabilize cellular membrane and also in so called vitrification. When there is water (with temperature below 0°C) turning into ice, non-penetrative cryoprotectants remain outside the cells, where they secure the creation interspaces between cellular membrane and extracellular environment. Electrolytes segregated from freezing solutions are being concentrated in these interspaces. As a consequence to change in osmotic ratio, extracellular hypertonicity removes water from a slowly freezing intracellular space. Moreover, the subsequent decrease in the osmotic differences does not damage the cell membrane. One needs to be cautious with the increase in hypertonicity of cooled cells as it may results in osmotic shock if the thawing process takes too long [5,18] .

3. Cryopreservation of red cells

Only recently the great limiting factor of cryopreservation of red blood cells has been at least partially solved - the life of erythrocytes after thawing was merely one day, which drastically limited the operational use of the given product. With the discovery of new technologies and resuspension solutions in the past years, the life of the blood after its thawing ("reconstitution") was extended to 1 - 3 weeks.

The current practice takes advantage of the erythrocytes cryopreservation and the intracellular cryoprotectant glycerol is used almost exclusively. Its cryoprotective effects has been known since 1949 when the sperm cells were frozen. Only a year later, in 1950, glycerol was firstly used for the freezing of erythrocytes. Thawed RBCs were first successfully transfused in 1951 by Mollison [13]. The method used low, 20% concentration of glycerol and quick freezing, discovered by A.U.Smith [17].

The routine clinical use of cryopreservation of erythrocytes was first implemented in the United States in early 1960's. Since the beginning, a method of cryopreservation was used freezing erythrocytes in high glycerol, i.e. with the addition of 40% glycerol to erythrocytic suspension. This method is now common in most departments dealing with RBC. The freezing process is slow, and it takes place at -80 °C in mechanical freezers. The frozen red cells are then stored in -65 °C. The method was first described by J.L.Tullis in 1958 [21,22].

Notwithstanding, the main reason for introducing this method was pragmatic - standard PVC bags were not applicable for this method and there were problems with obtaining license that would give way to the production of aluminum containers for the storage of RBC in liquid nitrogen. In other words, it was not the question of the quality of the erythrocytes that were frozen using this method. The complication of this method was caused by storage issues. Although special plastic bags for cryopreservation at -200 °C did appear on the market in the next 10 years, the already suffered massive investments into mechanical freezers, as well as high cost of liquid nitrogen in the U.S., meant that the method of freezing in high glycerol became the North American standard.

An alternative method of freezing and storing red blood cells in glycerol is rapid freezing in liquid nitrogen at -196 °C (40 °C / min) and subsequent storing in nitrogen vapors at -170°C. The method was first described by Pert et al. in 1963 [15]. In addition to lower concentrations of glycerol (5-20%) which is easier to wash off, the advantage of this method lies in its independence on the sources of electrical energy, thus reducing the risk of endangering the stored product. There are significant practical week points of this method: they are handling of liquid nitrogen containers, transport issues and also the scheme of Deward containers. This method had become widely used in Europe for some time, where cryopreservative procedures were being implemented into practice 10 years later than in the US, i.e. in early 1970's. At that time, plastic bags suitable for use in extremely cold temperatures were already available, liquid nitrogen was more affordable in Europe and, unlike in the US, mechanical deep-freeze boxes represented a very high investment.

There was another reason why the way of European practice headed towards this method. It was the simplicity of the deglycerolization process which can be, at low concentration, accomplished by manual methods, or by using special rinsing attachments in a centrifuge, such as the ADL cell-washing bowl (in contrast with rinsing of highly concentrated glycerol which requires more complex technique and more sophisticated technical equipment). The comparison of RBCs cryopreservation in high glycerol and low glycerol is displayed in Table 1.

Turning to the non-penetrative cryoprotectants, there is particularly the hydroxyethyl starch (HES) in the spotlight. Its usage in the field of erythrocytes cryopreservation was patented in the U.S. in 1991. Its benefits are the bio-compatible properties of macromolecular polysaccharides (including HES, which is commonly used as volume expander) at higher concentrations, that do not require any complex rinsing procedure during the process of thawing and reconstitution, and so the defrosted product may be directly transfused. Disadvantage of HES is the freezing and storage in liquid nitrogen and relative higher haemolysis after thawing.

	glycerol 40%	glycerol 20%
Freezing temperature	-80°C	-197°C
Freezing rate	slow	fast
Freezing technique	mechanically freezer	liquid Nitrogen
Storage temperature	min. -65°C	min.-120°C
Impact of temperature changes	thawing and refreezing is possible	critical
Containers	PVC, polyolefin	polyolefin
Transportation	dry ice	Nitrogen vapor
Time of deglycerolization	60 min.	30 min.
Hematocrit	55-70%	50-70%
Leucodepletion	94-99%	95%

Table 1. The comparison of RBCs cryopreservation in 40% glycerol and 20% glycerol

Despite the fact that deep-frozen tissues and cells (i.e. erythrocytes) can be preserved almost indefinitely (on condition they are provided with an appropriate storage temperature), it was necessary to determine an administratively acceptable storage time. Only in 1987 the United States Food and Drug Administration (FDA) set the life of at -80°C frozen RBCs to be 10 years. This time limit was adopted by other countries as well. In 2010, European legislation prolonged the frozen erythrocytes' administrative life up to 30 years, depending on the storage method (Directive 2044/33/EC). According to the *Guide to the Preparation, use and quality assurance of blood components* (No.R Recommendation (95) 15 Council of Europe), "the storage of frozen RBCs may be extended to at least ten years if the correct storage temperature can be guaranteed." [7,26,27].

From the practical point of view, the usability of erythrocytes after reconstitution, i.e. after defrosting and deglycerolization, is a more important parameter than their storage time in a frozen state. For a long time, reconstituted erythrocytes expired after 24 hours, which greatly limited their flexibility and possibilities of their usage. This did not change even after the introduction of semi-automated deglycerolization systems in 1970's (Haemonetics ACP-115, IBM Cell Washer, Elutramatic cell washer). There came a revolutionary breakthrough and significant prolongation of the erythrocytes life after thawing after the fully automated device (Haemonetics ACP-215) had been invented and homologated for general usage by FDA in 2011. This invention made the glycerolization as well as the deglycerolization possible in a fully closed manner, while locking it out of external environment and thus performing it out of contact with this external environment.

C. Robert Valery and his team from the Naval Research Blood Laboratory in particular proved the applicability of cryopreserved red blood cells 7 days after reconstitution when using conventional resuspension solutions (SAG-M), and 14 days after reconstitution when using

AS-3 solution (Nutricel) [4,24,25]. Subsequently, Bohonek et al. proved the applicability of cryopreserved erythrocytes 3 weeks after reconstitution, also when using AS-3 [1].

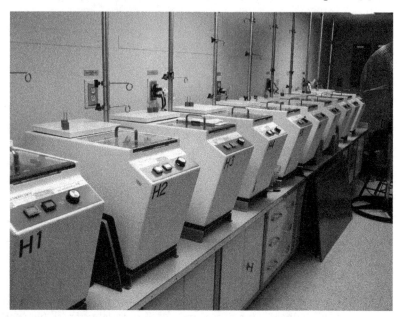

Fig. 1. The line of deglycerolization (washing) machines Haemonetics ACP-115 – first fully automated machines

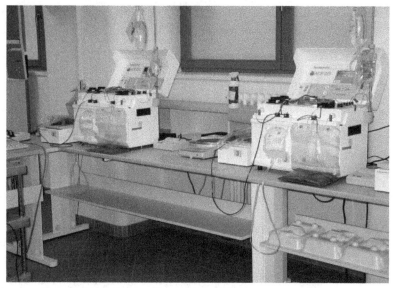

Fig. 2. Haemonetics APC-215, fully automated deglycerolisation (washing) machines with „close system"

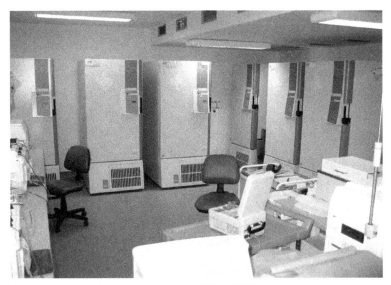

Fig. 3. Mechanical freezers for deep freezing (-65°C - -80°C)

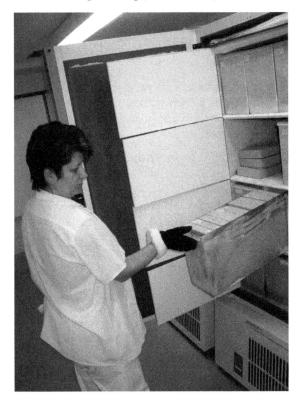

Fig. 4. Stock of frozen blood.

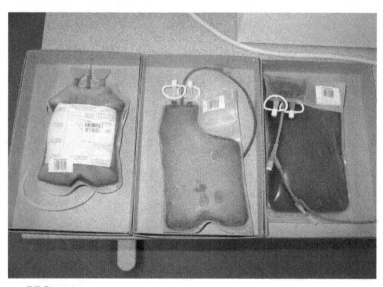

Fig. 5. Frozen RBCs units

4. Cryopreservation of platelets

Platelet could be cryopreserved in different cryoprotectives: intracellular (DMSO, glycerol) as well as in extracellular (HES, dextran).

The most widely used method for the platelets cryopreservation is freezing in 5-10% DMSO at -80 °C with their storage at -65 °C. This method is easy and does not need any technical equipment. After thawing, the platelets are suspended in thawed plasma and there is no need to wash out the cryoprotectant.

Although the platelets stored by cryopreservation are efficient in hemostasis, they are affected by a number of functional defects during storage and preparation for transfusion. Approximately 15% of cryopreserved platelets lost surface-bound GPIb, while there was no measurable loss of GPIIB/IIIa during cryopreservation. The cryopreserved platelets also showed a significant decrease in aggregation to ristocetin, but no loss of response to the stronger agonist, thrombin. Even though these defects are of a minor clinical relevance and the cryopreserved platelets were shown to be safe and effective for treatment of abnormal bleeding, it is still necessary to reckon with these changes [2,3,14,20].

5. Conclusion

The cryopreservation of blood is a method which solves various problems in blood transfusion service. The main application is in military medicine and blood crisis policy, but also in special transfusiology fields, such as the storage of rare red blood cells and long-term storage of autologous blood. Thanks to modern procedures, which allow for prolonged shelf time after thawing and reconstitution of frozen blood, the use of frozen blood is now more flexible and less limited.

6. References

[1] Bohonek M, Petras M, Turek I, Urbanova J, Hradek T, Chmatal P, Staroprazska V, Kostirova J, Horcickova D, Duchkova S, Svobodova J, Tejckova E., Quality evaluation of frozen apheresis red blood cell storage with 21-day postthaw storage in additive solution 3 and saline-adenine-glucose-mannitol: biochemical and chromium-51 recovery measures, Transfusion, 2010, 50:1007-1013

[2] Daly PA, Schiffer CA, Aisner J, Wierni PH, Successful transfusion of platelets cryopreserved for more than 3 years, Blood, 1979, 54:1023-1027

[3] Handin RI, Valeri CR, Improved Viability of Previously Frozen Platelets, Blood, 1972, 40:509-513

[4] Hess JR, Hill HR, Oliver CK, Lippert LE, Greenwalt TJ., The effect of two additive solutions on the postthaw storage of RBCs., Transfusion. 2001 Jul;41(7):923-7.

[5] Horn EP, Sputtek A, Standl T, Rudolf B, Kühnl P, Schulte Transfusion of autologous, hydroxyethyl starch-cryopreserved red blood cells, Anesthesia & Analgesia, 1997;85:739-745

[6] Huggins CE, Frozen Blood, Europ.surg.Res. 1969; 1: 3-12

[7] Lecak J, Scott K, Young C, Hannon J, Acker JP., Evaluation of red blood cells stored at -80 degrees C in excess of 10 years., Transfusion. 2004 Sep;44(9):1306-13.

[8] Lelkens CCM, Koning JG, de Kort B, Floot IBG, Noorman F, Experiences with frozen blood products in the Netherlands military, Tnasfus Apher Sci, 2006, 34:289-98

[9] Levin RL, Cravalho FG, Huggins CE, Effect of hydration on the water content of human erythrocytes, Biophys.J., 1976;16:1411-14260

[10] Lionetti, F. J. and Hunt, S. M., "Cryopreservation of Human Red Cells in Liquid Nitrogen with Hydroxyethyl Starch", Cryobiology, 1975; 12:110-118

[11] Lovelock JE, The Protective Action of Neutral Solutes aginst Haemolysis by Freezing and Thawing, Biochem.J., 1954; 56:265-270

[12] Meryman HT, Hornblower M, Red Cell Recovery and leukocyte Depletion Following Washing of Frozen-Thawed Red Cells, Transfusion, 1973; 13(6):388-393

[13] Mollison PL, Sloviter HA, Successful transfusion of previously frozen human red cells, Lancet, 1951; 261:862-864

[14] Owens M, Werner E, Holme S, Afferbach C, Membrane glycoproteins in cryopreserved platelets, Vox Sanguinis, 1994, 67:28-13

[15] Pert JH, Schork PK, Moore R, A new method of low temperature blood preservation using liquid nitrogen and glycerol sucrose additive, Clinical Research, 1963; 11:197

[16] Pouchet MFA, Recherches expérimentales sur la congélation des animaux, Journ..L´Anat. et Physiol, 1866;.iii:1-36

[17] Smith AT., Prevention during haemolysis during freezing and thawing of red blood cells, Lancet, 1950, 259: 910-911,

[18] Sputtek A, Singbartl G., Langer R., Schleinzer W., Henrich HA, Künl P., Cryoperervation of red blood cells with the non-penetrating cyoprotectant hydroxyethylstarch, Cryo Letters 16, 1995; 283-288

[19] Sputtek A, Kryokonservierung von Blutzellen, Transfusionsmedizin, 2nd.ed. (Ed.:C.Mueller-Eckhardt), 125-167, Springer, Berlin 1996

[20] Taylor MA, Cryopreservation of platelets: an in-vitro comparison of four methods, J Clin Pathol, 1981, 34:71-75

[21] Tullis JL, Ketchei MM, Pyle HM, Penneli GB, Gibson JG, Tinch RJ, Studies on the in vivo survival of glycerolized and frozen human red blood cells, J.of the Am.Med.Association, 1958; 168:399-404

[22] Tullis JL, Haynes L, Pyle H, Wallach S, Pennell R, Sproul M, Khoubesserian A, Clinical use of frozen blood, Arch.Surg., 1960, 81:169

[23] Valeri CR, Frozen Blood, New Engl.J.Med., 1966; 25:425-431

[24] Valeri CR., Pivace LE., Cassidy GP., Rango G., The survival, funktion, and hemolysis of human RBCs stored at 4°C in additive slution (AS-1, AS-3, or AS-5) for 42 days and then bochemimically modifie, frozen, thawe, washed, and stored at 4°C in sodium chloride and glucose solution for 24 hours, Transfusion, 2000, Nov; 40(11): 1341-5.

[25] Valeri CR, Ragno G, Pivacek LE, Srey R, Hess JR, Lippert LE, Mettille F, Fahie R, O'Neill EM, Szymanski IO., A multicenter study of in vitro and in vivo values in human RBCs frozen with 40-percent (wt/vol) glycerol and stored after deglycerolization for 15 days at 4 degrees C in AS-3: assessment of RBC processing in the ACP 215., Transfusion. 2001 Jul;41(7):933-9.

[26] Commission Directive 2004/33/EC of March 2004, Annex IV.

[27] Guide to the preparation, use and guality assurance of blood components, Council of Europe, Recommendation No.R(95) 15

Part 5

Immunomodulatory Effects of Blood Transfusion

15

Effect of Blood Transfusion on Subsequent Organ Transplantation

Puneet K. Kochhar[1], Pranay Ghosh[2] and Rupinder Singh Kochhar[2]
[1]*Lady Hardinge Medical College & SSK Hospital,*
[2]*Maulana Azad Medical College & Lok Nayak Hospital*
University of Delhi, New Delhi,
India

1. Introduction

In the current era, tissue and organ transplantation is an established specialty for treatment of multiple disorders. However, the chief immunological problem of organ transplantation is the risk of occurrence of acute or chronic rejection, initiated by host lymphocytes in response to graft alloantigens. Though the success of transplantation is attributed to the modern methods of immunosuppression, the role of pre-transplant blood transfusions cannot be ignored.

Since the beginning of clinical transplantation, there have been four phases in blood transfusion policies, swinging from liberal transfusions to avoidance of transfusions, followed by a repeat cycle of deliberate transfusions and again returning to abstinence (*Carpenter, 1990*). Pre-exposure to alloantigens has been discovered to have a dual effect: it is detrimental in some cases, while in others, it prolongs the graft survival.

Therefore, in this chapter, we would explore the mechanisms involved in both the detrimental and the beneficial effects of blood transfusion on graft survival and provide an overview of the current recommended practice.

2. Basics of HLA and graft rejection

2.1 *Human leukocyte antigens (HLA)* are a set of human major histocompatibility complex derived glycoproteins. These are expressed on cell surfaces and allow for discrimination of self from non-self. HLA have been classified into two major groups, Class I (HLA-A, HLA-B, and HLA-C) and Class II (HLA-DP, HLA-DQ, and HLA-DR). Recognition of the alloantigens (antigens displayed by the transplanted organ) is the prime event initiating the immune response against an allograft (*Gabardi, 2010*).

2.2 *Hyperacute rejection* is an immediate immune response in the recipient against an allograft, due to preformed recipient antibodies directed against the donor's HLA.

2.3 *Acute rejection* is a cell mediated process that usually occurs within 5 to 90 days after a transplant. Rarely, it can occur after this time.

2.4 *Humoral rejection* is characterized by B lymphocytes injuring the allograft through immunoglobulin and complement activities.

2.5 *Chronic rejection:* Although poorly understood, immunologic processes of chronic rejection may result from cell-mediated, humoral, or drug-induced allograft damage.

3. History of blood transfusion effect in clinical transplantation

Most patients with end-stage renal disease awaiting renal transplantation, sustained by dialysis machines, became profoundly anaemic and benefitted symptomatically from blood transfusions. Many required large numbers of blood transfusions, frequently exceeding 20 units over a period of months. Some even required as many as 50-100 units. Even those, who had some residual production of erythropoietin (EPO) by the remnant renal tissue, benefitted by transfusion of 2-5 units per year. Thus, the first phase in clinical transplantation was the high-volume use of blood to keep the patient's red cell mass in the 20-25% range (*Carpenter, 1990*).

In the second phase in the 1970s, efforts were made to avoid blood exposure. This trend began with the realization that blood exposure could be highly immunogenic leading to production of anti-HLA antibodies, which precluded transplantation at the time of cross-match (*Opelz, 1973*). This concept was originally described in the mouse by Medawar (*Medawar, 1946*). Subsequently, Hattler et al demonstrated that a single transfusion of whole blood can provoke sufficient immune response to induce accelerated rejection of a skin graft from the blood donor (*Hattler, 1966*). This policy of with-holding pre-transplant transfusions was reinforced by growing concerns about the serious long-term consequences of transfusion-induced hepatitis in the immunosuppressed graft recipient (*Parfrey, 1984*).

However, within a few years, it was reported that non-transfused patients receiving cadaveric donor grafts were at higher risk for graft rejection, having a 20-30% lower one-year graft survival rate (*Matas 1975, Opelz 1978*). In the pre-cyclosporine era, failure to transfuse a potential kidney recipient was the most important predictor of a poor outcome. It was shown that patients who had never received transfusions were not the optimal recipient population (*Opelz 1974*). Patients who had received blood transfusions prior to transplantation appeared to accept a significantly higher proportion of kidney transplants successfully (*Opelz 1976, Polesky 1976*). A similar trend in recipients of heart allografts was also noted (*Caves 1973*).

Thus, kidney transplant candidates received elective immunomodulatory red cell transfusions to improve graft survival. Survival of kidney graft from living related donors was enhanced by the pre-transplant conditioning of the recipient with several transfusions. However, the volume and timing of blood transfusion which was beneficial, was not established. This led to many attempts to define the optimal dose and timing for the transfusion effect. Opelz et al found a distinct dose effect, with the one-year survival rates being directly proportional to the numbers of units of blood transfused prior to transplantation (*Opelz 1978*). Some improvement was seen with a single transfusion, and survival rates increased with up to 10-20 units of blood. However, more recent studies have shown more than 5 transfusions to worsen graft survival (*Chavers 1997*) and patient survival (*Tang 2008*).

Though the duration of the favourable effect of blood transfusion was unknown, it was found that preoperative blood transfusion at the time of surgery was usually not effective, while blood received within a year or two had a beneficial effect (*Opelz 1981a*). Thus, it was recommended that blood should be given at least 3 to 6 months prior to transplant (*Radley 1986*).

It was also not clear which component of the transfused blood was responsible for the beneficial effect. Allogeneic blood containing leukocytes was shown to have an adverse effect in patients with aplastic anaemia undergoing bone marrow transplantation and in renal transplant patients. It was assumed that sensitisation to transplantation antigens could potentially be prevented by leukodepleting blood components that are to be used in pretransplantation transfusions. Thus, leukocyte poor red cells and frozen deglycerolized red cells were assumed to have low incidence of HLA immunization (*Sanfilippo 1985, Polesky 1977*).

The incidence of alloimmunization was also low when stored units, rather fresh units of blood were used for transfusion (*Light 1982*). One study suggested that the agglomeration method for blood preservation resulted in a product which was less immunogenic in terms of producing antibodies, while retaining its ability to improve graft results (*Fuller 1978*). Thus, preparations of frozen blood deglycerolized by agglomeration were found to be beneficial and relatively free of the hazards inherent in conventional blood support. While saline-washed, "leukocyte-poor" blood cells may be an alternative to frozen blood for reducing the rate of patient sensitization (*Miller 1975*), prolonged use of this apparently leads to a much higher sensitization incidence (Suarez-Ch 1972).

Thus, numerous studies indicated that blood transfusions may actually be beneficial in prolonging the survival of renal allografts (*Festenstein 1976, Opelz 1976, Polesky 1976*). As a result of these data, most transfusion services followed a deliberate transfusion policy of administering 2-5 units of blood to all new dialysis patients while awaiting transplantation. These were usually given in the form of whole blood, however red blood cells, deglycerilized RBC's and buffy coats were also used as effective alternatives to whole blood.

With the introduction of cyclosporine in 1980s, graft and patient survival improved. Since then, the question of the beneficial role of blood transfusions has been subject to ongoing re-evaluation. There has been an overall decline in the transfusion effect and an increase in the HLA matching effect, which is more clearly recognized now because of improved typing capabilities. The HLA effect is additive to that of cyclosporine, which itself produces a 15% increase in one year survival rates (*Opelz 1985*).

In addition, blood transfusion involves a risk of blood-borne infections, including HIV. Also, there has been an emergence of new factors in blood banking (e.g. use of EPO for supporting red cell production). These formed clear incentives to move away from use of pre-transplantation blood transfusions. This led to the fourth phase of transfusion policy, a return to the withholding of blood as possibly unnecessary, at least for the improvement of graft survival.

Some recent studies show that transfusion may cause severe acute rejection (*Waanders 2008*). Few programmes now use elective pre-transplant transfusions to improve graft survival. Patients with end stage liver diseases are being treated by drug octreotide, variceal banding, sclerotherapy, transjugular intrahepatic portosystemic shunt placements to relieve the effects of portal hypertension in order to have less gastrointestinal bleeding and to avoid transfusion (*Calcutti 2002*).

However, observations on patients having rejection episodes indicate that a beneficial blood transfusion effect still exists. Recent evidence suggests that the blood transfusion effect remains in certain circumstances, when one considers effects of HLA antigens, rejection episodes, and possibly the prospects of tolerance induction. In a single centre study of a no-transfusion policy, the non-transfused group had more early rejection episodes (*Lundgren 1986*). Another study on the relation of rejection activity to previous blood transfusions showed that 63% of the 231 non-transfused recipients had rejection episodes during the first 60 days after transplantation, while 48% of the transfused patients had rejection (*Toyotome 1987*). Additionally, it was found that if a rejection episode occurred, the one-year survival was 49% in those with no transfusions, and 70% in the transfused patients. Hence, the original deficit of 20% poorer survival in the absence of prior transfusions may still be discerned in those patients destined to reject.

Furthermore, though the change in the transfusion effect during the early 1980s (before the introduction of cyclosporine) is most marked by a disappearance of the graded response to increasing numbers of blood units, the deleterious effect of receiving no transfusions remains, with a 10% lower one-year survival rate (*Terasaki 1986*).

Unfortunately, there are no reliable predictive tests to know who would need to have transfusions prior to transplantation.

4. Possible mechanism of beneficial effects of pre-transplant transfusion

The exact mechanism by which blood transfusion enhances transplant survival remains unknown. However, several possible mechanisms have been postulated. These are as follows:

4.1 Pre-transplant blood transfusions may cause early immunization of some recipients to selected HLA antigens. This enables the pre-transplantation crossmatch to detect those cases where rejection of donor organ would be most likely to occur. Preformed HLA antibodies (presenting as incompatible crossmatch) are a major contraindication to transplantation. About 30% of cases who receive pre-transplant transfusions become highly immunized to HLA. This response may be beneficial by preventing an unsuccessful transplant.

4.2 The beneficial effect of transfusion may also be related to the immunosuppression induced by transfusion. This may occur through enhancement of suppressor T cell activity or induction of immune tolerance by some unknown mechanism.

5. Responses to allogenic blood transfusion and HLA senitization

There are several individual differences in the effects of allogenic blood exposure. Some of these are discussed here:

5.1 Most patients do not develop anti-HLA antibodies following transfusion. Overall, 30% of transfused individuals develop antibodies (with the rate being higher in previously pregnant females and lower in males) (*Opelz 1981b*). In non transfused multiparous females, about 10% develop such antibodies (the response being transient usually). Multiparous women challenged with blood transfusions show an increase in the responder rate to 30-40% (*Opelz 1981b*).

5.2 Some responders have a highly selective immune response directed to one to four HLA antigens, while others show sensitivity to better than 95% of a reference panel (*Carpenter 1990*).

Thus, even though a genetic control over responsiveness is evident, the responder status cannot be predicted from an individual's HLA phenotype.

The responder status to blood transfusions becomes evident very early after the initiation of blood transfusions. In the earlier days of frequent transfusions, many patients remained negative on antibody screens after more than 50 blood transfusions, and very few non-responders were found to convert after about six months.

The degree of sensitization is expressed as panel-reactive antibody (PRA). PRA testing evaluates who is most at risk of hyperacute or humoral rejection (*Cecka 2010*). A PRA of 80% reflects that the patient is crossmatch incompatible with 80% of donors. In general, patients with a PRA of more than 10% or more than 80% are considered sensitized or highly sensitized, respectively. However, different centres can use markedly different PRA cut-offs for determining sensitized and highly sensitized patients (*Cecka 2010*). On a typical waiting list for cadaveric renal transplantation, more than 50% of patients have antibodies to more than half of the reference panel, and 20% have antibodies to 90-100% (*Carpenter 1990*).

There are three types of assays used to determine PRA. The oldest is the Complement Dependent Cytotoxicity (CDC) test (*Cecka 2010, Hajeer 2006*). In this test, patient serum is tested against donor lymphocytes (B and T cells). Patients' antibodies will coat antigen expressing lymphocytes and upon administration of complement to the serum, lymphocytes are killed and detected by cell stain. The second type of assay is the Enzyme-Linked Immunoabsorbant Assay (ELISA), a solid phase assay which is more sensitive than the CDC. The third assay is the flow cytometry test. Also, there is the house method where locally acquired whole lymphocytes are used and a microbead method which uses purified HLA antigen coated microbeads. Commerical kits include the Flow PRA and Luminex tests. The CDC is thought to be inferior to the HLA Class I and II ELISA and microbead flow cytometry tests which are similar to each other (*Cecka 2010, Hajeer 2006, Worthington 2001*).

Though the superiority of one approach over another is debatable, it is important since PRA may be altered in response to stimuli. PRA response may be altered by the use of medications (rituximab, immune globulin, statins, cyclophosphamide/predisolone with plasmapheresis) or certain Angiotensin Converting Enzyme genotypes (*Vieira 2004, Vo 2008, Muhmoud 2007, Nurhan-Ozdemir 2004, Akcay 2004*).

As previously stated, patients with antibodies to a given donor are not suitable for that transplant. Thus, blood transfusions provide a process of negative selection such that transplants destined to early failure are avoided. However, immunosuppressive agents such as cyclosporine, anti-lymphocyte globulins (ALG), etc, may suppress the responses previously subject to negative selection by transfusion, and thus lead to a decline in the transfusion effect. Other factors, such as prompt diagnosis and treatment of early rejections and HLA matching, may also play a role in this decline observed in the transfusion effect.

Iwaki et al demonstrated a benefit from transfusions in HLA-DR mismatched cases. This benefit was not observed when there were no mismatches. In cases with no mismatches, one-year survival was reported as 80% in both transfused and non-transfused recipients, while transfusions added an 8-10% benefit in the one- and two-DR mismatched groups (*Iwaki 1990*).

6. Nonspecific Immune suppression after transfusion

Allogeneic blood transfusions produce generalized immunosuppression in the recipient. This is due to a variety of changes in the immunological functions, such as decreased function of natural killer cells, macrophage migration to sites of injury, lymphocyte proliferation, and cutaneous delayed hypersensitivity. Donor leukocytes in allogeneic blood may play a role in suppressing cellular immune function.

Serial measurements of cell-mediated responses in previously non-transfused end-stage renal disease patients showed marked reductions in response to mitogens and recall antigens (e.g. PPD, tetanus, mumps, vaccinia) after a single blood transfusion. This effect lasted for over two weeks (*Fischer 1980*). More profound and lasting depression was seen after a second transfusion given after 4 weeks.

Reports have also suggested that allogeneic blood transfusions increase the incidence of postoperative infection and the tumour recurrence rate (*Schriemer 1988, Wu 1988*). Such postoperative morbidities have been attributed to the immunomodulatory effects of blood transfusion. However, this association is unproven, and there is currently insufficient evidence to recommend the routine use of leukodepleted blood components for surgical patients to prevent either postoperative infection or tumour recurrence.

7. Antigen specific immune-suppression

The final objective in transplantation is the induction of specific unresponsiveness, or tolerance, so that patients do not need to take anti-rejection medications indefinitely. This unresponsiveness is specific for donor antigens; i.e. the recipients produce perfectly normal responses to cells bearing other HLA antigens.

Patients, who have received pre-transplant transfusions, have marked reductions in cells capable of killing donor cells (*Herzog 1987*). However, full activation by polyclonal mitogens will restore the expected cytotoxic T cells precursor frequency to the normal level (*Dallman 1989*). Thus, the possibility of clonal deletion is unlikely. Though the full T-cell repertoire is present, the individual is functionally unresponsive in the absence of stimuli which bypass inhibitory immunoregulatory influences.

When living donor kidney graft recipients are prepared by single-donor blood transfusions from the potential kidney donor, this is known as "donor-specific transfusions" (DST). Such blood transfusions (which share an HLA haplotype, or at least one DR antigen with the transfused recipient) do not produce an increase in cytotoxic T cells precursor frequency or cell mediated immunity. If such recipients do not develop a positive cross-match, they are still reported to have superior graft survival, close to that of an HLA identical donor (*Salvatierra 1980*).

8. Effect of in-utero (feto-maternal) transfusion in adult renal transplant

Many people behave as if they were clonally deleted for the HLA antigens of their mothers which they did not inherit. This was first observed in an analysis of end-stage renal disease patients having very high PRA, but consistently having no antibodies against a small number of HLA antigens (*Claas 1988*). This unresponsiveness to antibody response in some sensitized patients was found to be due to a failure to respond to non-inherited maternal HLA antigens. These findings are important as this may be applicable to selection of donors for transplant recipients.

9. Conditioning with blood transfusions for tolerance induction

There have been studies reporting selection of single blood donors from an unrelated population matched for one DR antigen only and not for a whole HLA haplotype (*Lagaaij 1989*). In recipients, anti-HLA antibodies were less frequent as result of one DR matched versus no DR matched transfusions. Such transfusions may induce production of anti-idiotypic antibodies which can prevent the response of T cells specific to the immunizing HLA antigens (*Phelan 1989, Kawamura 1989*).

Studies of renal and heart transplant recipients have shown a reduced rejection frequency and better graft survival when the only blood received prior to transplantation was 1-3 units from donors matched for one DR antigen with the recipient (*Lagaaij 1989*). Anti-HLA antibody production was also diminished in the one DR transfused group. This immunization effect could be due to suppression via some antigen-specific immunoregulatory pathway.

An alternative possibility could be that provision of self DR on transfused cells induces a different sort of systemic response similar to the autologous mixed lymphocyte response (AMLR) (*Sakane 1979*). However, additional confirmatory studies are needed, along with careful study of possibly different effects when alloantigens are presented in the context of self versus non-self class II HLA.

10. Conclusions and future research

Additional adequately powered multi-institutional studies should be conducted, because individual centre practices are variable. These studies should have adequate reporting of demographics and either use statistical means to account for confounders or use randomization. Patients receiving or being randomized to no transfusions should be screened to assure that this not only includes transfusions within the dialysis or transplant centre, but other transfusions as well.

The impact of different immunosuppressive regimens on outcomes in patients receiving transfusions should be studied to identify those regimens which can suppress the advantageous or detrimental effects of transfusion on outcomes. This should be specifically evaluated to determine whether transplants need to be encouraged, avoided, or matched with certain regimens.

Unlike the prior reports, where pre-transplant transfusions seemed to worsen renal allograft outcomes, transfusions generally have a beneficial to neutral effect on transplant outcomes.

There is not much support for the belief that transfusions increase the risk of graft rejection. There is evidence that patients receiving pre-transplant transfusions have increased levels of sensitization as assessed by PRA. With regard to rejection, the data are more ambiguous with some analyses showing benefit, some showing a neutral effect, and other analyses showing harm, although the number of studies evaluating more recent time periods is quite limited.

Thus, future application of deliberate HLA antigen exposure in conjunction with novel immunological manipulations may provide a more effective avenue to tolerance induction. However, the literature base is weak and future research is needed to assess the impact of transfusions on allograft and patient survival outcomes in renal transplant recipients.

11. References

Akcay A, Ozdemir FN, Atac FB, et al. Angiotensin-Converting Enzyme genotype is a predictive factor in the peak panel-reactive antibody response. Transplant Proc 2004;36:35-7.

Calcutti RA, Shah OJ, Khan NA, Dar MA, Farooq A. Role of Transfusion Services in Organ and Tissue Transplantation. JK Science 2002;4(4):163-168.

Carpenter CB. Blood Transfusion Effects in Kidney Transplantation. The Yale Journal of Biology & Medicine 1990;63:435-443.

Caves PK, Stinson EB, Griepp RB, et al. Results of 54 Cardiac Transplants. Surgery 1973;74:307.

Cecka JM. Calculated PRA (CPRA): the new measure of sensitization for transplant candidates. Am J Transplantation 2010;10:26-9.

Chavers BM, Sullivan EK, Tejani A, et al. Pre-transplant blood transfusion and renal allograft outcome: a report of the North American Pediatric Renal Transplant Cooperative Study. Pediatr Transplant 1997;1:22-8.

Claas FHJ, Gijbels Y, van der Velden-deMunck J, van Rood JJ. Induction of B cell unresponsiveness to maternal HLA antigens during fetal life. Science 1988;241:1815-1817.

Dallman MJ, Wood KJ, Morris PJ. Recombinant interleukin-2 (IL-2) can reverse the blood transfusion effect. Transplant Proc 1989;21:1165-1167.

Festenstein H, Sachs JA, Paris AMI, et al. Influence of HLA Matching and Blood-Transfusion on Outcome of 502 London Transplant Group Renal-graft Recipients. Lancet1976;1:157.

Fischer E, Lenhard V, Seifert P, Kluge A, Johanssen R. Blood transfusion-induced suppression of cellular immunity in man. Human Immunology 1980;3:187-194.

Fuller TC, Delmonico FL, Cosimi B, Huggins CE, King M, Russell PS. Impact of blood transfusions on renal transplantation. Ann Surg 1978;187:211-218.

Gabardi S and Olyaei AJ. Solid organ transplantation (chapter 55). In, Chisolm-Burns MA, Ed. Pharmacotherapy Principles and Practice, Second Edition. McGraw-Hill, NY. 2010: pgs 939-64.

Hajeer AH. Panel reactive antibody test (PRA) in renal transplantation. Saudi J Kidney Dis Transplant 2006;17:1-4.

Hattler BG, Young WG, Amos DB, et al. White Blood Cell Antibodies. Arch. Surg 1966;93:741.

Herzog W, Zanker B, Irschick E, Huber C, Franz HE, Wagner H, Kabelitz D. Selective reduction of donor-specific cytotoxic T lymphocyte precursors in patients with a well-functioning kidney allograft. Transplantation 1987;43:384-389.

Iwaki Y, Cecka M, Terasaki PI. The transfusion effect in cadaver kidney transplants-yes or no. Transplantation 1990;49:56-59.

Kawamura T, Sakagami K, Haisa M, Morisaki F, Takasu S, Inagaki M, Oiwa T, Toshihiko 0, Orita K. Induction of antiidiotypic antibodies by donor-specific blood transfusions. Transplantation 1989;48:459-463.

Lagaaij EL, Hennemann PH, Ruigrok M, deHaan MW, Persijn GG, Termijtelen A, Hendriks GFJ, Weimar W, Claas F, van Rood JJ. Effect of one HLA-DR antigen-matched and completely HLA-DR mismatched blood transfusions on survival of heart and kidney allografts. N Engl J Med 1989;321:701-705.

Light J A, Metz S, Oddenino K, et al. Fresh versus stored blood in donor specific transfusion. Transplant Proc 1982;14: 296-301.

Lundgren G, Groth CG, Albrechtsen D, et al. HLA matching and pretransplant blood transfusions in cadaveric renal transplantation-a changing picture with cyclosporine. Lancet 1986;i:66-69.

Matas AJ, Simmons RL, Buselmeier TJ, Najarian JS, Kjellstrand CM. Lethal complications of bilateral nephrectomy and splenectomy in hemodialyzed patients. Am J Surg 1975;129:616-620.

Medawar PB. Immunity to Homologous Grafted Skin. II. Relationship Between Antigens of Blood and Skin. Br J Exp Pathol 1946;27:15.

Miller WV, Schmidt R, Luke RG, et al. Effect of Cytotoxicity Antibodies in Potential Transplant Recipients of Leukocyte-poor Blood Transfusions. Lancet 1975;1:893.

Muhmoud KM, Sobh MA, el Shenawy F, et al. Management of sensitized patients awaiting renal transplantation: does sequential therapy with intravenous immunoglobulin and simvastatin offer a solution. Eur J Cancer Clin Oncol 2007;56:202-5.

Nurhan-Ozdemir F, Akcay A, Sezer S, et al. Effect of simvastatin in the treatment of highly sensitized dialysis patients: the pre and post-renal transplantation follow-up outcomes. Transplant immunology 2004;13:39-42.

Opelz G, Sengar DPS, Mickey MR, Terasaki PI. Effect of blood transfusions on subsequent kidney transplants. Transplant Proc 1973;5:253-259.

Opelz G and Terasaki PI. Poor Kidney-transplant Survival in Recipients with Frozen-blood Transfusions or no Transfusions. Lancet 1974;2:696.

Opelz G and Terasaki PI. Prolongation Effect of Blood Transfusions on Kidney Graft Survival. Transplantation 1976;22:380.

Opelz G, Terasaki PI. Improvement of kidney graft survival with increased numbers of blood transfusions. N Engl J Med 1978;299:799-803.

Opelz G, Terasaki PI. Importance of preoperative (not perioperative) transfusions for cadaveric kidney transplants. Transplantation 1981a;31:106-198.

Opelz G, Graver B, Mickey MR, Terasaki PI. Lymphocytotoxic antibody responses to transfusion in potential kidney transplant recipients. Transplantation 1981b;32:177-183.

Opelz G. The Collaborative Transplant Study: Correlation of HLA matching with kidney graft survival in patients with or without cyclosporine treatment. Transplantation 1985;40:240-243.

Parfrey PS, Forbes RDC, Hutchinson TA, Beaudoin JG, Dauphinee WD, Hollomby DJ, Guttmann RD. The clinical and pathological course of hepatitis B liver disease in renal transplant recipients. Transplantation 1984;37:461-466.

Phelan DL, Rodey GE, Anderson CB. The development and specificity of antiidiotypic antibodies in renal transplant recipients receiving single-donor blood transfusions. Transplantation 1989;48:57-60.

Polesky HF, McCullough JJ, Yunis EJ, et al. Re-evaluation of the Effects of Blood Transfusions on Renal Allograft Survival. Transfusion 1976;16:536.

Polesky HF, McCullough JJ, Yunis E et al. The effects of transfusion of frozen -thawed deglycerolized red cells on renal allograft survival. Transplantation 1977;24: 449-52.

Radley GE. Blood transfusion and their influence on renal allograft survival. In: Brown B E ed. Progress in hematology. *vol* XVI. Orlandu: Grune and Stratton Inc. 1986:99-122.

Sakane T, Green I. Specificity and suppressor function of human T cells responsive to autologous non-T cells. J Immunol 1979;123:584-589.

Salvatierra 0, Vincenti F, Amend W, Potter D, Iwaki Y, Opelz G, Terasaki PI, Duca R, Cochrum K, Hanes D, Stoney RJ, Feduska NJ. Deliberate donor-specific blood transfusions prior to living related renal transplantation-a new approach. Ann Surg 1980;192:543-552.

Sanfilippo FP, Bollinger RR, MacQueen JM, Brooks BJ, Koepke JA. A randomized study comparing leukocyte depleted versus packed red cell transfusion in prospective cadaver renal allograft recipient. Transfusion 1985; 25(2):116-19.

Schriemer PA, Longnecker DE, Mintz PD. The possible immunosuppresive effect of perioperative blood transfusions in cancer patients. Anesthesiology 1988;68:422-428.

Suarez-Ch R and Jonasson O. Isoimmunization of Potential Transplant Recipients: General Frequency and Some Associated Factors. Transplant. Proc. 1972; IV:577.

Tang H, Chelamcharla M, Baird BC, et al. Factors affecting kidney-transplant outcome in recipients with lupus nephritis. Clin Transplant 2008;22:263-72.

Terasaki PI, Himaya NS, Cecka M, Cicciarelli J, Cook DJ, Ito T, Iwaki Y, Mickey MR, Takiff H, Tiwari JL, Toyotome A. Overview. In: Clinical Transplants 1986. Edited by PI Terasaki. Los Angeles, CA, UCLA Tissue Typing Laboratory, 1986, pp 367-398.

Toyotome A, Terasaki PI, Salvatierra O, et al. Early graft function. In: Clinical Transplants 1987. Edited by PI Terasaki. Los Angeles, CA, UCLA Tissue Typing Laboratory, 1987:435-452.

Vieira CA, Agarwal A., Book BK, et al. Rituximab for reduction of anti-HLA antibodies in patients awaiting renal transplantation: safety, pharmacodynamics, and pharmacokinetics. Transplantation 2004;77:542-8.

Vo A.A., Lukovsky M, Wang J, et al. Rituximab and intravenous immune globulin for desensitization during renal transplantation. N Engl J Med 2008;359:242-51.

Waanders MM, Roelen DL, de Fijter JW, et al. Protocolled blood transfusions in recipients of a simultaneous pancreas-kidney transplant reduce severe acute graft rejection. Transplantation 2008;85:1668-70.

Worthington JE, Robson AJ, Sheldon S, et al. A comparison of enzyme-linked immunoabsorbent assays and flow cytometry techniques for the detection of HLA specific antibodies. Hum Immunol 2001;62:1178-84.

Wu H-S, Little AG. Perioperative blood transfusions and cancer recurrence. J Clin Oncol 1988;6:1348-1354.

Posthepatic Manipulative Blood Extraction with Blood Transfusion Alleviates Liver Transplant Ischemia/Reperfusion Injury and Its Induced Lung Injury

Changku Jia
Department of Hepatobiliary Surgery,
Affiliated Hospital of Hainan Medical college, Haikou, Hainan Province,
China

1. Introduction

Liver ischemia-reperfusion (I/R) occurs in a number of clinical syndromes, including liver transplantation (Huguet et al., 1994). Liver I/R is a major obstacle to liver transplantation (Rosen et al., 1998; Banga et al., 2005). It causes liver graft primary nonfunction, up to 10% of early liver transplant failures and higher incidence of acute and chronic rejection (Banga et al., 2005; Henderson et al., 1999; Farmer et al., 2008). Despite many experimental improvements and efforts have been made to attenuate liver I/R injury heretofore, clinical liver I/R was not effectively prevented (Olthoff., 2001; Lehmann et al., 2000; Clarke et al., 2009). And apart from the liver injury, extrahepatic factors like pulmonary injury also play an important role in the outcome of liver transplantation recipients (Sykes et al., 2007; Pereboom et al., 2009; Shimizu et al., 2005; Liu et al., 1996). The incidence rate of acute lung injury is about 40% and greatly threatens the lives of recipients and their quality of life after transplantion (Aduen et al., 2003). So it is meaningful to take strategy to protect the lung against liver transplantation induced injury.

Multiple mechanisms are involved in the pathogenesis of liver transplant I/R in which reactive oxygen species (ROS) have been shown to play a central role in aggravating tissue injury of the transplant (Zhang et al., 2007).

In previous study, using rat warm I/R injury model, we demonstrated that posthepatic ROS concentration elevated gradually with time after reperfusion. And in the early period of reperfusion posthepatic ROS concentration is higher than that in infrahepatic vena cava (IH-VC). Furthermore, we provided that 2% of body weight SH-VC manipulative blood extraction with blood transfusion at 10 min after reperfusion significantly alleviated liver warm I/R injury (Jia et al., 2008). In this study we evaluated the potential effects of posthepatic manipulative blood extraction and blood transfusion on the liver transplant cold I/R injury and the lung injury induced by liver cold I/R in rat.

2. Materials and methods

2.1 Animals and reagents

Male Sprague-Dawley rats, weighing 200-250 g, were supplied by the Shanghai Experimental Animal Center. Rats were housed under standard environmental conditions with a 12:12-h light-dark cycle. Before use in experiments, rats were fasted overnight with free access to water. All animals received humane care in accordance with the Guidelines of the Animal Care Committee of Zhejiang Medical University.

Reagents : (1) MDA and myeloperoxidase (MPO) assay kit (Jiancheng Bioengineering Co.Ltd, Nanjing, China). (2) Naphthol ASD chloroacetate esterase (Sigma Chemical Co., St. Louis, MO). (3) IL-6 ELISA assay kit (Quantikine · MN, USA). (4) TNF-α ELISA assay kit (Quantikine, MN, USA).

2.2 Part I: Liver transplantation and determination of peak production of posthepatic ROS after transplantation

2.2.1 Surgical procedures, experimental groups and sample harvesting

The animals were anesthetized with intraperitoneal injection of 4% chloral hydrate. Orthotopic liver transplantation was performed by Kamada's two-cuff technique (Huguet et al., 1994) (Kamada et al., 1983). Blood was taken at 5 min, 20 min, 30 min, 1 h, 2 h, 6 h after reperfusion respectively (n=7 for each time point). Pure posthepatic blood and IH-VC blood were sampled by the method described in previous study (Jia et al., 2008). Sera were separated for lipid peroxide detection. Median cold ischemia time in all transplantation procedures in this study including in Part I and Part II was 50.22 min.

2.2.2 Lipid peroxide assay

The amount of oxidative stress was assessed by determining serum levels of malonaldehyde (MDA). Serum MDA was determined by the thiobarbituric acid reaction. Sera were isolated then MDA was detected according to manufacturer's instructions.

2.3 Part II: Posthepatic manipulative blood extraction on liver transplant I/R injury and hepatic cold I/R induced lung injury

2.3.1 Surgical procedures, experimental groups and sample harvesting

Rats were randomly divided into four groups and subjected to the following treatments.

IR control group (IR, n=5): The first group involved liver transplantation but without any intervention after transplantation.

Two percent of body weight posthepatic manipulative blood extraction with blood transfusion group (PB, n=7): One hour after transplantation, two percent of body weight posthepatic manipulative blood extraction with blood transfusion was performed by the method described in previous study (Jia et al., 2008). After isolation of IH-VC, a 7# silk suture was placed just above the level of right adrenal vein behind the IH-VC. All the structures in the portal triad were clamped by a Bull-dog clamp. Fresh abdominal aorta blood was collected from other SD rats and was anti-coagulated using heparin. The syringe

Posthepatic Manipulative Blood Extraction with Blood Transfusion Alleviates Liver Transplant
Ischemia/Reperfusion Injury and Its Induced Lung Injury

257

containing fresh blood was connected to a 5.5# scalp needle and was place on microinfusion pump. Right external jugular vein of the tested rats was exposed and the scalp needle was inserted into it. The pipeline was maintained by small flow of blood transfusion (1 ml/h). To obtain pure and immediate SH-VC blood after 1 h of reperfusion, an indwelling intravenous line (BD Vialon Biomaterial) was cannulated in the IH-VC with the catheter tip positioned between the liver and diaphragm. A slipknot around the indwelling intravenous line was tied using the pre-placed 7# silk suture to separate blood between both sides of the suture. Then SH-VC was occluded at the level of diaphragm and blood transfusion was sped up to 90ml/h at the same time. Then pure SH-VC blood was drawn-out through the catheter with the speed matching that of transfusion. The bleeding volume is 2% of body weight. After the blood extraction SH-VC and IH-VC was orderly unblocked followed by the catheter withdrawn. A schematic representation for blood extraction and transfusion is shown in Figure 1.

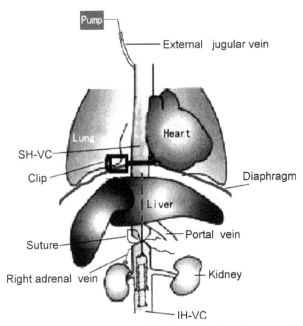

Fig. 1. Schema of blood extraction in SH-VC, blood transfusion in external jugular vein and sites of vascular occlusion.
To obtain pure and immediate SH-VC blood, the vena cava was occluded between the liver and the right atrium and between the liver and right adrenal vein. Pure SH-VC blood was drawn-out through the catheter with the speed matching that of transfusion.
(From Jia C, et al. Suprahepatic vena cava manipulative bleeding alleviates hepatic ischemia-reperfusion injury in rats. Dig Liver Dis, 2008, 40(4):285-292).

Two percent of body weight IH-VC manipulative blood extraction with blood transfusion group (IB, n=6): One hour after transplantation, two percent of body weight IH-VC manipulative blood extraction with blood transfusion was performed by the method described in previous study (Jia et al., 2008).

Two percent of body weight posthepatic manipulative blood extraction with Ringer's lactate solution transfusion group (PR, n=5): Ringer's lactate solution was used for transfusion while posthepatic manipulative blood extraction.

In IR group, a section of the liver was sampled and fixed in 10% formaldehyde, and blood samples were taken from IH-VC at 7 h after transplantation to meet the time course of other groups. In PB, IB and PR group, a section of the liver was sampled and fixed in 10% formaldehyde, and blood samples were taken from IH-VC at 6 h after blood extraction. A section of lung was sampled and fixed in 10% formaldehyde for pathological examination at 6 h after blood extraction. Another section of lung was sampled for the analysis of cytokine and tissue edema.

2.4 Myeloperoxidase and lipid peroxide assays

Sera were isolated and detected for MPO and MDA, an indicator of oxidative injury. Serum MPO contents were measured to analyze degree of neutrophil sequestration and activation. Serum MDA and MPO were assessed according to manufacturer's instructions.

2.5 Liver function

To assess hepatocellular injury in liver transplant, ALT and AST levels in Sera were measured using an Olympus AU600 Analyser (Olympus Optical, Tokyo, Japan).

2.6 Measurement of serum IL-6 level

We use commercially available ELISA kits for the determination of serum IL-6 level according to the manufacturer's instructions.

2.7 Measurement of TNF-α level in lung

We use commercially available ELISA kits for the determination of lung TNF-α level according to the manufacturer's instructions.

2.8 PMN infiltration in the transplant and in the lung

PMN infiltration in the transplant and lung was evaluated by staining for naphthol ASD chloroacetate esterase, a neutrophil specific marker. PMNs were identified by positive staining and were counted in 5 high-power fields under a light microscope (×400).

2.9 Lung edema assay

After resection, lung samples were weighed and then placed in an oven at 60°C until a constant weight was obtained. In this determination, edema is represented by an increase in the wet-to-dry weight ratios(Peralta et al., 1999).

2.10 Histopathological analysis

Liver and lung tissues were fixed with 10% neutral formalin and were stained with hematoxylin and eosin. The degrees of sinusoidal congestion, cytoplasmic vacuolization and necrosis of parenchymal cells were evaluated semiquantitatively according to Suzuki's criteria (Suzuki et al., 1993).

2.11 Statistical analysis

These data are expressed as mean ± SD. Calculations were made using the SPSS 13.0 for windows computer software (SPSS Inc., Chicago, IL). Statistical comparisons were performed using one-way analysis of variance (ANOVA) and the LSD t-test for blood MDA, IL-6, liver PMNs, TNF-α and enzyme levels. P-values less than 0.05 were considered statistically significant.

3. Results

3.1 Time course and peak level of posthepatic MDA after transplantation

Figure 2 represents the kinetic changes of MDA in all time points in experiment Part I. In this study MDA concentration within SH-VC peaked at 1 h after transplantation. MDA concentration at 1 h was significantly higher than that at other time points except for 5 min. Furthermore, MDA concentrations in SH-VC were significantly higher than that in IH-VC at 20 min，30 min，1h ($P<0.05$) and slightly higher at all other time points. MDA concentration within IH-VC peaked at 2 h after transplantation.

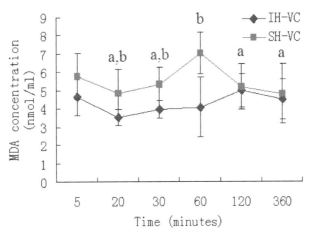

Fig. 2. Time course and peak level of MDA after liver transplantation in Part I
SH-VC represents the group that blood was taken form SH-VC. IH-VC represents the group that blood was taken form IH-VC. $^aP < 0.05$ vs. 60 min within SH-VC. $^bP < 0.05$ vs. IH-VC.

3.2 MDA and PMO levels in the sera

In experiment Part II, serum MDA level at 6 h after transplantation was slightly lower in PB, IB and PR group than in IR group but no statistically significant. Whereas serum MPO level in PB and PR groups (48.78±9.36 pg/ml and 49.36±18.32 pg/ml, respectively) were significantly lower than that in IR group (71.34±22.14) ($P=0.022$, $P=0.045$, respectively). Serum MPO level in IB group was not significantly lower than that in IR group (Figure 3).

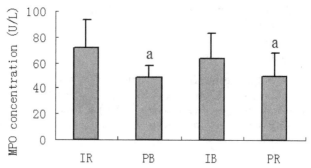

Fig. 3. Serum MPO level in all groups in Part II
IR: IR control group. PB: Two percent of body weight posthepatic manipulative blood
extraction with blood transfusion group. IB: Two percent of body weight IH-VC
manipulative blood extraction with blood transfusion group. PR: Two percent of body
weight posthepatic manipulative blood extraction with Ringer's lactate solution transfusion
group. aP < 0.05 vs. IR.

3.3 Serum IL-6 level

As shown in Figure 4, IL-6 level at 6 h in Part II were significantly lower in PB and IB group
(470.88±101.36 pg/ml and 392.71±259.80 pg/ml, respectively) than in IR group
(1067.42±547.91) (P=0.017, P=0.008, respectively). IL-6 level at 6 h in PR group was not
significantly lower than in IR group.

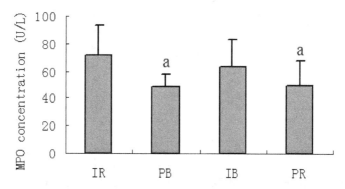

Fig. 4. Serum IL-6 level in all groups in Part II
IR: IR control group. PB: Two percent of body weight posthepatic manipulative blood
extraction with blood transfusion group. IB: Two percent of body weight IH-VC manipulative
blood extraction with blood transfusion group. PR: Two percent of body weight posthepatic
manipulative blood extraction with Ringer's lactate solution transfusion group. aP < 0.05 vs. IR.

3.4 Liver function

Figure 5 showed posthepatic manipulative blood extraction significantly attenuated
hepatocellular injury, as compared with I/R control group. ALT and AST levels at 6 h were

Posthepatic Manipulative Blood Extraction with Blood Transfusion Alleviates Liver Transplant
Ischemia/Reperfusion Injury and Its Induced Lung Injury

261

significantly lower in PB and IB group (460.00±126.65UI/L and 766.00±165.02 UI/L, respectively) than in IR group (1494.00±1015.05UI/L and 1976.00±1262.79 UI/L, respectively) (*P*=0.043, *P*=0.043, respectively). ALT and AST levels at 6 h in IB and PR group were not significantly lower than in IR group.

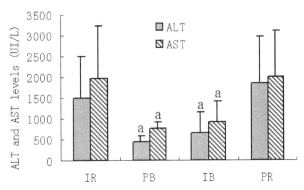

Fig. 5. ALT and AST levels in all groups in Part II
IR: IR control group. PB: Two percent of body weight posthepatic manipulative blood extraction with blood transfusion group. IB: Two percent of body weight IH-VC manipulative blood extraction with blood transfusion group. PR: Two percent of body weight posthepatic manipulative blood extraction with Ringer's lactate solution transfusion group. [a]*P* < 0.05 vs. IR.

3.5 TNF-α level in lung

As shown in Figure 6, lung TNF-α level at 6 h in Part II were significantly lower in PB group (21.01±7.87 pg/ml) than in IR group (47±19.62 pg/ml) (*P*=0.038). Lung TNF-α level in IB and PR group was not significantly lower than that in IR group.

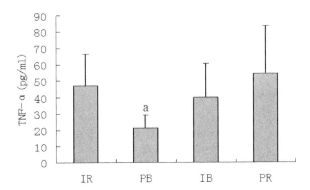

Fig. 6. Lung TNF-α level in all groups in Part II
IR: IR control group. PB: Two percent of body weight posthepatic manipulative blood extraction with blood transfusion group. IB: Two percent of body weight IH-VC manipulative blood extraction with blood transfusion group. PR: Two percent of body weight posthepatic manipulative blood extraction with Ringer's lactate solution transfusion group. [a]*P* < 0.05 vs. IR.

3.6 Lung edema assay

Wet-to-dry weight ratio of the lung tissue in group PB was 4.25±0.79, which was significnagly lower than that in IR group (7.0±4.03) (P=0.039). Wet-to-dry weight ratio of the lung tissue in IB and PR group were not significantly lower than that in IR group (Figure 7).

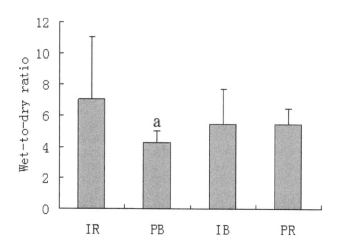

Fig. 7. Wet-to-dry weight ratio of the lung tissue in all groups in Part II
IR: IR control group. PB: Two percent of body weight posthepatic manipulative blood extraction with blood transfusion group. IB: Two percent of body weight IH-VC manipulative blood extraction with blood transfusion group. PR: Two percent of body weight posthepatic manipulative blood extraction with Ringer's lactate solution transfusion group. [a]P < 0.05 vs. IR.

3.7 PMN infiltration in the transplant and in the lung

To determine whether posthepatic manipulative blood extraction affected local leukocyte infiltration in transplant and lung, we assessed PMNs infiltration using naphthol ASD chloroacetate esterase staining. In this study, PMN counts in liver transplant were significantly lower in PB, IB and PR group (11.75±5.02 counts/HPF, 8.53±1.98 counts/HPF and 13.6±4.07 counts/HPF, respectively) than that in IR group (24.46±13.87 counts/HPF) (P=0.006, P=0.002, P=0.031, respectively) (Figure 8). PMN counts in lung were significantly lower in PB and IB group (44.13±19.29 counts/HPF and 56.57±9.10 counts/HPF, respectively) than that in IR group (82.8±25.01 counts/HPF) (P=0.001 and P=0.030, respectively). PMN infiltration in PR group was not significantly lower than that in IR group (Figure 9).

Posthepatic Manipulative Blood Extraction with Blood Transfusion Alleviates Liver Transplant
Ischemia/Reperfusion Injury and Its Induced Lung Injury

263

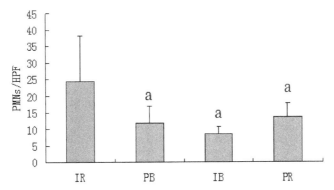

Fig. 8. PMN infiltrations in the transplants at 6 h after manipulation in Part II
PMN kinetics in the liver after reperfusion. IR: IR control group. PB: Two percent of body
weight posthepatic manipulative blood extraction with blood transfusion group. IB: Two
percent of body weight IH-VC manipulative blood extraction with blood transfusion group.
PR: Two percent of body weight posthepatic manipulative blood extraction with Ringer's
lactate solution transfusion group. [a]P<0.05 versus IR.

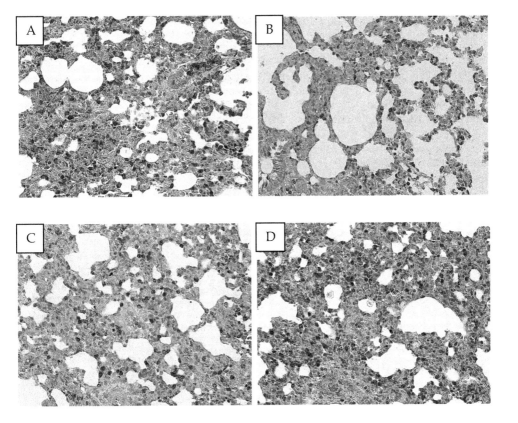

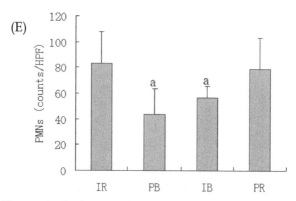

Fig. 9. PMN infiltration in the lung in all groups in Part II
PMNs were seen as deep-brown dots (original magnification ×400). A:IR group; B: PB group;
C:IB group; D: PR group. E: the comparison of PMN infiltration in the lung between groups.
IR: IR control group. PB: Two percent of body weight posthepatic manipulative blood
extraction with blood transfusion group. IB: Two percent of body weight IH-VC manipulative
blood extraction with blood transfusion group. PR: Two percent of body weight posthepatic
manipulative blood extraction with Ringer's lactate solution transfusion group. $^aP < 0.05$ vs. IR.

3.8 Histopathological findings in Part II

Histological changes of the transplant were in keeping with the aforementioned biochemical
observations. Liver sections of IR and PR rats at 6 h after manipulation showed sinusoidal
congestion, cytoplasmic vacuolization and conspicuously focal necrosis. Moderate severity
of necrosis and congestion were found in IB group. In marked contrast, liver sections in PB
rats showed significant preservation of the lobular architecture with ballooning of
parenchymal cells and minimal signs of hepatocyte necrosis (Figure 10). Four out of seven
rats in PB group showed + hepatic injury, 2 showed ++ and 1 showed +++, whereas rats in
other groups showed ++~+++ hepatic injury according to Suzuki's criteria. The histological
study of the lungs revealed a diffuse interstitial thickening with marked edema and
polymorphonuclear infiltration 6 h after liver transplant in IR group. In contrast, mild
lesions were seen in PB group with discrete thickening of the alveolar septa and the
presence of scattered inflammatory cells (Figure 11).

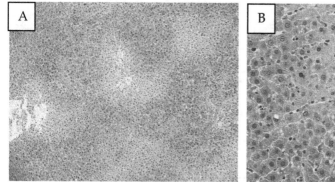
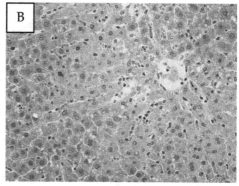

Posthepatic Manipulative Blood Extraction with Blood Transfusion Alleviates Liver Transplant
Ischemia/Reperfusion Injury and Its Induced Lung Injury

265

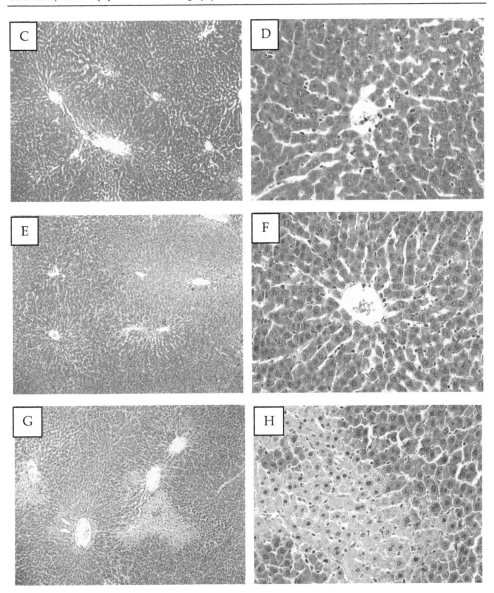

Fig. 10. Representative histologic findings in transplant at 6 h after manipulation.
At 6 h after transplantation, conspicuous necrosis and sinusoidal congestion were observed
in IR and PR group (A:IR group, original magnification ×100; B:IR group, original
magnification ×400; G:PR group, original magnification ×100; H:PR group, original
magnification ×400). Moderate severity of necrosis and congestion were found in IB group
(E:IB group, original magnification ×100; F:IB group, original magnification ×400). Only
ballooning of parenchymal cells and minimal necrosis were seen in PB group (C: original
magnification ×100; D: original magnification ×400).

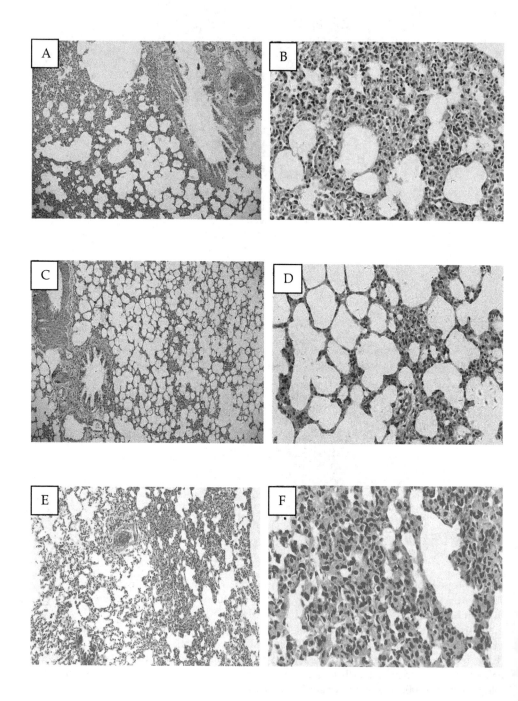

Posthepatic Manipulative Blood Extraction with Blood Transfusion Alleviates Liver Transplant
Ischemia/Reperfusion Injury and Its Induced Lung Injury

267

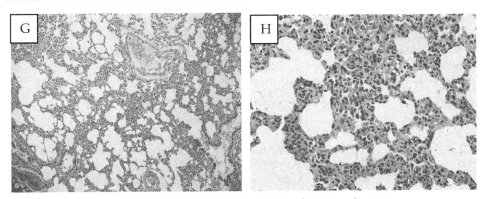

Fig. 11. Representative histologic findings in lung at 6 h after transplantation.
The histological study of the lungs revealed a diffuse interstitial thickening with marked
edema and polymorphonuclear infiltration in I/R, IB and PR group (A:IR group, original
magnification ×100; B:IR group, original magnification ×400; E:IB group, original
magnification ×100; F:IB group, original magnification ×400; G: PR group, original
magnification ×100; H:PR group, original magnification ×400). In contrast, mild lesions were
seen in PB group with discrete thickening of the alveolar septa and the presence of scattered
inflammatory cells (C: original magnification ×100; D: original magnification ×400).

4. Discussion

Our results provided evidence for the role of ROS in the pathogenesis of liver transplant
I/R. In Part I of this study, pure SH-VC and IH-VC blood were taken at multiple time points
to determine the peak production of posthepatic ROS after transplantation. We found that
serum MDA concentration in SH-VC increased and peaked at 1 h after transplantation. And
the MDA concentrations in SH-VC were significantly higher than that in IH-VC at 20
min，30 min，1h ($P<0.05$). The phenomenon that MDA concentration increased slowly in
the early stage after transplantation is due to its incomplete reflow and injured
microcirculation including endothelial cell swelling (Vollmar et al., 1994), vasoconstriction
(Marzi et al., 1994), leucocyte entrapment (Fondevila et al., 2003; Yadav et al., 1998) and
possibly intravascular haemoconcentration (Menger et al., 1988). This process prolongs the
period of hypoxia, with areas of the liver remaining ischemic after early period of
transplantation. In the later stage, neutrophils infiltrate into the liver increased with time, so
companied by increased ROS.

In Part II of this study, we evaluated the potential effects of posthepatic manipulative blood
extraction and blood transfusion at 1 h after reperfusion on the liver transplant cold I/R
injury and liver I/R induced lung injury. We found that 2% of body weight posthepatic
manipulative blood extraction with blood transfusion (PB) significantly reversed the
elevations in the serum MPO, IL-6, TNF-α, liver enzyme levels and dramatically decreased
PMNs in the liver and lung. Oxidative and other environmental stress lead to an
upregulation of proinflammatory mediators (Otterbein et al., 2000; Otterbein et al., 2003).
Increased production of IL-6 is thought to be involved in the pathogenesis of cold hepatic
I/R injury (Tomiyama et al., 2008; Uchida et al., 2009). IL-6 is considered a marker for liver

injury severity (Jin et al., 2006) and it has been demonstrated that IL-6 overexpression leads to detrimental effects in some studies (Monbaliu et al., 2007; Wustefeld et al., 2000). Here, prompt inflammatory response was evident in our model of cold hepatic I/R injury by the elevation of serum IL-6 level at 6 h of reperfusion. Then we have shown that posthepatic manipulative blood extraction reversed this elevation.

In Part II of this study, although serum MDA level was no statistically significant between groups, serum MPO levels in PB was significantly lower than that in IR group. Posthepatic manipulative blood extraction significantly reduced serum MPO level, indicating suppression of neutrophil accumulation and activation, which play important roles in I/R-induced ROS production (Parks et al., 1988; Zimmerman et al., 1990). This result shows the imbalance of oxidation/antioxidation and increase of lipid peroxide in vivo. So the protective effect of posthepatic manipulative blood extraction with blood transfusion was, in part, due to the inhibition of neutrophil infiltration and activation, which was further demonstrated by its suppression of PMNs accumulation in liver transplant and lung. Experimental evidence shows that there are two distinct phases of liver reperfusion injury (Jaeschke et al., 1990). The early phase covers the first 2 hours after reperfusion (Tamaki et al., 1996). So in the view of time course, we conclude that posthepatic manipulative blood extraction mainly alleviates liver IR injury in late phase in that it significantly decrease serum MPO, IL-6, liver enzyme levels and PMNs in the liver at 6 h after reperfusion.

Although IB group significantly reversed the elevations in the serum IL-6, liver enzymes and even PMN infiltrations in transplant, it did not exert significant protective effects in terms of serum MPO and did not improve transplant pathological injury. So we thought that the posthepatic manipulative blood extraction takes advantages over IH-VC manipulative blood extraction on attenuating hepatic cold I/R injury. Both blood/ROS extraction and fresh blood transfusion are indispensable in alleviating liver transplant I/R injury in our model. And the reason why PR group significantly decrease serum MPO and PMN infiltrations in the liver remains unclear. Blood dilution maybe at least one of the causes for this phenomenon.

The liver contains great concentration of Kupffer cells (Kamada et al., 1983). During the initial stage of hepatic ischemia, Kupffer cells are activated and these activated Kupffer cells released a lot of pro-inflammatory cytokines, and proteolytic enzymes. After reperfusion, activation products generated in the ischemic liver, including proinflammatory cytokines such as TNF-α, are released into the systemic circulation. Yoshidome et al demonstrated, in a rat hepatic I/R model, that hepatic-derived TNF-α plays a central role in the induction of lung neutrophil recruitment and tissue injury (Peralta et al., 1999). It initiates an inflammatory response both in liver and remote organs such as the lungs and kidneys (Rosen et al., 1998). These factors, after the reperfusion, can cause hepatocellular injury and hepatic microcirculation disorder. On the other hand, these active factors can reach to the pulmonary vascularity through systemic circulation to activate lung capillary endothelial cells, neutrophils and lead to the inflammatory reaction of the lung tissues, causing acute lung injury and increase the lung capillary permeability. This is because the pulmonary endothelium is sensitive to these cytokines, and because the pulmonary circulation represents the first vascular bed to which these mediators are delivered (Peralta et al., 1999). Furthermore, elevated levels of TNF-α are associated with neutrophil-dependent lung injury after hepatic I/R (Suzuki et al., 1993). In this study, as decreased in serum MPO, TNF-α, a pleiotropic pro-inflammatory cytokine which can induce liver and lung injuries, was also decreased via posthepatic blood diacharge in that the liver by itself is also an important source for TNF-α release during liver I/R (Vollmar et al., 1994).

So in this study, the protective effect of posthepatic manipulative blood extraction was, in part, due to the inhibition of neutrophil infiltration and activation via its inhibition of tissue TNF-a production, which was further demonstrated by its suppression of PMNs accumulation in lung. In addition, we found that water content of the lung significantly increases after reperfusion. TNF-a and activated neutrophils contribute to the damage through the release of ROS. Increased accumulation of pulmonary TNF-a and neutrophil results in increased lung capillary permeability in that it can damage both vascular endothelium cells and lung epithelial cells. And the toxic lipid peroxidation reaction products mediated by ROS will furthermore cause cell injury and death (Marzi et al., 1994).

The protective mechanisms involved in PB were the direct decreasing in circulating MPO and pulmonary TNF-α via manipulative blood extraction. And the lung pathological findings parallel with biochemistry parameters mentioned above. So it demonstrated that posthepatic manipulative blood extraction alleviates lung injury induced by liver ischemia-reperfusion. Although other groups, compared with IR group, slightly reversed the elevations in the some parameters, it was not statistically significant.

In conclusion, we provided the first evidence that posthepatic ROS concentration elevated with time and peaked at 1 h after transplantation. Posthepatic manipulative blood extraction and blood transfusion alleviates liver transplant cold IR injury and lung injury induced by liver cold IR injury through its marked decrease in serum PMO, IL-6, inhibition neutrophil infiltration in transplant, so significantly attenuating hepatocellular injury. Our data strongly support that targeting posthepatic manipulative blood extraction with blood transfusion represents a useful approach to prevent IR injury in rats and maybe a potential way in human. It is possible to use this strategy clinically due to its facility and practicability. In human liver transplantation, for example, the posthepatic manipulatively extracted blood can be re-transfused after re-oxygenation and removal of ROS and pro-inflammatory cytokines. It might improve the overall success of liver transplantation and should be further investigated.

5. References

Aduen JF, Stapelfeldt WH, Johnson MM, Jolles HI, Grinton SF, Divertie GD, Burger CD. Clinical relevance of time of onset,duration, and type of pulmonary edema after liver transplantation. Liver Transpl, 2003; 9: 764-771

Banga NR, Homer-Vanniasinkam S, Graham A, Al-Mukhtar A, White SA, Prasad KR.Ischaemic preconditioning in transplantation and major resection of the liver. Br J Surg 2005; 92:528–538.

Clarke CN, Kuboki S, Tevar A, Lentsch AB, Edwards M.CXC chemokines play a critical role in liver injury, recovery, and regeneration. Am J Surg 2009; 198:415-419.

Farmer DG, Kaldas F, Anselmo D, Katori M, Shen XD, Lassman C, Kaldas M, Clozel M, Busuttil RW, Kupiec-Weglinski J. Tezosentan, a novel endothelin receptor antagonist, markedly reduces rat hepatic ischemia and reperfusion injury in three different models. Liver Transpl. 2008;14:1737-1744.

Fondevila C, Busuttil RW, Kupiec-Weglinski JW. Hepatic ischemia/reperfusion injury-a fresh look. Exp Mol Pathol 2003;14:86-93.

Henderson JM. Liver transplantation and rejection: an overview. Hepatogastroenterology 1999;46(Suppl 2):1482-1484.

Huguet C, Gavelli A, Bona S. Hepatic resection with ischemia of the liver exceeding one hour. J Am Coll Surg 1994;178: 454-458.

Jaeschke H, Farhood A, Smith CW. Neutrophils contribute to ischemia/reperfusion injury in rat liver in vivo. FASEB J 1990; 4:3355-3359.

Jia C, Wang W, Zhu Y, Zheng S. Suprahepatic vena cava manipulative bleeding alleviates hepatic ischemia-reperfusion injury in rats. Dig Liver Dis 2008; 40:285-292.

Jin X, Zimmers TA, Perez EA, Pierce RH, Zhang Z, Koniaris LG. Paradoxical effects of short- and long-term interleukin-6 exposure on liver injury and repair. Hepatology 2006;43:474 -484.

Kamada N · Calne RY · A surgical experience with five hundred thirty liver transplants in the rat · Surgery 1983;93:64-69 ·

Lehmann TG, Wheeler MD, Schwabe RF, Connor HD, Schoonhoven R, Bunzendahl H, Brenner DA, Jude Samulski R, Zhong Z, Thurman RG. Gene delivery of Cu/Zn-superoxide dismutase improves graft function after transplantation of fatty livers in the rat. Hepatology 2000; 32:1255-1264.

Liu DL, Jeppsson B, Hakansson CH, Odselius R. Multiple-system organ damage resulting from prolonged hepatic inflow interruption. Arch Surg, 1996;131:442-447.

Marzi I, Takei Y, Rücker M, Kawano S, Fusamoto H, Walcher F, Kamada T. Endothelin-1 is involved in hepatic sinusoidal vasoconstriction after ischemia and reperfusion. Transpl Int 1994; 7:S503-506.

Menger MD, Sack FU, Barker JH, Feifel G, Messmer K. Quantitative analysis of microcirculatory disorders after prolonged ischemia in skeletal muscle: therapeutic effects of prophylactic isovolaemic haemodilution. Res Exp Med 1988;188:151-165.

Monbaliu D, van Pelt J, De Vos R, Greenwood J, Parkkinen J, Crabbé T, Zeegers M, Vekemans K, Pincemail J, Defraigne JO, Fevery J, Pirenne J. Primary graft nonfunction and Kupffer cell activation after liver transplantation from non-heart-beating donors in pigs. Liver Transpl 2007 ; 13(2):239-247.

Olthoff KM. Can reperfusion injury of the liver be prevented? Trying to improve on a good thing. Pediatr Transplant 2001; 5:390-393.

Otterbein LE, Bach FH, Alam J, Soares M, Tao Lu H, Wysk M, Davis RJ, Flavell RA, Choi AM. Carbon monoxide has anti-inflammatory effects involving the mitogen-activated protein kinase pathway. Nat Med 2000;6: 422-428.

Otterbein LE, Otterbein SL, Ifedigbo E, Liu F, Morse DE, Fearns C, Ulevitch RJ, Knickelbein R, Flavell RA, Choi AM. MKK3 mitogen-activated protein kinase pathway

Posthepatic Manipulative Blood Extraction with Blood Transfusion Alleviates Liver Transplant
Ischemia/Reperfusion Injury and Its Induced Lung Injury

271

mediates carbon monoxide-induced protection against oxidant-induced lung injury. Am J Pathol 2003;163: 2555–2563.

Parks DA, Granger DN. Ischemia-reperfusion injury: a radical view. Hepatology 1988; 8: 680-682.

Peralta C, Prats N, Xaus C, Gelpí E, Roselló-Catafau J. Protective effect of liver ischemic preconditioning on liver and lung injury induced by hepatic ischemia-reperfusion in the rat. Hepatology, 1999, 30:1481-1489

Pereboom IT, de Boer MT, Haagsma EB, Hendriks HG, Lisman T, Porte RJ. Platelet transfusion during liver transplantation is associated with increased postoperative mortality due to acute lung injury. Anesth Analg, 2009;108(4):1083-1091.

Rosen HR, Martin P, Goss J, Donovan J, Melinek J, Rudich S, Imagawa DK, Kinkhabwala M, Seu P, Busuttil RW, Shackleton CR. Significance of early aminotransferase elevation after liver transplantation. Transplantation 1998; 65:68–72.

Shimizu H, Kataoka M, Ohtsuka M, Ito H, Kimura F, Togawa A, Yoshidome H, Kato A,Miyazaki M. Extended cold preservation of the graft liver enhances neutrophil-mediated pulmonary injury after liver transplantation. Hepatogastroenterology, 2005;52:1172–1175.

Suzuki S, Toledo-Pereyra LH, Rodriguez FJ, Cejalvo D. Neutrophil infiltration as an important factor in liver ischemia and reperfusion injury. Modulating effects of FK506 and cyclosporine. Transplantation 1993; 55:1265–1272.

Sykes E, Cosgrove JF, Nesbitt ID, O'Suilleabhain CB. Early noncardiogenic pulmonary edema and the use of PEEP and prone ventilation after emergency liver transplantation. Liver Transpl, 2007; 13: 459-462.

Tamaki S, Ueno T, Torimura T, Sata M, Tanikawa K. Evaluation of hyaluronic acid binding ability of hepatic sinusoidal endothelial cells in rats with liver cirrhosis. Gastroenterology 1996; 111:1049-1057.

Tomiyama K, Ikeda A, Ueki S, Nakao A, Stolz DB, Koike Y, Afrazi A, Gandhi C, Tokita D, Geller DA, Murase N.Inhibition of Kupffer cell-mediated early proinflammatory response with carbon monoxide in transplant-induced hepatic ischemia/reperfusion injury in rats. Hepatology 2008; 48:1608-1620.

Uchida Y, Freitas MC, Zhao D, Busuttil RW, Kupiec-Weglinski JW.The inhibition of neutrophil elastase ameliorates mouse liver damage due to ischemia and reperfusion. Liver Transpl 2009;15:939-947.

Vollmar B, Glasz J, Leiderer R, Post S, Menger MD. Hepatic microcirculatory perfusion failure is a determinant for liver dysfunction in warm ischemia-reperfusion. Am J Pathol 1994; 145:1421-1431.

Wustefeld T, Rakemann T, Kubicka S, Manns MP, Trautwein C. Hyperstimulation with interleukin 6 inhibits cell cycle progression after hepatectomy in mice. Hepatology 2000; 32: 514

Yadav SS, Howell DN, Gao W, Steeber DA, Harland RC, Clavien PA. L-selectin and ICAM-1 mediate reperfusion injury and neutrophil adhesion in the warm ischemic mouse liver. Am J Physiol 1998; 275:G1341-1352.

Zhang W, Wang M, Xie HY, Zhou L, Meng XQ, Shi J, Zheng S.Role of Reactive Oxygen Species in Mediating Hepatic Ischemia-Reperfusion Injury and Its Therapeutic Applications in Liver Transplantation. Transplant Proc 2007; 39:1332-1327.

Zimmerman BJ, Grisham MB, Granger DN. Role of oxidants in ischemia/reperfusion-induced granulocyte infiltration.Am J Physiol 1990; 258: G185-190.

Permissions

The contributors of this book come from diverse backgrounds, making this book a truly international effort. This book will bring forth new frontiers with its revolutionizing research information and detailed analysis of the nascent developments around the world.

We would like to thank Dr. Puneet Kaur Kochhar, for lending his expertise to make the book truly unique. He has played a crucial role in the development of this book. Without his invaluable contribution this book wouldn't have been possible. He has made vital efforts to compile up to date information on the varied aspects of this subject to make this book a valuable addition to the collection of many professionals and students.

This book was conceptualized with the vision of imparting up-to-date information and advanced data in this field. To ensure the same, a matchless editorial board was set up. Every individual on the board went through rigorous rounds of assessment to prove their worth. After which they invested a large part of their time researching and compiling the most relevant data for our readers. Conferences and sessions were held from time to time between the editorial board and the contributing authors to present the data in the most comprehensible form. The editorial team has worked tirelessly to provide valuable and valid information to help people across the globe.

Every chapter published in this book has been scrutinized by our experts. Their significance has been extensively debated. The topics covered herein carry significant findings which will fuel the growth of the discipline. They may even be implemented as practical applications or may be referred to as a beginning point for another development. Chapters in this book were first published by InTech; hereby published with permission under the Creative Commons Attribution License or equivalent.

The editorial board has been involved in producing this book since its inception. They have spent rigorous hours researching and exploring the diverse topics which have resulted in the successful publishing of this book. They have passed on their knowledge of decades through this book. To expedite this challenging task, the publisher supported the team at every step. A small team of assistant editors was also appointed to further simplify the editing procedure and attain best results for the readers.

Our editorial team has been hand-picked from every corner of the world. Their multi-ethnicity adds dynamic inputs to the discussions which result in innovative outcomes. These outcomes are then further discussed with the researchers and contributors who give their valuable feedback and opinion regarding the same. The feedback is then collaborated with the researches and they are edited in a comprehensive manner to aid the understanding of the subject.

Apart from the editorial board, the designing team has also invested a significant amount of their time in understanding the subject and creating the most relevant covers. They scrutinized every image to scout for the most suitable representation of the subject and create an appropriate cover for the book.

The publishing team has been involved in this book since its early stages. They were actively engaged in every process, be it collecting the data, connecting with the contributors or procuring relevant information. The team has been an ardent support to the editorial, designing and production team. Their endless efforts to recruit the best for this project, has resulted in the accomplishment of this book. They are a veteran in the field of academics and their pool of knowledge is as vast as their experience in printing. Their expertise and guidance has proved useful at every step. Their uncompromising quality standards have made this book an exceptional effort. Their encouragement from time to time has been an inspiration for everyone.

The publisher and the editorial board hope that this book will prove to be a valuable piece of knowledge for researchers, students, practitioners and scholars across the globe.

List of Contributors

Emili Cid, Sandra de la Fuente, Miyako Yamamoto and Fumiichiro Yamamoto
Institut de Medicina Predictiva I Personalitzada del Càncer (IMPPC), Badalona, Barcelona, Spain

Saqeb B. Mirza
Specialist Registrar, University Hospital Southampton, UK

Sukhmeet S. Panesar
Special Advisor, National Patient Safety Agency, UK

Douglas G. Dunlop
Consultant Orthopedic Surgeon, University Hospital Southampton, UK

Ruud H.G.P. van Erve and Alexander C. Wiekenkamp
Beter Lopen, Deventer, the Netherlands

João Manoel Silva Junior
Anesthesiology and intensive care Department, Hospital do Servidor Público Estadual, São Paulo, Brazil

Alberto Mendonça P. Ferreira
Intensive Care Department from Hospital do Servidor Público Estadual, São Paulo, Brazil

Subhayu Bandyopadhyay
Ninewells Hospital, Dundee, UK

Pei Shan Lim
Universiti Kebangsaan Malaysia Medical Center, Universiti Kebangsaan Malaysia, Malaysia

Ebrahim Mikaniki, Mohammad Mikaniki and Amir Hosein Shirzadian
Babol University of Medical Sciences, Iran

S. Gowri Sankar
Department of Biotechnology, Anna University of Technology, Tiruchirappalli, Tamil Nadu, India

A. Alwin Prem Anand
Institute of Anatomy, University of Tuebingen, Tubingen, Germany

Pankaj Abrol
Post Graduate Institute of Medical Sciences, University of Health Sciences, Rohtak (Haryana), India

Harbans Lal
Maharaja Agrasen Medical College, Agroha, Hissar (Haryana), India

Marina Lobato Martins
Gerência de Desenvolvimento Técnico Científico, Centro de Hematologia e Hemoterapia de Minas Gerais (Fundação HEMOMINAS), Brazil
Interdisciplinary HTLV Research Group (GIPH), Brazil

Rafaela Gomes Andrade, Bernardo Hinkelmann Nédir and Edel Figueiredo Barbosa-Stancioli
Laboratório de Virologia Básica e Aplicada, Departamento de Microbiologia, Universidad Federal de Minas Gerais, Brazil
Interdisciplinary HTLV Research Group (GIPH), Brazil

A.W.M.M. Koopman-van Gemert
Department of Anesthesiology, Albert Schweitzer Hospital, 3300AK Dordrecht, the Netherlands

Nathaniel I. Usoro
Department of Surgery, University of Calabar Teaching Hospital, Calabar, Nigeria

D.A. Otsuki, D.T. Fantoni and J.O.C. Auler Junior
LIM08-Anesthesiology, Faculdade de Medicina da Universidad de São Paulo, Brazil

Miloš Bohoněk
Department of Hematology, Biochemistry and Blood Transfusion, Central Military Hospital Prague, Praha, Czech Republic

Puneet K. Kochhar
Lady Hardinge Medical College & SSK Hospital, University of Delhi, New Delhi, India

Pranay Ghosh and Rupinder Singh Kochhar
Maulana Azad Medical College & Lok Nayak Hospital, University of Delhi, New Delhi, India

Changku Jia
Department of Hepatobiliary Surgery, Affiliated Hospital of Hainan Medical College, Haikou, Hainan Province, China

Printed in the USA
CPSIA information can be obtained
at www.ICGtesting.com
JSHW011453221024
72173JS00005B/1061

9 781632 410597